MORE 4U!

the clinics.com

The ~~~~~~ available online.

Here's what you get:

- Full text of EVERY issue from 2002 to NOW
- Figures, tables, drawings, references and more
- Searchable: find what you need fast

Search [All Clinics ▼] for [   ] [GO]

~nals

INDIVIDUAL SUBSCRIBERS

LOG ON TODAY. IT'S FAST AND EASY.

Click **Register** and follow instructions

You'll need your account number

Your subscriber account number → is on your mailing label

This is your copy of:

THE CLINICS OF NORTH AMERICA

CXXX   **2296532-2**   2   Mar 05

J.H. DOE, MD
531 MAIN STREET
CENTER CITY, NY 10001-001

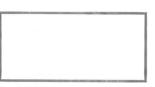

DATE DUE

~UE? Sorry, you won't be able ~lease subscribe today to get ~ting customer service at ~ada) or 407 345 4000 (outside ~il at elsols@elsevier.com.

NEW!

~e for INSTITUTIONS

Works/Integrates with MD Consult
Available in a variety of packages: Collections containing
14, 31 or 50 Clinics titles
Or Collection upgrade for existing MD Consult customers

Call today! 877-857-1047 or e-mail: mdc.groupinfo@elsevier.com

ELSEVIER

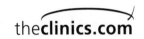

PHYSICAL MEDICINE AND REHABILITATION CLINICS

OF NORTH AMERICA

Current Trends in Neuromuscular Research: Assessing Function, Enhancing Performance

GUEST EDITOR
Gregory T. Carter, MD

CONSULTING EDITOR
George H. Kraft, MD, MS

November 2005 • Volume 16 • Number 4

SAUNDERS

An Imprint of Elsevier, Inc.
PHILADELPHIA   LONDON   TORONTO   MONTREAL   SYDNEY   TOKYO

W.B. SAUNDERS COMPANY
A Division of Elsevier Inc.

1600 John F. Kennedy Blvd. • Suite 1800 • Philadelphia, Pennsylvania 19103

http://www.theclinics.com

PHYSICAL MEDICINE AND REHABILITATION
CLINICS OF NORTH AMERICA
November 2005
Editor: Molly Jay

Volume 16, Number 4
ISSN 1047-9651
ISBN 1-4160-3470-6

The ideas and opinions expressed in *Physical Medicine and Rehabilitation Clinics of North America* do not necessarily reflect those of the Publisher. The Publisher does not assume any responsibility for any injury and/or damage to persons or property arising out of or related to any use of the material contained in this periodical. The reader is advised to check the appropriate medical literature and the product information currently provided by the manufacturer of each drug to be administered to verify the dosage, the method and duration of administration, or contraindications. It is the responsibility of the treating physician or other health care professional, relying on independent experience and knowledge of the patient, to determine drug dosages and the best treatment for the patient. Mention of any product in this issue should not be construed as endorsement by the contributors, editors, or the Publisher of the product or manufacturers' claims.

Physical Medicine and Rehabilitation Clinics of North America (ISSN 1047-9651) is published quarterly by W.B. Saunders Company, Corporate and Editorial Offices: 1600 John F. Kennedy Blvd., Suite 1800, Philadelphia, PA 19103-2899. Accounting and Circulation Offices: 6277 Sea Harbor Drive, Orlando, FL 32887-4800. Periodicals postage paid at Orlando, FL 32862, and additional mailing offices. Subscription price per year is $160.00 (US individuals), $250.00 (US institutions), $80.00 (US students), $195.00 (Canadian individuals), $320.00 (Canadian institutions), $110.00 (Canadian students), $225.00 (foreign individuals), $320.00 (foreign institutions), and $110.00 (foreign students). Foreign air speed delivery is included in all *Clinics* subscription prices. All prices are subject to change without notice. POSTMASTER: Send address changes to *Physical Medicine and Rehabilitation Clinics of North America*, W.B. Saunders Company, Periodicals Fulfillment, Orlando, FL 32887-4800. **Customer Service: 1-800-654-2452 (US). From outside of the US, call 1-407-345-4000.**

Physical Medicine and Rehabilitation Clinics of North America is indexed in *Excerpta Medica, Index Medicus, Cinahl,* and *Cumulative Index to Nursing and Allied Health Literature.*

Printed in the United States of America.

CONSULTING EDITOR

GEORGE H. KRAFT, MD, MS, Professor, Department of Rehabilitation Medicine; Adjunct
Professor of Neurology; Director, Electrodiagnostic Medicine, Western Multiple Sclerosis
Center; and Co-Director, Muscular Dystrophy Clinic, The University of Washington,
Seattle, Washington

GUEST EDITOR

GREGORY T. CARTER, MD, Clinical Professor, Department of Rehabilitation Medicine,
University of Washington, Seattle, Washington

CONTRIBUTORS

SIMONE ABMAYR, PhD, Senior Fellow, Department of Neurology, University of
Washington, Seattle, Washington

R. TED ABRESCH, MS, Director of Research, Department of Physical Medicine and
Rehabilitation, University of California, Davis, Davis, California

FRANCISCO H. ANDRADE, PhD, Associate Professor, Department of Physiology,
University of Kentucky Medical Center, Lexington, Kentucky

C. WILLIAM BALKE, MD, FACP, Professor, Departments of Internal Medicine and
Physiology; and Director, Institute for Molecular Medicine, University of Kentucky
Medical Center, Lexington, Kentucky

JOSHUA O. BENDITT, MD, Professor of Medicine, University of Washington School of
Medicine, Seattle, Washington

LOUIS BOITANO, RRT, MS, Respiratory Care Services, University of Washington
Medical Center, Seattle, Washington

BAOHONG CAO, MD, PhD, Assistant Professor, Department of Orthopaedic Surgery,
University of Pittsburgh, Growth and Development Laboratory, Children's Hospital
of Pittsburgh, Pittsburgh, Pennsylvania

GREGORY T. CARTER, MD, Clinical Professor, Department of Rehabilitation Medicine,
University of Washington, Seattle, Washington

JEFFREY S. CHAMBERLAIN, PhD, Professor, Departments of Neurology, Biochemistry,
and Medicine, Senator Paul D. Wellstone Muscular Dystrophy Cooperative Research
Center, University of Washington School of Medicine, Seattle, Washington

BRIDGET M. DEASY, PhD, Research Assistant Professor, Department of Orthopaedic Surgery, University of Pittsburgh, Growth and Development Laboratory, Children's Hospital of Pittsburgh, Pittsburgh, Pennsylvania

B. JANE DISTAD, MD, Assistant Professor, Department of Neurology, University of Washington, School of Medicine, Seattle, Washington

MARK E. DOMROESE, MD, PhD, Department of Rehabilitation Medicine, University of Washington, Seattle, Washington

JOYCE M. ENGEL, OT, PhD, Professor, Department of Rehabilitation Medicine, Division of Occupational Therapy, University of Washington, Seattle, Washington

KARYN A. ESSER, PhD, Associate Professor, Department of Physiology, University of Kentucky Medical Center, Lexington, Kentucky

MORRIS A. FISHER, MD, Department of Neurology, Hines Veterans Administration Hospital, Hines; Loyola University, Stritch School of Medicine, Maywood, Illinois

RUSSELL C. FRITZ, MD, National Orthopaedic Imaging Associates, Greenbrae; Department of Radiology, University of California, San Francisco, San Francisco, California

WALTER R. FRONTERA, MD, PhD, Professor and Chair of Physical Medicine and Rehabilitation, Harvard Medical School, Spaulding Rehabilitation Hospital, Boston, Massachusetts

SHAI N. GOZANI, MD, PhD, NeuroMetrix, Inc., Waltham, Massachusetts

PAUL GREGOREVIC, PhD, Senior Fellow, Department of Neurology, Senator Paul D. Wellstone Muscular Dystrophy Cooperative Research Center, University of Washington School of Medicine, Seattle, Washington

JAY J. HAN, MD, Assistant Professor, Departement of Physical Medicine and Rehablitation, University of California, Davis, Sacramento, California

AMY J. HOFFMAN, MPH, Research Coordinator, Department of Rehabilitation Medicine, University of Washington School of Medicine, Seattle, Washington

JOHNNY HUARD, PhD, Henry Mankin Associate Professor, Department of Orthopaedic Surgery, University of Pittsburgh, Growth and Development Laboratory, Children's Hospital of Pittsburgh, Pittsburgh, Pennsylvania

KENNETH M. JAFFE, MD, Professor, Department of Rehabilitation Medicine, University of Washington; Adjunct Professor, Pediatrics and Neurological Surgery; Director, Rehabilitation Medicine, Children's Hospital & Regional Medical Center, Seattle, Washington

MARK P. JENSEN, PhD, Hughes M. and Katherine G. Blake Endowed Professor in Health Psychology, Department of Rehabilitation Medicine, University of Washington School of Medicine; and Multidisciplinary Pain Center, University of Washington Medical Center–Roosevelt, Seattle, Washington

DEBORAH KARTIN, PT, PhD, Associate Professor, Department of Rehabilitation Medicine, Division of Physical Therapy, University of Washington, Seattle, Washington

DAVID D. KILMER, MD, Professor and Chair, Department of Physical Medicine and Rehabilitation, University of California, Davis Medical Center; and VA Northern California Health Care System, Sacramento, California

XUAN KONG, PhD, NeuroMetrix, Inc., Waltham, Massachusetts

JOSEPH N. KORNEGAY, DVM, PhD, Dean, College of Veterinary Medicine, University of Missouri Columbia, Columbia, Missouri

LISA S. KRIVICKAS, MD, Assistant Professor of Physical Medicine and Rehabilitation, Harvard Medical School, Spaulding Rehabilitation Hospital, Boston, Massachusetts

PATRICK LAURIE, BS, Research Associate, Neurogenomics Laboratory, Benaroya Research Institute at Virginia Mason, Seattle, Washington

JAU-SHIN LOU, MD, PhD, Co-Director, MDA Clinic; Director, ALS Center of Oregon; Director, EMG Laboratory; and Associate Professor, Department of Neurology, Oregon Health & Science University, Portland, Oregon

DOUGLAS J. MAHONEY, PhD, Postdoctoral Fellow, Apoptosis Research Center, Children's Hospital of Eastern Ontario Research Institute, Ottawa, Ontario, Canada

GREGG D. MEEKINS, MD, Assistant Professor, Department of Neurology, University of Washington School of Medicine, Seattle, Washington

J. THOMAS MEGERIAN, MD, PhD, NeuroMetrix, Inc., Waltham; Department of Neurology, Children's Hospital, Boston, Massachusetts

THOMAS MÖLLER, PhD, Research Associate Professor, Department of Neurology; Center for Neurogenetics and Neurotherapeutics, University of Washington, Seattle, Washington

JONATHAN POLLETT, PhD, Postdoctoral Research Associate, Department of Orthopaedic Surgery, University of Pittsburgh, Growth and Development Laboratory, Children's Hospital of Pittsburgh, Pittsburgh, Pennsylvania

JOHN RAVITS, MD, FAAN, Affiliate Investigator and Director, Neurogenomics Laboratory, Benaroya Research Institute at Virginia Mason; Staff Neurologist, Virginia Mason Medical Center; Clinical Associate Professor, Department of Neurology, University of Washington School of Medicine; Seattle, Washington

MICHAEL B. REID, PhD, Professor and Chair, Department of Physiology, University of Kentucky Medical Center, Lexington, Kentucky

SEWARD B. RUTKOVE, MD, Department of Neurology, Beth Israel Deaconess Medical Center, Boston, Massachusetts

CHANDRA SHEKAR, MD, Neuromuscular Research Fellow, Departement of Rehablitation Medicine, University of Washington, Seattle, Washington

BRAD STONE, PHD, Principal Investigator and Director, Microarray Laboratory, Benaroya Research Institute at Virginia Mason, Seattle, Washington

MARK A. TARNOPOLSKY, MD, PhD, Professor, Department of Pediatrics and Medicine, Division of Neurology and Rehabilitation, McMaster University Medical Center, Hamilton, Ontario, Canada

MICHAEL D. WEISS, MD, Assistant Professor, Department of Neurology, University of Washington, School of Medicine, Seattle, Washington

PATRICK WEYDT, MD, Senior Fellow, Department of Laboratory Medicine, University of Washington, Seattle, Washington

HOLLY H. ZHAO, MD, Assistant Professor, Department of Physical Medicine and Rehabilitation, University of California, Davis Medical Center; and VA Northern California Health Care System, Sacramento, California

CONTENTS

Foreword   xv
George H. Kraft

Preface   xvii
Gregory T. Carter

**Understanding Skeletal Muscle Adaptation to Exercise
Training in Humans: Contributions from Microarray
Studies**   859
Douglas J. Mahoney and Mark A. Tarnopolsky

A period of endurance or resistance exercise training leads to physiologic adaptations that have important treatment and rehabilitation implications for many patient populations. The underlying molecular and cellular mechanisms responsible for exercise training–mediated adaptations are beginning to be unraveled. Studies examining the global gene expression response from skeletal muscle of healthy subjects after a single bout of endurance-type and resistance-type exercise have been completed. Most of the transcripts are induced and not repressed, and the large response seen 3 hours after an acute bout is largely abolished by 48 hours. The results of these studies offer new insights into the regulation of skeletal muscle adaptations in response to exercise, which hold promise for future treatment targets in disease.

**Functional Enhancement of Skeletal Muscle by Gene
Transfer**   875
Paul Gregorevic and Jeffrey S. Chamberlain

Impaired muscle function is a significant factor in determining patient prognosis for many serious diseases and disorders. This article considers the development of gene transfer technology as a source of promising new interventions to treat the muscular dystrophies and severe muscle-wasting states. Although much of the current technology remains experimental, a growing body of evidence suggests that recombinant adeno-associated viral vectors designed to deliver a therapeutic expression cassette to affected muscle fibers may prove useful in slowing or halting disease progression and enhancing muscle function. Application of this technology is discussed with particular reference to Duchenne muscular dystrophy. It is hoped that further work will improve expression cassette design and gene transfer efficiency and help to develop interventions with clinical potential.

Cell Therapy for Muscle Regeneration and Repair   889
Baohong Cao, Bridget M. Deasy, Jonathan Pollett, and Johnny Huard

Duchenne muscular dystrophy is a muscle disease characterized by a lack of dystrophin in the sarcolemma of muscle fibers. Many researchers have investigated myoblast transplantation as a potential approach to deliver dystrophin and alleviate muscle weakness in this condition. Although myoblast transplantation has led to the regeneration of dystrophin-positive muscle fibers within dystrophic skeletal muscle, this technology has been limited by poor survival and limited dissemination of the injected cells and inducement of an immune response. Researchers have made extensive efforts to eliminate these hurdles. This article summarizes current knowledge pertaining to muscle cell transplantation and discusses recent achievements in stem cell transplantation and impediments to their overall use for muscle regeneration and repair.

Amyotrophic Lateral Sclerosis Microgenomics   909
John Ravits, Patrick Laurie, and Brad Stone

Amyotrophic lateral sclerosis (ALS) has unique features that lend itself to a new paradigm of molecular research made possible by recent advances in biotechnology that bridge histopathology and molecular biology. These biotechnologies include laser-based tissue microdissection, chip-based microelectrophoresis, linear amplification of RNA by in vitro transcription, and oligonucleotide microarray. They allow isolation and collection of cells from tissues with complex architecture such as the nervous system for direct and comprehensive profiling of gene expression: microgenomics. Microgenomics may overcome the main difficulties investigating ALS, which are limited access to the targets of investigation, motor neurons, due to reduction caused by the disease; their location in the central nervous system; variable location of pathology along the neuraxis; cell isolation; and low pathogenic-to-nonpathogenic signal-to-noise ratio. Microgenomics may bring molecular research directly to bear on human sporadic neurodegenerative disease; key directly on the neuronal and glial compartments of importance; perform comprehensive molecular exploration; objectively acquire a list of candidate genes and gene pathways to characterize molecular pathogenesis; examine hypotheses; open new directions for genomic and proteomic research; and identify rational therapeutic targets by such new technologies as RNA-interference and molecular Trojan horses.

Redox Mechanisms of Muscle Dysfunction in Inflammatory Disease   **925**

Michael B. Reid, Francisco H. Andrade, C. William Balke, and Karyn A. Esser

Oxidative stress is a fundamental element of muscle pathology that occurs in a wide variety of inflammatory diseases. This stress reflects an imbalance between the production of muscle-derived reactive oxygen species (ROS) and buffering by endogenous anti-oxidants. This article addresses redox biology as a cause of muscle dysfunction under these conditions and reviews cellular mechanisms by which ROS are likely to act. Concepts are outlined in four areas: (1) role of ROS in cachexia, (2) effect of ROS on growth and repair of striated muscle as illustrated by muscle responses to angiotensin II, (3) oxidative stress as a cause of cardiac dysfunction in sleep-disordered breathing, and (4) skeletal muscle dysfunction in heart failure and the putative role of ROS.

Single Muscle Fiber Physiology in Neuromuscular Disease   **951**

Lisa S. Krivickas and Walter R. Frontera

The skinned single muscle fiber preparation allows investigators to directly assess the impact of neuromuscular disease on contractile function of muscle at the cellular level. It is complementary to other measurement techniques that assess muscle function on a larger scale. The single fiber technique allows one to assess the impact of disease and/or treatment differentially on Type I, IIa, IIx, and hybrid fibers, as well as on atrophic and hypertrophic fibers. Thus far, single-fiber contractile properties of patients with prior polio, amyotrophic lateral sclerosis, myotonic and facioscapulohumeral muscular dystrophies, inflammatory myopathy, and critical illness myopathy have been studied. The findings from these studies have been summarized in this article, and future research applications suggested.

Electrodiagnostic Studies in a Murine Model of Demyelinating Charcot-Marie-Tooth Disease   **967**

Gregg D. Meekins and Michael D. Weiss

Functional studies of murine models for neuromuscular disease are of importance in helping to elucidate the human conditions they resemble. Such studies are also of value in determining the benefit of different therapeutic agents in preclinical trials. The *trembler-j* mouse is a demyelinating mutant that carries a peripheral myelin protein-22 point mutation seen in patients with Charcot-Marie-Tooth disease Type 1A. This article summarizes the findings of motor nerve conduction studies performed in these mutants, which emphasize the relative degree of demyelination in these animals compared with that in the human disease. The technique and findings of stimulated single-fiber electromyography performed on *trembler-j* mice, as a tool for assessing axonal degeneration, is also described.

Using Electromyography to Assess Function in Humans and Animal Models of Muscular Dystrophy 981
Jay J. Han, Gregory T. Carter, Michael D. Weiss,
Chandra Shekar, and Joseph N. Kornegay

This article reviews of the available studies in animal models of muscular dystrophy and describes a newly developed protocol for using needle electromyography to perform quantitative motor unit analysis in the mdx mouse. This makes a possible role for electromyography as an in vivo, objective measurement tool to assess neuromuscular function without endangering the patient or requiring sacrifice of the animal model being studied, making it ideally suitable for therapeutic intervention trials in this setting.

Neurotrophic Factors in Neuromuscular Disease 999
B. Jane Distad and Michael D. Weiss

Neurotrophic factors have been shown to support the growth and differentiation of neurons in the developing nervous system and the maintenance of neurons in the adult nervous system. A number of neurotrophic factors have been studied for several years and found to have overlapping and unique functions. Many support the survival of neurons after injury and allow for axonal sprouting and regeneration. As a result of these findings, many researchers are actively exploring the therapeutic potential of such factors in human neuromuscular disease, especially in peripheral neuropathy and motor neuron disease. In this article, we describe the characteristics of a number of neurotrophic factors, evidence for their survival effect on neurons or peripheral nerve in vitro and in vivo, and response to treatment in a number of human clinical trials.

Electrodiagnostic Automation: Principles and Practice 1015
Shai N. Gozani, Morris A. Fisher, Xuan Kong, J. Thomas
Megerian, and Seward B. Rutkove

Automation is an integral component of nearly all nerve conduction studies (NCS) performed using modern instrumentation. In this review, the definition, history, and examples of electrodiagnostic automation are provided with a particular focus on NCS. Recent advances are described, along with limitations and appropriate clinical use of automation technology. Finally, future directions and the potential impact on physicians and patients are discussed.

Physiological and Anatomical Basis of Muscle Magnetic Resonance Imaging 1033
Russell C. Fritz, Mark E. Domroese, and Gregory T. Carter

This article describes the current state of the technology in magnetic resonace (MR) imaging of muscle, with comparision to electrophysiogic testing. Functional MR as well as MR spectroscopic techniques are also reviewed and discussed.

Obesity, Physical Activity, and the Metabolic Syndrome in Adult Neuromuscular Disease   1053
David D. Kilmer and Holly H. Zhao

There is an epidemic in the United States of obesity and the development of cardiovascular disease and type 2 diabetes mellitus. With increased life span of individuals with slowly progressive neuromuscular diseases, there is increased interest in secondary conditions related to disability. Cardiovascular disease, type 2 diabetes mellitus, and their precursor, the metabolic syndrome, are significant potential concerns in this population because of decreased physical activity and obesity. This article presents evidence addressing these issues in adult neuromuscular diseases and discusses potential methods to improve quality of life for patients with these diseases.

Approaching Fatigue in Neuromuscular Diseases   1063
Jau-Shin Lou

Fatigue is a complex phenomenon that is understudied. Fatigue may affect quality of life in patients with neuromuscular diseases. It is crucial for physicians to assess subjective fatigue and objective fatigue simultaneously. Questionnaires are useful in assessing the severity of subjective fatigue, and exercise protocols are useful in assessing objective physical fatigue. Physiologic techniques are now available for researchers to measure central and peripheral physical fatigue.

The Role of Microglial Cells in Amyotrophic Lateral Sclerosis   1081
Patrick Weydt and Thomas Möller

Neuroinflammation is a significant pathogenic factor in amyotrophic lateral sclerosis. Current data suggest that microglial activation is detrimental for motor neurons and might be a driving force in the rapid progression of the disease. The emerging data on the detrimental impact of neuroinflammation on the generation of endogenous stem cells raises the possibility that control of microglial activation in amytrophic lateral sclerosis might be critical for implementing stem cell therapies. Co-culture systems and tissue-specific expression of amytrophic lateral sclerosis–relevant transgenes are the most promising approaches toward this goal. Once better understood, interfering with the microglia-mediated inflammatory process might contain the spread of the disease and help pave the way for regenerative therapies.

Skeletal Muscle in Amyotrophic Lateral Sclerosis: Emerging Concepts and Therapeutic Implications   1091
Simone Abmayr and Patrick Weydt

Amyotrophic lateral sclerosis (ALS) is the most common adult-onset motor neuron disorder. We summarize recent insights emerging from clinical studies and transgenic animal research that suggest that skeletal muscle is more autonomously involved in the pathogenesis of ALS than previously thought. The implications of this new perspective for developing innovative therapies directly targeted at the muscle are discussed.

Chronic Pain in Persons with Neuromuscular Disease   1099
Amy J. Hoffman, Mark P. Jensen, R. Ted Abresch, and Gregory T. Carter

This article reviews what is known concerning the nature and scope of pain in persons with neuromuscular diseases and discusses possible mechanisms of neuromuscular disease–related pain, including neuropathic and musculoskeletal components. Much of the information presented comes from the initial results of a multicenter neuromuscular research program that has been conducted as part of a National Institutes of Health Program Project grant and from a review of the current literature. Treatment strategies for treating pain in persons with neuromuscular diseases also are discussed.

Exploring Chronic Pain in Youths with Duchenne Muscular Dystrophy: A Model for Pediatric Neuromuscular Disease   1113
Joyce M. Engel, Deborah Kartin, and Kenneth M. Jaffe

There is a striking lack of research on pain in children with neuromuscular disease (NMD). Given that Duchenne muscular dystrophy (DMD) is the most common NMD in childhood, we have chosen to use it as a model to explore pain in children with NMD. We provide an overview of DMD and discuss pain in the context of this NMD. Strategies for pediatric pain assessment and possible pain treatments are reviewed. Direction for future research and clinical implications for addressing pain in children with NMD are recommended.

Respiratory Support of Individuals with Duchenne Muscular Dystrophy: Toward a Standard of Care   1125
Joshua O. Benditt and Louis Boitano

Excellent respiratory assessment and support are necessary to maintain quality of life, extend duration of survival, and avoid emergency situations for individuals with DMD. This article outlines a program of assessment and intervention at appropriate points during the progression of the disease that should help standardize respiratory management across centers. All individuals with DMD need to have access to proper ongoing assessment and the full range of respiratory support methods.

Cumulative Index 2005   1141

FORTHCOMING ISSUES

February 2006
Orthotics and Prosthetics
Mark H. Bussell, MD, *Guest Editor*

May 2006
Pain Rehabilitation
James Robinson, MD, *Guest Editor*

August 2006
Sports Medicine
Gregory A. Strock, MD, *Guest Editor*

RECENT ISSUES

August 2005
Running Injuries
Venu Akuthota, MD, Mark A. Harrast, MD
Guest Editors

May 2005
Multiple Sclerosis: A Paradigm Shift
Theodore R. Brown, MD, MPH,
George H. Kraft, MD, MS, *Guest Editors*

February 2005
Aging with a Disability
Adrian Cristian, MD, *Guest Editor*

PHYSICAL MEDICINE
AND REHABILITATION
CLINICS OF
NORTH AMERICA

ELSEVIER
SAUNDERS

Phys Med Rehabil Clin N Am
16 (2005) xv–xvi

Foreword

Current Trends in Neuromuscular Research: Assessing Function, Enhancing Performance

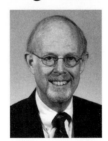

George H. Kraft, MD, MS
Consulting Editor

Much has happened in the field of neuromuscular disease in the past few decades. Until recently, these diseases were characterized by their physical presentation (phenotype), electromyographic findings, and biopsy characteristics. Many of these diseases are now identifiable by genetic analysis (genotype). Now we are on the threshold of using genetic engineering to actually correct the dysfunction seen in these disorders.

Dr. Greg Carter—a familiar contributor to this series—accepted the challenge of pulling together a wealth of useful information on this topic. He has recruited leading researchers to write articles ranging from basic science, through applications of assessment techniques, to practical treatments for these diseases.

Applicable basic sciences are reviewed, and the role of oxidative stress and microglial cells are explained. Metabolic syndrome and abnormalities in muscle in ALS are discussed, along with the animal model of hereditary neuropathy.

Application of familiar assessment techniques such as electromyography and single-fiber EMG to neuromuscular research is explained. In addition, there is an innovative discussion of MRI in muscle disease.

However, because the *Physical Medicine and Rehabilitation Clinics of North America* is a series for practitioners, application of these innovative treatments to neuromuscular diseases is emphasized. Gene transfer, stem cell

doi:10.1016/j.pmr.2005.09.001

treatments, and the use of neurotrophic factors are discussed as potential treatments. Fundamental concepts of therapeutic exercise are also discussed. Ventilatory and pain management are discussed.

Dr. Carter has recruited a truly distinguished group of authors: Drs. Tarnopolsky, Chamberlain, Huard, Ravits, Reid, Krivickas, Frontera, Weiss, Han, Fritz, Distad, Kilmer, Lou, Muller, Jensen, Aberesh, Engel, Abmayr, Weydt, and Benditt have all contributed to this excellent issue. My thanks and those of the readers must go to them for this outstanding and lasting contribution.

George H. Kraft, MD, MS
Department of Rehabilitation Medicine
University of Washington School of Medicine
1959 NE Pacific Avenue, Box 356490
Seattle, WA 98195-6490, USA

E-mail address: ghkraft@u.washington.edu

PHYSICAL MEDICINE
AND REHABILITATION
CLINICS OF
NORTH AMERICA

ELSEVIER
SAUNDERS

Phys Med Rehabil Clin N Am
16 (2005) xvii–xviii

Preface

Current Trends in Neuromuscular Research: Assessing Function, Enhancing Performance

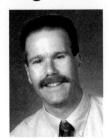

Gregory T. Carter, MD
Guest Editor

It is my distinct honor to be a Guest Editor for this issue of the *Physical Medicine and Rehabilitation Clinics of North America* on "Current Trends in Neuromuscular Research: Assessing Function, Enhancing Performance." I would like to thank Dr. George Kraft, for inviting me to undertake this task. In addition to being my mentor and role model, I am fortunate to have George as a close personal friend.

My goal with this text is to provide the reader with an up-to-date synopsis of where we are now in neuromuscular disease (NMD) treatment and research. I also requested that the authors discuss the theoretic implications of their research, with the hope that this body of articles will serve as a catalyst to spur new research ideas. The authors in this volume are all doing some of the very best research and clinical work in this field, and this book is evidence of that.

Although there have been tremendous strides achieved in the field of NMD over the past decade, we still have a ways to go before there are safe, effective treatments. Research requires long hours in lab or clinic, and some days end with no useful data. I am grateful for the inspiration that our patients who struggle with these disorders provide for us. I am also thankful for organizations like the Muscular Dystrophy Association (MDA). The MDA continues to prod us along, pushing for better treatments, while supporting clinics that strive for excellence in treating people with NMDs.

1047-9651/05/$ - see front matter © 2005 Elsevier Inc. All rights reserved.
doi:10.1016/j.pmr.2005.08.010

Finally, I would like to dedicate this book to Dr. Barbara Horwitz, professor of Physiology at the University of California, Davis. Barbara was my undergraduate mentor and graduate school advisor, and had a tremendously positive impact on me. She has dedicated her life to teaching thousands of students over the years, all the while doing cutting-edge research in cellular metabolism. Despite all her achievements, she remains a kind and humble soul, thoroughly dedicated to her students, as well as the art of teaching and the discipline of science. Thank you, Barbara!

Gregory T. Carter, MD
1809 Cooks Hill Road
Centralia, WA 98531, USA

E-mail address: gtcarter@u.washington.edu

PHYSICAL MEDICINE
AND REHABILITATION
CLINICS OF
NORTH AMERICA

Phys Med Rehabil Clin N Am
16 (2005) 859–873

ELSEVIER
SAUNDERS

Understanding Skeletal Muscle Adaptation to Exercise Training in Humans: Contributions from Microarray Studies

Douglas J. Mahoney, PhD[a],
Mark A. Tarnopolsky, MD, PhD[b],*

[a]Apoptosis Research Center, Children's Hospital of Eastern Ontario Research Institute,
Room 3121, 401 Smyth Road, Ottawa, Ontario, Canada, K1H 8L1
[b]Department of Pediatrics and Medicine, Division of Neurology and Rehabilitation,
Room 4U4, McMaster University Medical Center, Hamilton Health Sciences,
1200 Main Street, West Hamilton, Ontario, Canada, L8N 3Z5

Physical exercise represents a potent stimulus for physiologic adaptation. It has been known since the time of the ancient Olympics that repetitively lifting heavy weights results in muscle hypertrophy and progressively running longer distances allows individuals to complete long-distance runs such as the marathon (Fig. 1). At the cellular level, resistance exercise results in muscle fiber hypertrophy through an increase in contractile protein accumulation [1] and net myofibrillar protein synthesis [2]. In contrast, endurance exercise induces mitochondrial biogenesis and capillary proliferation, without muscle hypertrophy [3–5]. The study of exercise adaptations in skeletal muscle is important to the field of rehabilitation. Resistance exercise commonly is used in the postimmobilization period after orthopedic procedures, such as joint replacement or ligament surgery [6], or as a countermeasure to age-associated sarcopenia [7,8]. Endurance exercise commonly is used in the rehabilitation of patients with cardiovascular disease [9–11], peripheral vascular disease [12], or chronic obstructive pulmonary disease [13]. Although the apparent link between exercise-enhanced recovery in the aforementioned disease states and exercise-mediated adaptations in healthy individuals may not be immediately apparent, the fundamental signals

This work was supported by NSERC, Canada.
* Corresponding author.
E-mail address: tarnopol@mcmaster.ca (M.A. Tarnopolsky).

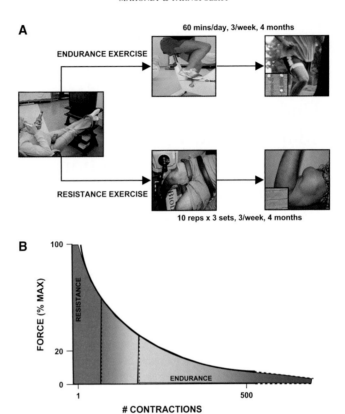

Fig. 1. Adaptation to endurance and resistance training. (*A*) The progression from a non-trained, sedentary individual to an exercise-trained individual is depicted. In the upper pictures, a period of endurance exercise training (eg, 60 min/d three times per week for 4 months) leads to physiologic adaptations in skeletal muscle and other tissues that enables the formerly sedentary individual to complete long-distance endurance activities (eg, marathon). An electron micrograph of skeletal muscle from a highly trained endurance athlete shows an accumulation of mitochondria and intramyocellular triglycerides. In the lower pictures, a period of resistance exercise training (eg, three sets of 10 repetitions three times a week for 4 months) leads to physiologic adaptation that culminates in muscle hypertrophy in the formerly nontrained individual. An electron micrograph shows highly ordered sarcomeres that do not have mitochondrial and intramyocellular triglyceride proliferation as is seen after endurance training. (*B*) Endurance-type versus resistance-type exercise is defined largely by the muscle force that is generated with each contraction and the number of contractions that can be performed before fatigue. Endurance exercise consists of many low-force contractions, whereas resistance exercise consists of a few high-force contractions.

involved are likely similar, and it is much easier to evaluate adaptation in healthy volunteers under controlled conditions as opposed to individuals with comorbidities and multiple medication interactions. The knowledge gained under controlled conditions can be used to identify targets for therapy or "genetic signatures" that could predict successful rehabilitation of a patient with a given disorder.

The protein adaptations in response to endurance exercise training have been well characterized and include increases in proteins involved in mitochondrial ATP production [14–16]; mobilization, transport, and oxidation of fatty acids [17,18]; glucose transport and glycogen synthesis [19–21]; antioxidant defenses [22,23]; and oxygen delivery to, and extraction from, skeletal muscle [24,25]. Collectively, these adaptations lead to enhanced fatigue resistance during submaximal exercise, via an increase in maximal oxygen consumption, a greater reliance on lipid and lower protein and glycogen use during exercise, and higher stores of glycogen and intramyocellular lipid (IMCL) (Fig. 2A) [16,21,26,27]. The protein adaptations to repeated resistance exercise have been less well characterized, but in general proteins involved in the contractile apparatus [28,29], and antioxidant and stress-responsive enzymes [30,31] show the most robust changes, with glucose transporter GLUT-4 also increasing [32]. The resultant hypertrophy of muscle fibers leads to a greater ability to develop absolute force or to perform more contractions against a given resistance (Fig. 2B).

How different types of muscular contraction patterns can lead to such divergent cellular adaptations is still not entirely understood. In general, factors such as strain on the sarcolemma, reductions in phosphocreatine, increases in lactate, remodeling of exercise-induced damage, and inflammation are believed to be important in the induction of the hypertrophy signal [33–38]. Endurance exercise adaptations occur in response to reductions in cellular fuel sources (glycogen and IMCL), increased electron flux through the mitochondria, and relative cellular hypoxemia [39–42]. These "cellular alterations" can engage pathways involved in cellular adaptation at many levels, including transcriptional, post-transcriptional, translational, and post-translational, ultimately to influence protein content or regulation. Generally, the adaptation to any type of exercise includes the

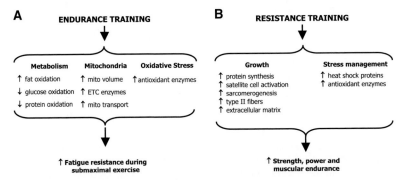

Fig. 2. The major adaptations that occur in response to endurance and resistance training. (*A*) Endurance training elicits, among others, adaptations in fuel selection, mitochondrial content, and protection from oxidant stress that leads to increased fatigue resistance during endurance-type exercise. (*B*) Resistance training elicits, among others, adaptations in contractile and stress-related proteins that lead to elevated strength, power, and muscular endurance.

following factors (Fig. 3): (1) stimulus (eg, endurance exercise); (2) cellular alteration (eg, increase in intracellular calcium); (3) sensor/signaling mechanism (eg, calcium/calmodulin-dependent protein kinase IV); (4) transcriptional, post-transcriptional, translational, or post-translational modification (eg, transcription factor–mediated transcriptional activation of peroxisome proliferator activated receptor [PPAR] γ coactivator 1 α [*PGC1α*]); and (5) adaptation to attenuate future threats to homeostasis (eg, mitochondrial biogenesis leading to an enhanced capacity to generate ATP aerobically).

Although it is difficult to ascertain definitively the level of regulation that is responsible for adaptation, the most accepted generalized hypothesis is that adaptation is mediated largely at the transcriptional level. It is believed that "pulses" of elevated mRNA expression after individual exercise bouts within a training program lead to long-term increases in protein abundance,

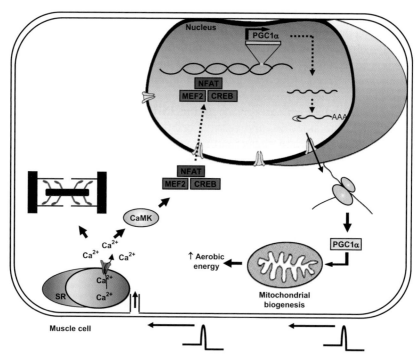

Fig. 3. Skeletal muscle regulation of exercise-mediated adaptation. Endurance exercise induces alterations in the muscle cell environment (eg, intracellular calcium accumulation) that are "sensed" by various kinases and phosphatases (eg, CaMKIV). These cell sensors transmit information to transcriptional regulatory proteins (eg, CREB, MEF2, NFAT), which can induce gene-specific transcriptional activation (eg, PGC1α). Translation of the gene products into proteins can induce a functional response that contributes to adaptation (eg, PGC1α-mediated transcription of mitochondrial genes, which contribute to mitochondrial biogenesis).

which culminates in physiologic adaptations (Fig. 4) [43,44]. As such, a major directive of molecular exercise physiology is to elucidate the transcriptional response to exercise in an attempt to understand the underpinnings of exercise-mediated adaptation. A relatively recent approach termed *genomics* allows for the simultaneous evaluation of the abundance of tens of thousands of mRNA species in response to a stimulus. This evaluation is possible through the use of technology called *microarray analysis* with the global mRNA response to a stimulus called the *transcriptome* [45,46]. In essence, thousands of cDNAs or oligonucleotides are spotted or synthesized directly onto a platform. After extraction from tissue or cells, the mRNA from a control sample is labeled with a fluorescent dye such as Cy3, and the mRNA from the experimental sample is labeled with a different dye (eg, Cy5) and hybridized onto the "chip." The chip is scanned using a laser scanner, and the relative abundance of the experimental transcriptome is compared with the control. Because the many thousands of mRNA species that are evaluated simultaneously can lead to false-positive results, numerous statistical tests have been developed exclusively for microarray data analysis, such as significance analysis of microarrays [47] and others [48]. Usually microarray data are reported with some analysis of the fold induction/repression, data from an alternative method for measuring mRNA (ie, reverse transcriptase polymerase chain reaction), a measure of the statistical significance, and some attempt at clustering or organizing the data. Most journals now require that microarray data conform to the guidelines set forth on the "Minimal Information About Microarray Experiments (MIAME)" website (http://www.mged.org/Workgroups/MIAME/miame.html) [49]. With numerous technical and conceptual issues taken into account, microarray data can provide powerful information regarding pathways that are important to cellular adaptation in response to exercise. This article reviews more recent studies of global gene expression in human skeletal muscle in response to endurance and resistance exercise, with a focus

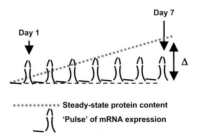

Fig. 4. Hypothesis for transcriptional contributions to adaptation. It is postulated that repetitive pulses of elevated mRNA expression in response to each individual exercise bout within a training program leads to long-term increases in protein expression, which is the basis of adaptation.

on how these array studies have advanced understanding of exercise-mediated adaptation in human skeletal muscle.

Endurance exercise

The authors published a study in which they examined global gene expression profiles in human skeletal muscle after a single bout of endurance exercise (approximately 75 minutes of moderate-intensity to high-intensity cycle ergometry) [50]. In this study, the authors identified many genes that were differentially expressed, some being "classic" exercise-responsive genes and others being genes that have not been shown previously to respond to exercise.

Endurance exercise activates transcriptional regulators of aerobic ATP generation

Endurance exercise rapidly induced a cluster of regulatory genes involved in aerobic ATP production and fuel selection (Fig. 5). This general response was expected because mitochondrial proliferation and elevated reliance on fat as a fuel source during exercise are two of the most pronounced adaptations to endurance exercise training [15,41,51–53]. Included within this cluster of genes were *PGC1α* and pyruvate dehydrogenase kinase 4 (*PDK4*), the "master regulators" of skeletal muscle mitochondrial biogenesis and glucose sparing [54,55]. The authors were not the first to observe these expression changes after exercise; a recurrent theme is that the expression of *PCG1α* and *PDK4* is robustly increased in response to endurance exercise [56,57]. *PGC1α* is thought to engage the coordinate induction of the nuclear and

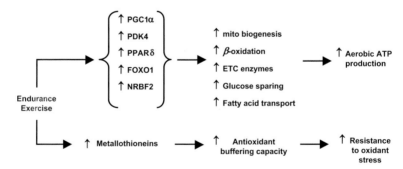

Fig. 5. Schematic representation of important DNA microarray results after endurance exercise study. Endurance exercise rapidly activated *PGC1α, PDK4, PPARδ, FOXO1,* and *NRBF2,* which seem to be important for exercise-mediated mitochondrial expansion and altered fuel selection, which enhances aerobic ATP-generating capacity in skeletal muscle. Endurance exercise also rapidly activated the metallothionein gene family, which seems to have a role in oxidant management and may confer protection from exercise-induced oxidant stress.

mitochondrial-encoded proteins required for mitochondrial proliferation, electron transport chain (ETC) and β-oxidation expansion, whereas *PDK4* activation represses the activity of the pyruvate dehydrogenase complex, attenuating the use of glucose as a fuel substrate. Collectively, exercise-mediated induction of these proteins is thought to lead to enhanced aerobic capacity and lipid oxidation, which improves performance in athletes, whereas the same adaptations can improve insulin sensitivity in individuals with metabolic syndrome and insulin resistance [58–60].

Endurance exercise also rapidly induced *PPARδ*, forkhead transcription factor O1 (*FOXO1*), and nuclear receptor binding factor-2 (*NRBF-2*) expression. These genes are known transcriptional regulators that are emerging as potential mediators of mitochondrial and metabolic adaptations to endurance exercise. *PPARδ* is an important regulator of fat metabolism, mitochondrial biogenesis, and fiber type determination in skeletal muscle [61]. Transgenic mice overexpressing *PPARδ* have elevated oxidative fibers, mitochondrial DNA content, and mitochondrial enzymes [62,63]. These mice performed better on a treadmill test and were protected from obesity. *PPARδ* overexpression in skeletal muscle recapitulates the important adaptations that occur with endurance exercise training, as was observed in mice overexpressing *PGC1α* [64]. Two other groups also have reported *PPARδ* upregulation in response to endurance exercise and endurance training [41,62].

FOXO1 is a transcription factor that positively regulates fatty acid metabolism and mitochondrial content and negatively regulates glucose metabolism, via activating lipoprotein lipase [65], *PGC1α* [66], and *PDK4* [67] transcription. In support of the authors' data, two studies also observed a dramatic increase in *FOXO1* skeletal muscle expression after endurance exercise [41,65]. Based on these observations and its known function in skeletal muscle, the authors had speculated that *FOXO1* might be involved in the mitochondrial and metabolic adaptations that occur in response to endurance training. Data from animal models overexpressing *FOXO1* in skeletal muscle do not support this speculation, however. Constitutive *FOXO1* overexpression leads to a loss of type I fibers and decreased exercise, glucose, and insulin tolerance [68]. These observations are in direct contrast to the adaptations that occur after endurance training and raise the important point that acute alterations in mRNA expression after a single bout of exercise are *not necessarily* involved in the adaptive program to exercise training (see later).

An important point, particularly when considering possible therapeutic implications, is that the mitochondria-related and metabolism-related genes that responded most robustly to exercise were *regulatory* genes (eg, transcription factors, transcriptional coactivators, nuclear receptors), not *effector* genes (eg, components of the ETC, β-oxidation). Therapeutically, it would be advantageous to target genes that assert widespread effects on the multitude of cellular events that compose adaptation (eg, mitochondrial biogenesis *and* elevated fat oxidation *and* glucose transport) as opposed to targeting individual genes within a given facet of adaptation.

Endurance exercise activates genes involved in antioxidant defenses

One of the most striking observations from the authors' study was the rapid, coordinate, and robust increase in all seven metallothionein genes measured on the array. Although the definitive cellular function of metallothioneins is not known, there is growing interest in their potential antioxidant function. Studies have shown that oxygen free radicals can induce MTI-III mRNA expression [69,70], particularly mitochondrial-derived free radicals [71], and that MTI-III proteins can protect cells from oxidant damage [72]. Because free radical production is a known sequela of endurance exercise [73], the authors hypothesized that metallothioneins may represent novel biologic mediators of free radical management in skeletal muscle (Fig. 5). Other investigators recently have observed a coordinate induction of oxidant stress and metallothionein gene expression and protein abundance after a bout of cycling [74] and have suggested a similar role for metallothioneins in muscle.

Expression changes observed after endurance exercise do not necessarily propagate throughout a period of endurance training

Timmons et al [75] have reported global gene expression profiles in human skeletal muscle in response to 4 weeks of endurance exercise training, in which there were several notable differences in gene expression patterns compared with the authors' acute study. The cluster of mitochondrial and metabolic regulatory genes that were activated after exercise was not elevated after training. Only a few genes involved in aerobic ATP production were elevated after training. Given that the protein products of these genes were surely elevated (this is the basis of exercise-mediated adaptation), these discrepant data indicate that mRNA itself does not need to accumulate to affect a training-induced increase in its protein product. Additionally, several genes that were activated after exercise were repressed after exercise training (eg, *PDK4*, metallothionein, *ras*-related associated with diabetes, uncoupling protein 3, and *FOXO*). This repression suggests that these genes are not involved in adaptation and respond to exercise for different reasons. It is possible that these genes are involved in restoring muscle cell homeostasis during the recovery period after exercise or are part of a generalized stress response that is triggered in "uninitiated skeletal muscle" before a more specific response can be "fine-tuned" throughout the training period. Regardless, the major "take-home" messages from these divergent data sets are: (1) Genes that are not elevated after exercise training still may be involved in adaptation, and (2) acutely responsive genes do not necessarily participate in adaptation.

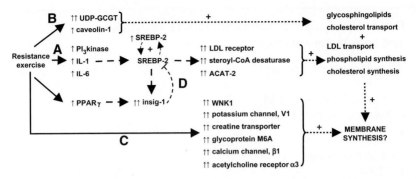

Fig. 6. Schematic representation of important DNA microarray results after resistance exercise study. (*A*) Resistance exercise rapidly activated *SREBP-2,* perhaps via PI₃kinase, IL-1, or IL-6 signaling. Resistance exercise also activated many *SREBP-2* downstream targets involved in cholesterol and lipid synthesis, uptake, and modification, such as the low-density lipoprotein receptor, stearoyl-CoA desaturase, and acetyl-CoA acetyltransferase 2 (ACAT-2). (*B*) Resistance exercise induced the expression of other genes involved in cholesterol and lipid homeostasis, such as caveolin-1 and UDP glucose ceramide glucosyl transferase (*UDP-GCGT*). (*C*) Resistance exercise induced the expression of genes that encode for membrane proteins, such as protein kinase lysine deficient 1 (*WNK1*), potassium channel VI, creatine transporter, glycoprotein M6A, calcium channel β1, and acetylcholine receptor α3. Collectively, activating these three "arms" may contribute to a program for de novo biosynthesis of a functional plasma membrane in muscle. (*D*) The delayed activation of insulin-induced gene 1 (*insig-1*) may provide negative feedback control over this response. De novo membrane biosynthesis may be activated in skeletal myofibers in response to either membrane damage or a stimulus for muscle growth. → denotes that resistance exercise induced mRNA expression of ... ; — → denotes that the given proteins may have been responsible for the induction of ... based on existing literature; ---→ denotes the likely biologic outcome of the given expression changes; ↑ denotes that mRNA expression was rapidly (3 hours) increased after resistance exercise; ↑↑ denotes the delayed (48 hours) induction of mRNA expression after resistance exercise.

Resistance exercise

The authors have examined global gene expression in human skeletal muscle after a bout of eccentrically biased resistance exercise in humans and observed the coordinate induction of an interested set of cholesterol and lipid-related genes (Mahoney DJ, 2005, unpublished observations). Resistance exercise induced a rapid increase in the expression of the transcription factor sterol regulatory element binding protein (SREBP)–2, which was followed by a delayed increase in a number of *SREBP-1* and *SREBP-2* gene targets, including the low-density lipoprotein receptor, stearoyl-CoA desaturase, acetyl-CoA acetyl transferase 2, and insulin-induced gene 1. These expression changes, together with the observed elevation in expression of caveolin-1 and UDP glucose ceramide glucosyl transferase, are characteristic of an established transcriptional program geared toward increasing cholesterol and lipid synthesis, uptake, and modification [76]. The expression of several potential upstream regulators of this *SREBP-2* program also rapidly increased after eccentric exercise, such as phosphotidyl inositol 3 kinase

---

Box 1. Upregulated genes common to resistance and endurance exercise

Immediate early genes
- c-*myc*
- Nuclear receptor 4A1
- Nuclear receptor 4A3
- v-*abl* homolog 1

Cell stress genes
- *HSF4*
- Proenkephalin
- Anion exchanger 2
- Tyrosyl-DNA phosphodiestase 1

Hypertrophy regulation
- *CARP1*
- *GSK 3 β*

Metabolism and mitochondria
- IL-6 receptor
- Mitochondrial ribosomal protein L2
- Mitochondrial ribosomal protein L32
- *PDK4*
- *PPAR*γ

Miscellaneous
- Keratin 5
- NMDA receptor
- Paralemmin
- Polymerase ε
- Pyridoxal kinase
- Splicing factor 1
- Testis zinc finger protein
- Transmembrane protein induced by TNF-α

(PI$_3$kinase)–γ, interleukin (IL)-1 receptor, IL-6 receptor, and *PPAR*γ. Together with a delayed increase in the expression of numerous plasma membrane transport proteins, the authors' results point toward an *SREBP-2*-mediated program of de novo membrane biosynthesis after eccentric exercise (Fig. 6) [77,78]. The authors speculate this *SREBP-2*-mediated transcriptional program is activated in response to either sarcolemmal damage or in anticipation of the need for sarcolemmal growth, hypotheses that currently are being evaluated. Given that sarcolemmal damage is pervasive in many types of muscle diseases, in particular the dystrophinopathies, this

SREBP-2 transcriptional program may represent a potential therapeutic target for the induction of de novo membrane biosynthesis in disease.

Signals and pathways common to endurance and resistance exercise

The authors' two studies were designed specifically with muscle sampling at the same time points so that a direct comparison could be made of genes that responded to endurance versus resistance exercise. Such a comparison yielded a group of 54 common genes that were differentially expressed after both exercise bouts, of which 36 responded to a similar extent and in a similar timeline (Box 1). This result was surprising, given the vastly different stresses faced by muscle during each of these protocols [26,79] and the different adaptations that occur after a period of endurance versus resistance training [26,80]. These genes may belong to a class of "exercise-responsive" genes, which respond to common signals and stresses inherent in both exercise modes. Many of these are immediate early genes or genes involved in the cell stress response, which supports this speculation. It would be interesting to test whether common differential expression would persist after each exercise bout throughout a period of exercise training. The number of common genes probably would decrease throughout a period of training, as the muscle fine-tunes the transcriptional response to meet the needs of the specific stresses placed on it more accurately (Fig. 7). This hypothesis is supported indirectly by a more recent microarray study in mice, in which a single bout of endurance exercise elicited the expression of many genes involved in muscle proliferation (a stress-related paradigm more commonly observed after resistance exercise), a response that was not observed after a period of endurance training [81].

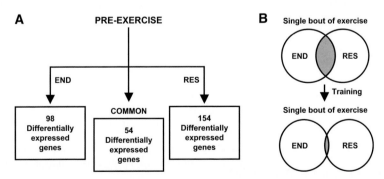

Fig. 7. Common and exercise type–specific gene expression. (*A*) A bout of endurance and resistance exercise induced the expression of 98 and 154 exercise type–specific genes. After both exercise bouts, 54 common genes were differentially expressed, which seem to be involved largely in stress management. (*B*) It is hypothesized that the number of common genes expressed after each individual exercise session within a training program would decrease throughout the progression of the program, as the muscle fine-tunes its transcriptional response to meet its needs more appropriately. ECC, eccentric; END, endurance; RES, resistance.

Summary

The authors' two studies using cDNA microarrays to profile the transcriptome pattern in response to endurance and resistance exercise have shed new light on exercise-mediated adaptation in skeletal muscle. Given that the two modes of exercise that the authors used represented the "extremes" of the exercise continuum, most forms of therapeutic exercise likely fall somewhere between them. One potential value of the data would be to provide transcriptome "signatures" that could be used to screen a variety of interventions that may enhance the pattern, including nutritional, pharmacologic, or alternative exercise paradigms. The data also could be used as a standard by which to compare the exercise response from a variety of patient populations to identify which components of the response could be altered by the disease in question. Future work is needed to map out the timeline of the response and to determine whether specific transcriptome patterns lead to idiosyncratic proteomic and phenotypic responses after a period of exercise training.

References

[1] MacDougall JD, Sale DG, Moroz JR, et al. Mitochondrial volume density in human skeletal muscle following heavy resistance training. Med Sci Sports 1979;11:164.

[2] Phillips SM, Tipton KD, Aarsland A, et al. Mixed muscle protein synthesis and breakdown after resistance exercise in humans. Am J Physiol 1997;273:E99.

[3] Henriksson J. Effects of physical training on the metabolism of skeletal muscle. Diabetes Care 1992;15:1701.

[4] Hoppeler H, Fluck M. Plasticity of skeletal muscle mitochondria: structure and function. Med Sci Sports Exerc 2003;35:95.

[5] Proctor DN, Sinning WE, Walro JM, et al. Oxidative capacity of human muscle fiber types: effects of age and training status. J Appl Physiol 1995;78:2033.

[6] Stanish WD, Lai A. New concepts of rehabilitation following anterior cruciate reconstruction. Clin Sports Med 1993;12:25.

[7] Yarasheski KE. Managing sarcopenia with progressive resistance exercise training. J Nutr Health Aging 2002;6:349.

[8] Yarasheski KE, Pak-Loduca J, Hasten DL, et al. Resistance exercise training increases mixed muscle protein synthesis rate in frail women and men $> / = 76$ yr old. Am J Physiol 1999;277:E118.

[9] Edwards DG, Schofield RS, Lennon SL, et al. Effect of exercise training on endothelial function in men with coronary artery disease. Am J Cardiol 2004;93:617.

[10] Lloyd-Williams F, Mair FS, Leitner M. Exercise training and heart failure: a systematic review of current evidence. Br J Gen Pract 2002;52:47.

[11] McConnell TR, Mandak JS, Sykes JS, et al. Exercise training for heart failure patients improves respiratory muscle endurance, exercise tolerance, breathlessness, and quality of life. J Cardiopulm Rehabil 2003;23:10.

[12] Gokce N, Vita JA, Bader DS, et al. Effect of exercise on upper and lower extremity endothelial function in patients with coronary artery disease. Am J Cardiol 2002;90:124.

[13] Harpa Arnardottir R, Sorensen S, Ringqvist I, et al. Two different training programmes for patients with COPD: a randomised study with 1-year follow-up. Respir Med 2005.

[14] Carter SL, Rennie CD, Hamilton SJ, et al. Changes in skeletal muscle in males and females following endurance training. Can J Physiol Pharmacol 2001;79:386.

[15] Holloszy JO, Booth FW. Biochemical adaptations to endurance exercise in muscle. Annu Rev Physiol 1976;38:273.

[16] McKenzie S, Phillips SM, Carter SL, et al. Endurance exercise training attenuates leucine oxidation and BCOAD activation during exercise in humans. Am J Physiol Endocrinol Metab 2000;278:E580.

[17] Bonen A, Dyck DJ, Ibrahimi A, et al. Muscle contractile activity increases fatty acid metabolism and transport and FAT/CD36. Am J Physiol 1999;276:E642.

[18] Johnson NA, Stannard SR, Thompson MW. Muscle triglyceride and glycogen in endurance exercise: implications for performance. Sports Med 2004;34:151.

[19] Houmard JA, Hickey MS, Tyndall GL, et al. Seven days of exercise increase GLUT-4 protein content in human skeletal muscle. J Appl Physiol 1995;79:1936.

[20] Phillips SM, Han XX, Green HJ, et al. Increments in skeletal muscle GLUT-1 and GLUT-4 after endurance training in humans. Am J Physiol 1996;270:E456.

[21] Richter EA, Derave W, Wojtaszewski JF. Glucose, exercise and insulin: emerging concepts. J Physiol 2001;535:313.

[22] Ookawara T, Haga S, Ha S, et al. Effects of endurance training on three superoxide dismutase isoenzymes in human plasma. Free Radic Res 2003;37:713.

[23] Ookawara T, Suzuk K, Haga S, et al. Transcription regulation of gene expression in human skeletal muscle in response to endurance training. Res Commun Mol Pathol Pharmacol 2002;111:41.

[24] Hickson RC. Skeletal muscle cytochrome c and myoglobin, endurance, and frequency of training. J Appl Physiol 1981;51:746.

[25] Vogt M, Puntschart A, Geiser J, et al. Molecular adaptations in human skeletal muscle to endurance training under simulated hypoxic conditions. J Appl Physiol 2001;91:173.

[26] Adhihetty PJ, Irrcher I, Joseph AM, et al. Plasticity of skeletal muscle mitochondria in response to contractile activity. Exp Physiol 2003;88:99.

[27] Schrauwen-Hinderling VB, Schrauwen P, Hesselink MK, et al. The increase in intramyocellular lipid content is a very early response to training. J Clin Endocrinol Metab 2003;88:1610.

[28] Balagopal P, Schimke JC, Ades P, et al. Age effect on transcript levels and synthesis rate of muscle MHC and response to resistance exercise. Am J Physiol Endocrinol Metab 2001;280:E203.

[29] Willoughby DS, Rosene J. Effects of oral creatine and resistance training on myosin heavy chain expression. Med Sci Sports Exerc 2001;33:1674.

[30] Parise G, Brose AN, Tarnopolsky MA. Resistance exercise training decreases oxidative damage to DNA and increases cytochrome oxidase activity in older adults. Exp Gerontol 2005;40:173.

[31] Parise G, Phillips SM, Kaczor JJ, et al. Antioxidant enzyme activity is up-regulated after unilateral resistance exercise training in older adults. Free Radic Biol Med 2005;39:289.

[32] Tabata I, Suzuki Y, Fukunaga T, et al. Resistance training affects GLUT-4 content in skeletal muscle of humans after 19 days of head-down bed rest. J Appl Physiol 1999;86:909.

[33] Bamman MM, Shipp JR, Jiang J, et al. Mechanical load increases muscle IGF-I and androgen receptor mRNA concentrations in humans. Am J Physiol Endocrinol Metab 2001;280:E383.

[34] Folland JP, Chong J, Copeman EM, et al. Acute muscle damage as a stimulus for training-induced gains in strength. Med Sci Sports Exerc 2001;33:1200.

[35] Fowles JR, MacDougall JD, Tarnopolsky MA, et al. The effects of acute passive stretch on muscle protein synthesis in humans. Can J Appl Physiol 2000;25:165.

[36] Hornberger TA, Esser KA. Mechanotransduction and the regulation of protein synthesis in skeletal muscle. Proc Nutr Soc 2004;63:331.

[37] Komulainen J, Kalliokoski R, Koskinen SO, et al. Controlled lengthening or shortening contraction-induced damage is followed by fiber hypertrophy in rat skeletal muscle. Int J Sports Med 2000;21:107.

[38] Thompson HS, Maynard EB, Morales ER, et al. Exercise-induced HSP27, HSP70 and MAPK responses in human skeletal muscle. Acta Physiol Scand 2003;178:61.

[39] Ji LL, Gomez-Cabrera MC, Steinhafel N, et al. Acute exercise activates nuclear factor (NF)-kappaB signaling pathway in rat skeletal muscle. FASEB J 2004;18:1499.

[40] Nielsen JN, Mustard KJ, Graham DA, et al. 5′-AMP-activated protein kinase activity and subunit expression in exercise-trained human skeletal muscle. J Appl Physiol 2003;94:631.

[41] Russell AP, Hesselink MK, Lo SK, et al. Regulation of metabolic transcriptional co-activators and transcription factors with acute exercise. FASEB J 2005;19:986.

[42] Wu H, Kanatous SB, Thurmond FA, et al. Regulation of mitochondrial biogenesis in skeletal muscle by CaMK. Science 2002;296:349.

[43] Neufer PD, Dohm GL. Exercise induces a transient increase in transcription of the GLUT-4 gene in skeletal muscle. Am J Physiol 1993;265:C1597.

[44] Pilegaard H, Ordway GA, Saltin B, et al. Transcriptional regulation of gene expression in human skeletal muscle during recovery from exercise. Am J Physiol Endocrinol Metab 2000;279:E806.

[45] Melov S, Hubbard A. Microarrays as a tool to investigate the biology of aging: a retrospective and a look to the future. Sci Aging Knowledge Environ 2004;42:re7.

[46] Nair PN, Golden T, Melov S. Microarray workshop on aging. Mech Ageing Dev 2003;124: 133.

[47] Tusher VG, Tibshirani R, Chu G. Significance analysis of microarrays applied to the ionizing radiation response. Proc Natl Acad Sci U S A 2001;98:5116.

[48] Zhao Y, Pan W. Modified nonparametric approaches to detecting differentially expressed genes in replicated microarray experiments. Bioinformatics 2003;19:1046.

[49] Brazma A, Hingamp P, Quackenbush J, et al. Minimum information about a microarray experiment (MIAME)-toward standards for microarray data. Nat Genet 2001;29:365.

[50] Mahoney DJ, Parise G, Melov S, et al. Analysis of global mRNA expression in human skeletal muscle during recovery from endurance exercise. FASEB J 2005;19(11):1498–500.

[51] Holloszy JO. Adaptations of skeletal muscle mitochondria to endurance exercise: a personal perspective. Exerc Sport Sci Rev 2004;32:41.

[52] Holloszy JO, Kohrt WM, Hansen PA. The regulation of carbohydrate and fat metabolism during and after exercise. Front Biosci 1998;3:D1011.

[53] Pilegaard H, Keller C, Steensberg A, et al. Influence of pre-exercise muscle glycogen content on exercise-induced transcriptional regulation of metabolic genes. J Physiol 2002;541:261.

[54] Puigserver P, Spiegelman BM. Peroxisome proliferator-activated receptor-gamma coactivator 1 alpha (PGC-1 alpha): transcriptional coactivator and metabolic regulator. Endocr Rev 2003;24:78.

[55] Sugden MC, Holness MJ. Recent advances in mechanisms regulating glucose oxidation at the level of the pyruvate dehydrogenase complex by PDKs. Am J Physiol Endocrinol Metab 2003;284:E855.

[56] Baar K. Involvement of PPARgamma co-activator-1, nuclear respiratory factors 1 and 2, and PPARalpha in the adaptive response to endurance exercise. Proc Nutr Soc 2004;63:269.

[57] Pilegaard H, Darrell Neufer P. Transcriptional regulation of pyruvate dehydrogenase kinase 4 in skeletal muscle during and after exercise. Proc Nutr Soc 2004;63:221.

[58] Dumortier M, Brandou F, Perez-Martin A, et al. Low intensity endurance exercise targeted for lipid oxidation improves body composition and insulin sensitivity in patients with the metabolic syndrome. Diabetes Metab 2003;29:509.

[59] Short KR, Vittone JL, Bigelow ML, et al. Impact of aerobic exercise training on age-related changes in insulin sensitivity and muscle oxidative capacity. Diabetes 2003;52:1888.

[60] Teran-Garcia M, Rankinen T, Koza RA, et al. Endurance training-induced changes in insulin sensitivity and gene expression. Am J Physiol Endocrinol Metab 2005;288:E1168.

[61] Holst D, Luquet S, Nogueira V, et al. Nutritional regulation and role of peroxisome proliferator-activated receptor delta in fatty acid catabolism in skeletal muscle. Biochim Biophys Acta 2003;1633:43.

[62] Luquet S, Lopez-Soriano J, Holst D, et al. Peroxisome proliferator-activated receptor delta controls muscle development and oxidative capability. FASEB J 2003;17:2299.

[63] Wang Y-X, Zhang C-L, Ruth TY, et al. Regulation of muscle fiber type and running endurance by PPARdelta. PLos Biol 2004;2(10):E294.

[64] Lin J, Wu H, Tarr PT, et al. Transcriptional co-activator PGC-1 alpha drives the formation of slow-twitch muscle fibres. Nature 2002;418:797.

[65] Kamei Y, Mizukami J, Miura S, et al. A forkhead transcription factor FKHR up-regulates lipoprotein lipase expression in skeletal muscle. FEBS Lett 2003;536:232.

[66] Daitoku H, Yamagata K, Matsuzaki H, et al. Regulation of PGC-1 promoter activity by protein kinase B and the forkhead transcription factor FKHR. Diabetes 2003;52:642.

[67] Kwon HS, Huang B, Unterman TG, et al. Protein kinase B-alpha inhibits human pyruvate dehydrogenase kinase-4 gene induction by dexamethasone through inactivation of FOXO transcription factors. Diabetes 2004;53:899.

[68] Kamei Y, Miura S, Suzuki M, et al. Skeletal muscle FOXO1 (FKHR)-transgenic mice have less skeletal muscle mass, down-regulated type I (slow twitch / red muscle) fiber genes, and impaired glycemic control. J Biol Chem 2004;279(39):41114–23.

[69] Bauman JW, Liu J, Liu YP, et al. Increase in metallothionein produced by chemicals that induce oxidative stress. Toxicol Appl Pharmacol 1991;110:347.

[70] Dalton TP, Li Q, Bittel D, et al. Oxidative stress activates metal-responsive transcription factor-1 binding activity: occupancy in vivo of metal response elements in the metallothionein-I gene promoter. J Biol Chem 1996;271:26233.

[71] Kondoh M, Inoue Y, Atagi S, et al. Specific induction of metallothionein synthesis by mitochondrial oxidative stress. Life Sci 2001;69:2137.

[72] You HJ, Oh DH, Choi CY, et al. Protective effect of metallothionein-III on DNA damage in response to reactive oxygen species. Biochim Biophys Acta 2002;1573:33.

[73] Ji LL. Exercise-induced modulation of antioxidant defense. Ann N Y Acad Sci 2002;959:82.

[74] Penkowa M, Keller P, Keller C, et al. Exercise-induced metallothionein expression in human skeletal muscle fibres. Exp Physiol 2005;90(4):477–86.

[75] Timmons JA, Larsson O, Jansson E, et al. Human muscle gene expression responses to endurance training provide a novel perspective on Duchenne muscular dystrophy. FASEB J 2005;19:750.

[76] Brown MS, Goldstein JL. The SREBP pathway: regulation of cholesterol metabolism by proteolysis of a membrane-bound transcription factor. Cell 1997;89:331.

[77] Demoulin JB, Ericsson J, Kallin A, et al. Platelet-derived growth factor stimulates membrane lipid synthesis through activation of phosphatidylinositol 3-kinase and sterol regulatory element-binding proteins. J Biol Chem 2004;279:35392.

[78] Porstmann T, Griffiths B, Chung YL, et al. PKB/Akt induces transcription of enzymes involved in cholesterol and fatty acid biosynthesis via activation of SREBP. Oncogene 2005.

[79] Clarkson PM, Hubal MJ. Exercise-induced muscle damage in humans. Am J Phys Med Rehabil 2002;81:S52.

[80] Schroeder ET, Hawkins SA, Jaque SV. Musculoskeletal adaptations to 16 weeks of eccentric progressive resistance training in young women. J Strength Cond Res 2004;18:227.

[81] Choi S, Liu X, Li P, et al. Transcriptional profiling in mouse skeletal muscle following a single bout of voluntary running: evidence of increased cell proliferation. J Appl Physiol 2005.

PHYSICAL MEDICINE
AND REHABILITATION
CLINICS OF
NORTH AMERICA

Phys Med Rehabil Clin N Am
16 (2005) 875–887

Functional Enhancement of Skeletal Muscle by Gene Transfer

Paul Gregorevic, PhD[a],
Jeffrey S. Chamberlain, PhD[a,b,c],*

[a]Department of Neurology, Senator Paul D. Wellstone Muscular Dystrophy Cooperative Research Center, University of Washington School of Medicine, 1959 NE Pacific Street, Seattle, WA 98195-7720, USA
[b]Department of Biochemistry, Senator Paul D. Wellstone Muscular Dystrophy Cooperative Research Center, University of Washington School of Medicine, 1959 NE Pacific Street, Seattle, WA 98195-7720, USA
[c]Department of Medicine, Senator Paul D. Wellstone Muscular Dystrophy Cooperative Research Center, University of Washington School of Medicine, 1959 NE Pacific Street, Seattle, WA 98195-7720, USA

Maintaining adequate skeletal muscle strength is key for not only quality of life, but also longevity. Limb muscle function is important for locomotion and daily manipulative tasks, but muscles of the trunk, neck, and head are instrumental in the maintenance of posture and breathing and the mechanisms of eating and swallowing. Many diseases and disorders result in, or are exacerbated by, impaired muscle function. Particularly critical conditions, such as severe muscular dystrophies and neuropathies, and extreme muscle wasting (eg, aging-associated sarcopenia and cachexia related to cancer and HIV/AIDS) ultimately can cause premature death. In light of the prevalence and severity of conditions that affect skeletal muscles, it is essential to develop therapeutic interventions to preserve and improve skeletal muscle function.

Gene therapy and gene transfer technology

Research advances are helping clinicians to understand the factors responsible for conditions that affect skeletal muscles and the mechanisms

This work was supported by a Research Development Grant from the Muscular Dystrophy Association (to P. Gregorevic) and by grants from the National Institutes of Health (AG015434) and the Muscular Dystrophy Association (to J.S. Chamberlain).

* Corresponding author. Department of Neurology, Senator Paul D. Wellstone Muscular Dystrophy Cooperative Research Center, University of Washington School of Medicine, 1959 NE Pacific Street, Seattle, WA 98195-7720.

E-mail address: jsc5@u.washington.edu (J.S. Chamberlain).

by which interventions promote adaptations in skeletal muscle function. In parallel, technologic developments are identifying valuable new biologic targets for existing pharmaceutical agents and the design of new drugs for established targets. The advent of so-called gene therapies may prove most valuable, however, in the development of new interventions to combat the life-threatening symptoms of severe muscle diseases and disorders. In stereotypical terms, gene therapies involve the introduction into the affected cells of a gene or gene fragment under the control of elements that regulate its expression. To deliver expression cassettes of interest to target muscle fibers, interventions generally employ either synthetic "vectors" incorporating small DNA fragments or circularized plasmids (some of which may be naked or complexed with lipophilic compounds to facilitate cellular uptake) or engineered recombinant vectors of viral origin that have been created by substituting the expression cassette for the viruses' regular genomic payload during controlled virion assembly [1]. Each strategy has advantages and shortcomings that make it better suited to particular applications [2].

In brief, nonviral technologies are generally cheaper to produce, are less restrictive regarding the size of the expression cassette that can be packaged, may be subject to reduced probability of a reactionary immunologic response after administration, but usually achieve only short-term transgene expression before being cleared from the targeted cells and requiring repeat administration. By comparison, recombinant viral vectors are more involved to produce and more restrictive in terms of packaging constraints, but usually offer considerably enhanced gene transfer efficiency by taking advantage of mechanisms for cell entry and gene transfer that have been fine-tuned over untold years of virus evolution and longer term transgene expression. Some of the earliest viral vectors developed were founded on retroviruses and adenoviruses, which although in certain guises remain in use today have been largely replaced with lentivirus-based and adeno-associated virus (AAV)–based vectors as the preferred viral vectors for gene transfer to muscle [1].

Lentiviral vector designs rely on configuration of their envelope protein assembly to endow them with the features required to enter mature skeletal muscle fibers, but by far their most valuable asset concerns their ability to facilitate integration of an expression cassette into the host cell's genome. This feature is used to particularly good effect for the transduction of skeletal muscle progenitor cells because multiple proliferative events completed by a single satellite cell can give rise to many new muscle cells that all inherit the integrated transgene [3]. Proliferative expansion of a transduced cell population in vivo, as might be expected with repeated cycles of skeletal muscle regeneration after injury, can increase progressively the efficiency of a single gene transfer event and may prove useful in the treatment of conditions in which frequent fiber degeneration and regeneration is a feature of pathology, such as Duchenne muscular dystrophy (DMD) (discussed in further detail later). Presently, lentiviral vectors are used most effectively in the transduction of muscle progenitor cells ex vivo before population expansion and targeted engraftment. This technology is discussed in more detail in another article in this issue. Principal limitations of lentiviral vectors concern the potential for immunologic reaction to the envelope proteins of the vector, challenges associated with controlling the genomic sites of integration and the production of sufficient highly pure vector, and difficulty in achieving widespread gene transfer to mature skeletal muscle fibers.

Compared with other vector systems, recombinant adeno-associated virus (rAAV) vectors would seem to be the presently favored means of extensively transducing mature skeletal muscle fibers. rAAV vectors appear comparatively immunoprivileged and currently are not associated with any known human pathology; they can achieve stable transgene expression on the order of years without requiring genomic integration; they can be generated in large, highly pure quantities; and they have been shown to transduce most of the mature skeletal musculature of mammals via systemic delivery routes.

Adeno-associated viral vectors for gene transfer

AAV are nonpathogenic members of the parvovirus family [4–6]. At least nine serotypes of AAV have been identified from primates, referred to as AAV1–AAV9 [7–9], and the different serotypes display various tropisms in vivo [10–13]. Serotypes 1, 5, and 6 have been reported to be particularly effective at transducing muscle fibers from mice and humans [10,12,14,15]. rAAV vectors support stable, long-term gene expression [16] from noninte- grated episomes after infection of muscle cells, and to date, rAAV vector in- tegration has not been detected in muscle tissue [17,18]. Stable gene expression after rAAV injection into muscle has been reported for 2 years in mice and more than 5 years in dogs and rhesus monkeys [19–23]. Al- though an inflammatory response has been observed in rare cases after de- livery of rAAV vectors that express an immunogenic protein, such as *Escherichia coli* βgal, under the control of a ubiquitously active promoter, such as cytomegalovirus [24–26], this response often can be blocked by the use of a muscle-specific promoter [25–27]. Other proteins derived from mammalian genomes have not elicited an immune response when adminis- tered to mice, even when employed with a ubiquitous promoter [26–30]. As a demonstration of vector tolerance, a phase 1 human trial for hemophilia b with rAAV2 did not produce any adverse events in patients even after in- jection of 10^{14} vector genomes [23], and the investigators reported that pre- existing antibodies to AAV2 in patients had no effect on myofiber transduction.

rAAV vectors package a 4.7-kb single-stranded genome flanked by short, inverted terminal repeats [4,5] and are grown to high yields by cotransfecting a transfer plasmid with a helper plasmid into human 293 cells [5,16,31–35]. The transfer plasmid contains the gene expression cassette flanked by the ter- minal repeats from wild-type AAV. The helper plasmid encodes the AAV genes *rep* and *cap* and adenoviral genes for genome replication [13,32,34].

Recombinant AAV "pseudotyped" vectors may be prepared using an AAV2 genome, the *rep* gene from AAV2, and the *cap* gene from the particular serotype of interest [36], the result being that the tropism of pseudotyped rAAV vector is derived from the nature of the capsid gene used [7,13].

Although the most commonly used rAAV vectors are based on the AAV serotype 2, the authors have characterized transduction of the skeletal musculature with rAAV vectors pseudotyped with the serotype 6 capsid and have shown that rAAV6 transduces skeletal muscle extremely efficiently compared with rAAV2 (Fig. 1) [35]. rAAV6 vectors yield transduction levels more than 500-fold greater than is achievable with rAAV2 vectors. With rAAV6, transduction levels peak 2 to 4 weeks before rAAV2 in fast and slow muscles, an important advantage in muscular dystrophy, in which the target tissue undergoes degeneration and regeneration cycles and must express the exogenous therapeutic transgene before the transduced myofibers degenerate. These characteristics of rAAV6-mediated transduction of skeletal muscle enable efficient transduction of the diaphragm and intercostal muscles after a single

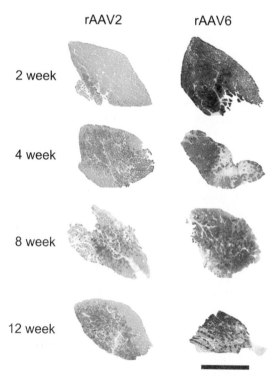

Fig. 1. Comparison of rAAV serotypes 2 and 6 for transduction of skeletal muscles. Mouse soleus muscles were injected at 6 weeks of age with 2×10^9 vector genomes (vg) of rAAV2-CMV/*lacZ* or rAAV6-CMV/*lacZ* vectors and analyzed for β-galactosidase activity (blue) in transverse cryosections 2, 4, 8, or 12 weeks after injection. The rAAV6 vectors expressed higher levels of gene product at all time points examined. Scale bar = 500 μM.

intrathoracic or intraperitoneal injection—muscles that are vital to respiration, yet historically difficult to transduce [35].

The impressive ability of rAAV6 to transduce muscle prompted the authors to ask if a systemic delivery system could be developed for adult mice. The authors found that rAAV6 vectors traverse the microvascular endothelium and transduce cardiac and skeletal muscles throughout an entire mouse after a single intravenous injection into adults and that coadministration of vector with VEGF-A$_{165}$ dramatically increases transgene expression at vector doses otherwise too low to yield detectable gene expression (Fig. 2) [26]. The effect of VEGF is dose dependent, but is not observed at high

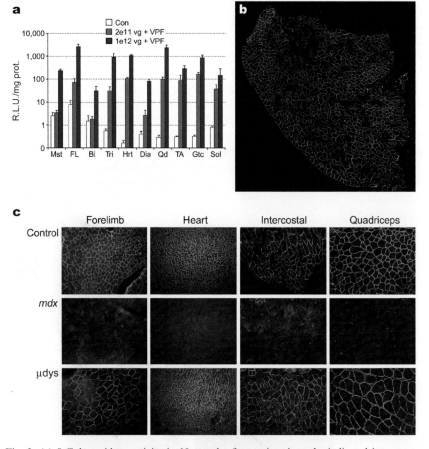

Fig. 2. (*a*) β-Galactosidase activity in 10 muscles from mice given the indicated intravenous dose of rAAV6/CMV-βgal and VPF (ie, VEGF). Mean ± SEM. (*b*) Dystrophin immunostaining in the *tibialis anterior* muscle of a mouse injected with 1×10^{13} vg of rAAV6/CK6-µDys via the tail vein. The mouse was injected at 6 weeks of age and analyzed 8 weeks later. (*c*) Immunostaining in representative muscles for dystrophin in 8-week-old *mdx* mice administered 1×10^{12} vg rAAV6/CMV-µDys via the tail vein. Analysis was 8 weeks postinjection.

($> 10^{12}$ vg) vector doses. Further investigation is required to enhance these techniques to scale gene transfer up for larger animal models approaching the size of human patients. The authors have performed an initial evaluation of these techniques in a ramped-dose safety study using a canine model, which established a vector dose that is readily tolerated by subjects, yet achieves encouraging levels of transduction in the myocardium and diaphragm (Fig. 3). Ongoing experiments are focused on identifying the mechanisms that influence gene transfer on a systemic scale.

Rational expression cassette and transgene design

In devising intervention strategies for a given condition, it is important to establish the specific cause of the clinical symptoms when possible. DMD is caused when genetic mutations disrupt production of the protein dystrophin, which is involved in structural organization and intracellular signaling within muscle fibers [37–40]. Consequently, dystrophin-deficient muscle fibers exhibit destabilization of the intracellular architecture and increased susceptibility to mechanical damage, leading to continued muscle fiber degeneration and muscle weakness [41]. An intervention designed to promote muscle growth (or hypertrophy) may have the potential to increase muscle fiber size and strength, but in the case of DMD, does not compensate for an inherent deficiency in a key structural protein and may aggravate the underlying pathology if muscles are subjected to more mechanical loading than they can withstand. In this instance, such an intervention may offer minimal

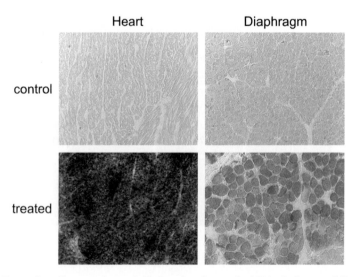

Fig. 3. Expression of human placental alkaline phosphatase (hpAP) in the heart and diaphragm of a 2-month-old beagle injected with 4×10^{13} vg/kg of rAAV6/RSV-hpAP into the jugular vein. Analysis was at 3 weeks.

benefit if not coadministered with an intervention designed to restore expression of the otherwise deficient/nonfunctional protein.

The major isoform of dystrophin is encoded on a 14-kb mRNA that generates a 427-kDa protein containing an N-terminal actin-binding domain, 24 spectrin-like repeats separated by two "hinges," a cysteine-rich domain that binds β-dystroglycan, and a C-terminal domain that binds the syntrophins and dystrobrevins [42]. Large deletions in the dystrophin gene found in some mildly affected patients with the related, although clinically milder Becker muscular dystrophy have spurred efforts to make highly functional "mini" and "micro" versions of dystrophin [28,29,43–47]. Through an extensive analysis of transgenic mice, the authors have observed that two large regions of dystrophin can be truncated with minimal functional impact: most of the spectrin-like repeats and the C-terminal domain. Microdystrophins with four or more repeats display surprisingly high function [28,29,46]. The most active 4-repeat clone that the authors designed (ΔR4-R23) contains the first 3 and the last of the 24 repeats and almost fully prevents dystrophy in transgenic *mdx* mice [29]. The most functional microdystrophin (ΔR4-R23) was modified for expression in AAV. The authors trimmed most of the 5′ and 3′ untranslated regions, mutated the Kozak sequence to boost translation, removed the C-terminal domain, and added the muscle-specific CK6 promoter developed in the Hauschka laboratory [30]. This 3.8-kb ΔR4-R23/ΔCT microdystrophin is able to reverse many of the morphologic abnormalities of dystrophic muscle when delivered to young adult mice by AAV2 [29]. Current opinion suggests, however, that existing microdystrophins still lack the complete functionality of full-length dystrophin. In this regard, the authors are continuing to examine the roles of specific regions of the dystrophin protein and their implications for construct design.

Expression of particular functional dystrophin constructs in transgenic *mdx* mice largely prevents development of the dystrophic phenotype if greater than 20% of wild-type dystrophin levels are produced [37,44,48]. Although dystrophin-positive fibers have a partially protective effect on neighboring dystrophin-negative fibers, most fibers in important muscle groups need to be targeted for optimal effect [44,48–51]. Because a major obstacle to applying gene therapy for DMD and other muscle disorders is the need for a systemic gene delivery system able to target all of the muscles of the body [52], the authors have been optimizing their rAAV vector–mediated gene transfer techniques for the expression of dystrophin genes in mouse models of muscular dystrophy. To consider the applicability of these novel delivery techniques as a treatment for muscular dystrophy, the authors have administered intravenously rAAV6 vectors expressing microdystrophin to *mdx* mice. Treated mice express functional dystrophin-based proteins in various limb muscles at levels sufficient to increase significantly the resistance of these muscles to contraction-induced injury (Fig. 2). Increased vector doses (4×10^{13} vg/kg with CK6) or use of the cytomegalovirus promoter (4×10^{12} vg) leads to essentially wild-type levels of dystrophin in all striated muscles. Although this systemic delivery has a striking effect on the dystrophic phenotype, treated muscles do not display a significant increase in mass, especially in older animals (discussed later). Additional methods that increase mass and strength may complement the ability of microdystrophins to halt further muscle damage and reverse partially the dystrophic phenotype. These exciting results establish a method for systemically administering a therapeutic vector without surgery or anesthesia that can improve the phenotype of a model of muscular dystrophy. Further investigation now is addressing the extent to which this therapeutic technique can be adapted for larger animal models of DMD, such as dogs, and the extent of phenotypic change in relation to the state of disease progression at the time of intervention. Because evidence suggests that treated animals show improvement but incomplete phenotypic reversal to the wild-type state, the authors also have begun to address the scope for combination treatment strategies using coadministration of other vectors designed to promote skeletal muscle hypertrophy.

Combination gene therapy to enhance muscle function

In considering an intervention strategy for a condition that includes symptoms of muscle weakness, it also is crucial to appreciate the cellular mechanisms exploited to enhance muscle function. An intervention that promotes muscle growth by stimulating protein synthesis may offer little benefit to a patient presenting with cachectic wasting if the principal cause of the condition involves profound stimulation of degradative proteolytic enzymes. This scenario might be considered analogous to pouring water (instead of protein) into a container (instead of a muscle fiber) with a hole at the bottom. A sufficient increase in the rate of water added may overcome the rate of water loss and achieve a net gain in the volume within the container at a given moment, but may consume more energy (and in the case of a muscle fiber, nutrients required for protein production) to sustain compared with devising a strategy to "slow or plug the leak," reducing (or halting) the loss of already hard-won resources.

Because DMD is associated with recurring cycles of muscle fiber degeneration and regeneration rather than merely excessive overactivity of degradative proteolytic processes, the authors have been exploring whether codelivery of microdystrophin with genes that could enhance muscle hypertrophy or regeneration might prove more beneficial for improving the dystrophic phenotype. One such gene is the insulin-like growth factor–I (IGF-I) gene, which expresses a specific isoform in skeletal muscle (mIgf-I). To determine if the beneficial effects of IGF-I on *mdx* muscles [53] are synergistic with the protective effect of dystrophin [26,29], the authors compared delivering mIgf-I alone versus codelivering mIgf-I and dystrophin to *mdx* muscles. Expression vectors in rAAV6 that expressed either microdystrophin or mIgf-I were injected into *tibialis anterior* (TA) muscles of 9-month-old adult *mdx* mice separately or together, then analyzed 4 months postinjection.

Immunostaining showed persistent expression of dystrophin that reached an average of 40% of the muscle cross-sectional area. The authors also observed persistent expression of Igf-I mRNA at levels 200 to 400 fold greater than endogenous *mdx* Igf-I levels in coinjected muscles. In contrast, injection of rAAV-Igf-I alone resulted in a fourfold decline of Igf-I mRNA levels in 4 months, suggesting that dystrophin protects muscle fibers from loss of vector DNA. Central nucleation was reduced by 20% in animals treated with AAV-μDys and animals cotreated with AAV-Igf-I and AAV-μDys relative to *mdx*. Muscles treated with AAV-Igf-I displayed an increase in muscle mass, but were not significantly protected from contraction-induced injuries (Fig. 4). In contrast, AAV-μDys-treated animals showed increased protection from contraction-induced injury, but did not display increases in mass or specific force. The combined treatment of AAV-Igf-I and AAV-μDys showed an increase in mass and strength, however, together with protection from contraction-induced injury, such that cotreatment was more beneficial than treatment with either vector alone (see Fig. 4). These studies show great potential for codelivering Igf-I and dystrophin to dystrophic muscle [54].

Another, less studied modulator of muscle regeneration and hypertrophy is myostatin (GDF-8). Myostatin is a member of the transforming growth factor–β protein family that has been identified as a potent negative regulator of muscle fiber size during myogenesis and after birth [55]. The biologically active component consists of a protein homodimer generated after secretion into the extracellular space that interacts with membrane-bound activin receptors present on skeletal muscle cells. The availability of biologically active myostatin is regulated by (1) transcription and mRNA accumulation; (2) protein synthesis and secretion of the precursor protein; (3) cleavage and dissociation of the myostatin propeptide to liberate the active, ligand-binding molecule; (4) interaction between the active dimer and other proteins that negatively regulate its activity, such as follistatin, follistatin-related gene, and growth and differentiation–associated serum protein-1 [56]; and (5) negative feedback of signal transduction elements stimulated by myostatin. In an attempt to regulate myostatin activity negatively, groups have sought to reduce translation of myostatin transcripts via expression of short interfering RNA sequences [57], reduce circulating protein levels via infusion of myostatin-specific antibodies [58,59], and inhibit proteolytic activation of myostatin by overexpressing a modified, noncleaving synthetic precursor peptide [60]. Overexpression of myostatin binding proteins in transgenic mice also has proved capable of increasing muscle mass [60]. These observations suggest perturbation of endogenous myostatin signaling is possible via many different methods, several of which could lead to a significant increase in muscle mass and might prove beneficial for the treatment of genetic or acquired muscle diseases characterized by muscle wasting and weakness. Although it is unclear how the inhibition of myostatin specifically elicits increases in muscle size, several groups have begun to consider the role of the myostatin pathway with

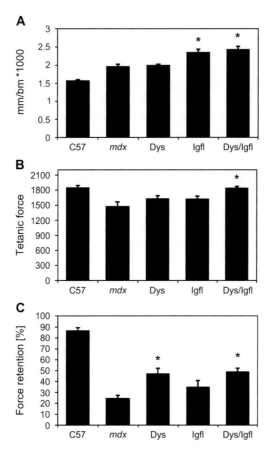

Fig. 4. Effect of AAV-Igf-I-treated and AAV-μDys-treated *mdx* muscles on functional proper-ties. *Tibialis anterior* (TA) muscles from 9-month-old *mdx* mice injected with AAV-μDys, AAV-Igf-I, AAV-μDys and AAV-Igf-I combined, or saline were analyzed 4 months postinjection. (*A*) Muscle mass/body mass (×1000). (*B, C*) TA muscles were analyzed in situ by measuring max-imum force production (*B*) and force after one lengthening contraction (*C*). Protection from contraction-induced injury is measured as the percentage of force-generating capacity after each lengthening contraction. Mean ± SEM; n = 9–12.

regards to events of factors affecting the dystrophic phenotype and the mech-anisms that regulate skeletal muscle regeneration [61]. This is an exciting av-enue for further research, and it is hoped that novel approaches are developed that may prove beneficial as interventions to enhance muscle function in dis-ease states such as the muscular dystrophies.

Summary

This article considers the development of gene therapies as a potentially viable means of enhancing skeletal muscle function for the treatment of dystrophin-related muscular dystrophies. As has been discussed, however, a clearer understanding of the causative mechanisms of muscle weakness in a given disease model and identification of the precise mechanisms of action associated with promising interventions may enable the rational design of gene therapies for many additional conditions characterized by impaired muscle function. The authors anticipate that these developments also would benefit from continuing improvements in vector design that enhance gene transfer efficiency and intervention safety. Assessing technical improvements in animal disease models of varying size and physiology would be crucial for verifying their efficacy and safety and should provide solid platforms from which to identify promising intervention strategies that warrant translation to clinical application. As with all experimental approaches being devised for life-threatening conditions for which no cure currently exists, thorough but sympathetic oversight of the development process by responsible regulatory agencies will prove invaluable for the ultimate realization of what it is hoped will be the next generation of therapies for serious neuromuscular disorders.

References

[1] Chamberlain JS. Gene transfer to skeletal muscle. In: Danos O, editor. Encylcopedia of genetics, genomics, proteomics and bioinformatics. Chicester: John Wiley & Sons; 2005.

[2] Thomas CE, Ehrhardt A, Kay MA. Progress and problems with the use of viral vectors for gene therapy. Nat Rev Genet 2003;4:346–58.

[3] Li S, Kimura E, Fall BM, Reyes M, et al. Stable transduction of myogenic cells with lentiviral vectors expressing a minidystrophin. Gene Ther 2005;12:1099–108.

[4] Atchison RW, Casto BC, Hammon WM. Adenovirus-associated defective virus particles. Science 1965;149:754–6.

[5] Muzyczka N. Use of adeno-associated virus as a general transduction vector for mammalian cells. Curr Top Microbiol Immunol 1992;158:97–129.

[6] Muzyczka N, Berns KI. Parvoviridae: The viruses and their replication. In: Knipe DM, Howley PM, editors. Fundamental virology. 4th ed. Philadelphia: Lippincott Williams & Wilkins; 2001. p. 1089–122.

[7] Rutledge EA, Halbert CL, Russell DW. Infectious clones and vectors derived from adeno-associated virus (aav) serotypes other than aav type 2. J Virol 1998;72:309–19.

[8] Xiao W, Chirmule N, Berta SC, et al. Gene therapy vectors based on adeno-associated virus type 1. J Virol 1999;73:3994–4003.

[9] Gao GP, Alvira MR, Wang L, et al. Novel adeno-associated viruses from rhesus monkeys as vectors for human gene therapy. Proc Natl Acad Sci U S A 2002;99:11854–9.

[10] Chao H, Liu Y, Rabinowitz J, et al. Several log increase in therapeutic transgene delivery by distinct adeno-associated viral serotype vectors. Mol Ther 2000;2:619–23.

[11] Halbert CL, Allen JM, Miller AD. Adeno-associated virus type 6 (aav6) vectors mediate efficient transduction of airway epithelial cells in mouse lungs compared to that of aav2 vectors. J Virol 2001;75:6615–24.

[12] Duan D, Yan Z, Yue Y, et al. Enhancement of muscle gene delivery with pseudotyped adeno-associated virus type 5 correlates with myoblast differentiation. J Virol 2001;75:7662–71.

[13] Grimm D, Kay MA, Kleinschmidt JA. Helper virus-free, optically controllable, and two-plasmid-based production of adeno-associated virus vectors of serotypes 1 to 6. Mol Ther 2003;7:839–50.

[14] Scott JM, Li S, Harper SQ, et al. Viral vectors for gene transfer of micro-, mini-, or full-length dystrophin. Neuromusc Disord 2002;12:S23–9.

[15] Hildinger M, Auricchio A, Gao G, et al. Hybrid vectors based on adeno-associated virus serotypes 2 and 5 for muscle-directed gene transfer. J Virol 2001;75:6199–203.

[16] Rabinowitz JE, Samulski J. Adeno-associated virus expression systems for gene transfer. Curr Opin Biotechnol 1998;9:470–5.

[17] Schnepp BC, Clark KR, Klemanski DL, et al. Genetic fate of recombinant adeno-associated virus vector genomes in muscle. J Virol 2003;77:3495–504.

[18] Vincent-Lacaze N, Snyder RO, Gluzman R, et al. Structure of adeno-associated virus vector DNA following transduction of the skeletal muscle. J Virol 1999;73:1949–55.

[19] Xiao X, Li J, Samulski RJ. Efficient long-term gene transfer into muscle tissue of immuno-competent mice by adeno-associated virus vector. J Virol 1996;70:8098–108.

[20] Fisher KJ, Jooss K, Alston J, et al. Recombinant adeno-associated virus for muscle directed gene therapy. Nat Med 1997;3:306–12.

[21] Song S, Morgan M, Ellis T, et al. Sustained secretion of human alpha-1-antitrypsin from murine muscle transduced with adeno-associated virus vectors. Proc Natl Acad Sci U S A 1998; 95:14384–8.

[22] Herzog RW, Yang EY, Couto LB, et al. Long-term correction of canine hemophilia b by gene transfer of blood coagulation factor ix mediated by adeno-associated viral vector. Nat Med 1999;5:56–63.

[23] Manno CS, Chew AJ, Hutchison S, et al. AAV-mediated factor IX gene transfer to skeletal muscle in patients with severe hemophilia b. Blood 2003;101:2963–72.

[24] Yuasa K, Sakamoto M, Miyagoe-Suzuki Y, et al. Adeno-associated virus vector-mediated gene transfer into dystrophin-deficient skeletal muscles evokes enhanced immune response against the transgene product. Gene Ther 2002;9:1576–88.

[25] Cordier L, Guang-Ping G, Hack A, et al. Muscle-specific promoters may be neccesary for adeno-associated virus-mediated gene transfer in the treatment of muscular dystrophies. Hum Gene Ther 2001;12:205–15.

[26] Gregorevic P, Blankinship MJ, Allen JM, et al. Systemic delivery of genes to striated muscles using adeno-associated viral vectors. Nat Med 2004;10:828–34.

[27] Hartigan-O'Connor D, Kirk CJ, Crawford R, et al. Immune evasion by muscle-specific gene expression in dystrophic muscle. Mol Ther 2001;4:525–33.

[28] Wang B, Li J, Xiao X. Adeno-associated virus vector carrying human minidystrophin genes effectively ameliorates muscular dystrophy in mdx mouse model. Proc Natl Acad Sci U S A 2000;97:13714–9.

[29] Harper SQ, Hauser MA, DelloRusso C, et al. Modular flexibility of dystrophin: implications for gene therapy of duchenne muscular dystrophy. Nat Med 2002;8:253–61.

[30] Hauser MA, Robinson A, Hartigan-O'Connor D, et al. Analysis of muscle creatine kinase regulatory elements in recombinant adenoviral vectors. Mol Ther 2000;2:16–25.

[31] Collaco RF, Cao X, Trempe JP. A helper virus-free packaging system for recombinant adeno-associated virus vectors. Gene 1999;238:397–405.

[32] Xiao X, Li J, Samulski RJ. Production of high-titer recombinant adeno-associated virus vectors in the absence of helper adenovirus. J Virol 1998;72:2224–32.

[33] Trempe JP. Packaging systems for adeno-associated virus vectors. Curr Top Microbiol Immunol 1996;218:35–50.

[34] Grimm D, Kern A, Rittner K, et al. Novel tools for production and purification of recombinant adenoassociated virus vectors. Hum Gene Ther 1998;9:2745–60.

[35] Blankinship MJ, Gregorevic P, Allen JM, et al. Efficient transduction of skeletal muscle using vectors based on adeno-associated virus serotype 6. Mol Ther 2004;10:671–8.

[36] Rabinowitz JE, Rolling F, Li C, et al. Cross-packaging of a single adeno-associated virus (aav) type 2 vector genome into multiple aav serotypes enables transduction with broad specificity. J Virol 2002;76:791–801.

[37] Cox GA, Phelps SF, Chapman VM, et al. New *mdx* mutation disrupts expression of muscle and nonmuscle isoforms of dystrophin. Nat Genet 1993;4:87–93.

[38] Brooks SV, Faulkner JA. Contractile properties of skeletal muscles from young, adult and aged mice. J Physiol 1988;404:71–82.

[39] Campbell KP. Three muscular dystrophies: loss of cytoskeleton-extracellular matrix linkage. Cell 1995;80:675–9.

[40] Petrof BJ, Shrager JB, Stedman HH, et al. Dystrophin protects the sarcolemma from stresses developed during muscle contraction. Proc Natl Acad Sci U S A 1993;90:3710–4.

[41] Emery AE, Muntoni F. Duchenne muscular dystrophy. 3rd ed. Oxford: Oxford University Press; 2003.

[42] Abmayr S, Chamberlain J. The structure and function of dystrophin. In: Winder SJ, editor. The molecular mechanisms in muscular dystrophy. Georgetown: Landes Biosciences; 2004.

[43] England SB, Nicholson LV, Johnson MA, et al. Very mild muscular dystrophy associated with the deletion of 46% of dystrophin. Nature 1990;343:180–2.

[44] Phelps SF, Hauser MA, Cole NM, et al. Expression of full-length and truncated dystrophin mini-genes in transgenic *mdx* mice. Hum Mol Genet 1995;4:1251–8.

[45] Crawford GE, Faulkner JA, Crosbie RH, et al. Assembly of the dystrophin-associated protein complex does not require the dystrophin cooh-terminal domain. J Cell Biol 2000;150: 1399–410.

[46] Sakamoto M, Yuasa K, Yoshimura M, et al. Micro-dystrophin cDNA ameliorates dystrophic phenotypes when introduced into mdx mice as a transgene. Biochem Biophys Res Commun 2002;293:1265–72.

[47] Chamberlain JS. Gene therapy of muscular dystrophy. Hum Mol Genet 2002;11:2355–62.

[48] Rafael JA, Sunada Y, Cole NM, et al. Prevention of dystrophic pathology in mdx mice by a truncated dystrophin isoform. Hum Mol Genet 1994;3:1725–33.

[49] Chamberlain JS. Dystrophin levels required for correction of duchenne muscular dystrophy. Basic Appl Myol 1997;7:251–5.

[50] DelloRusso C, Scott J, Hartigan-O'Connor D, et al. Functional correction of adult mdx mouse muscle using gutted adenoviral vectors expressing full-length dystrophin. Proc Natl Acad Sci USA 2002;99:12979–84.

[51] Dunant P, Larochelle N, Thirion C, et al. Expression of dystrophin driven by the 1.35-kb mck promoter ameliorates muscular dystrophy in fast, but not in slow muscles of transgenic mdx mice. Mol Ther 2003;8:80–9.

[52] Gregorevic P, Chamberlain JS. Gene therapy for muscular dystrophy—a review of promising progress. Exp Opin Biol Ther 2003;3:803–14.

[53] Barton ER, Morris L, Musaro A, et al. Muscle-specific expression of insulin-like growth factor I counters muscle decline in mdx mice. J Cell Biol 2002;157:137–48.

[54] Abmayr S, Gregorevic P, Allen JM, et al. Phenotypic improvement of dystrophic muscles by raav/microdystrophin vectors is augmented by igfi codelivery. Mol Ther 2005;12:441–50.

[55] McPherron AC, Lawler AM, Lee SJ. Regulation of skeletal muscle mass in mice by a new TGF-beta superfamily member. Nature 1997;387:83–90.

[56] Lee SJ. Regulation of muscle mass by myostatin. Annu Rev Cell Dev Biol 2004;20:61–86.

[57] Acosta J, Carpio Y, Borroto I, et al. Myostatin gene silenced by RNAi show a zebrafish giant phenotype. J Biotechnol 2005; in press.

[58] Whittemore LA, Song K, Li X, et al. Inhibition of myostatin in adult mice increases skeletal muscle mass and strength. Biochem Biophys Res Commun 2003;300:965–71.

[59] Bogdanovich S, Krag TO, Barton ER, et al. Functional improvement of dystrophic muscle by myostatin blockade. Nature 2002;420:418–21.

[60] Lee SJ, McPherron AC. Regulation of myostatin activity and muscle growth. Proc Natl Acad Sci U S A 2001;98:9306–11.

[61] McCroskery S, Thomas M, Platt L, et al. Improved muscle healing through enhanced regeneration and reduced fibrosis in myostatin-null mice. J Cell Sci 2005;118(pt 15): 3531–41.

ELSEVIER
SAUNDERS

Phys Med Rehabil Clin N Am
16 (2005) 889–907

PHYSICAL MEDICINE
AND REHABILITATION
CLINICS OF
NORTH AMERICA

Cell Therapy for Muscle Regeneration and Repair

Baohong Cao, MD, PhD, Bridget M. Deasy, PhD,
Jonathan Pollett, PhD, Johnny Huard, PhD*

*Department of Orthopaedic Surgery, University of Pittsburgh, Growth and
Development Laboratory, Children's Hospital of Pittsburgh, 4100 Rangos
Research Center, 3460 Fifth Avenue, Pittsburgh, PA 15213, USA*

Muscle cell transplantation is a possible treatment for skeletal muscle diseases, such as Duchenne muscular dystrophy (DMD). Research and clinical trials have revealed that the success of this technique is limited by several factors, including poor cell survival, inadequate dissemination of transplanted cells, and inducement of an immune response against the donor cells. Researchers have attempted to use various immunosuppressive regimens to reduce the host immune response and prolong donor cell survival, and some recent results are promising (ie, inducement of immune tolerance by chimerism). Researchers continue to make efforts to identify more cell populations that might be useful for transplantation-related applications. Although stem cells derived from various tissues have exhibited myogenic potential, readily accessible satellite cells and multipotent muscle stem cells remain the best choices for use in efforts to promote muscle regeneration and repair. Cell delivery to skeletal muscle is challenging because the proper distribution of transplanted cells is integral to achieving the desired therapeutic outcome. Although systemic delivery would ensure that the donor cells reach all the targets, it is not yet an efficient method for delivery of muscle cells. The posttransplantation microenvironment also has influenced cell differentiation strongly. To optimize the chances of successful treatment, researchers who

This work was supported by the National Institutes of Health (R01AR 49684-01), the William F. and Jean W. Donaldson Chair at Children's Hospital of Pittsburgh, and the Henry J. Mankin Endowed Chair at the University of Pittsburgh.

* Corresponding author. 4100 Rangos Research Center, 3460 Fifth Avenue, Pittsburgh, PA 15213.

E-mail address: jhuard@pitt.edu (J. Huard).

perform cell transplantation must work to understand and learn to control the in vivo microenvironment.

One of the most promising potential applications of cell transplantation is for the treatment of DMD, a congenital muscle disease caused by the lack of dystrophin in the membrane-associated cytoskeleton complex of muscle fibers [1–4]. Traditionally, most researchers who attempted to perform cell transplantation in muscle have used myoblasts. Transplantation of normal myoblasts into dystrophin-deficient muscle can create a reservoir of normal myoblasts capable of fusing with dystrophic muscle fibers and restoring dystrophin [5]. Previous experiments have shown that normal myoblasts fuse with dystrophic myoblasts to form hybrid myotubes that express dystrophin and that the transplantation of normal myoblasts into mice that model DMD (*mdx* mice) results in dystrophin expression at the muscle fiber plasma membrane in the injected dystrophic muscle [6–9]. The results of initial clinical trials focused on myoblast transfer to DMD patients demonstrated transient restoration of dystrophin-positive muscle fibers and improved muscle strength in patients who received injections [10–17]. The relatively poor outcome of myoblast transfer in these clinical trials was at least partially the result of the inadequate dissemination and poor survival of the injected myoblasts and immune rejection of the injected cells [18–24].

Recently, researchers have focused more and more attention on the types of cells used for transplantation. The results of many studies show that muscle may contain multipotent stem cells, which can generate not only muscle but also tissue of other lineages, including bone, cartilage, blood vessels, and hematopoietic lineages [25–31]. We discuss these novel muscle stem cells in detail in the remainder of this article.

The use of cell therapy in muscle has two advantages: the cells can deliver normal gene products to myofibers and can support muscle regeneration. When a transplanted myogenic cell fuses with a host myofiber, the hybrid myofiber expresses proteins coded by the donor and the host nuclei. Using cell therapy, researchers can induce the expression of a protein whose absence or low level of expression in the myofiber causes a disease (eg, the expression of dystrophin in patients who have DMD and in *mdx* mice) [9,17,32,33]. The results of some mouse experiments suggest that donor myoblasts also can serve as a permanent source of precursor cells in the host muscles [34–36]. The following sections describe the limitations that face researchers who study myoblast transplantation (MT) and present possible approaches to overcoming these challenges.

Challenge 1: immune response

The first major challenge encountered after delivering donor cells to the desired location is the possibility of triggering a host immune response. An immune response induced by cell therapy typically comprises two components: early response (which occurs within hours or days of the transplantation) and later response (which occurs after the early response).

Early immune response

The early immune response is poorly understood. Some observations seem to implicate immune cells in the death of many donor myoblasts [22]. The expression of various immunomodulatory substances by transplanted myoblasts has led to different degrees of improvement in donor cell survival [24,37]. Some research has shown that inflammatory cells are responsible for killing the donor cells [22]. The results of other recent studies indicate that natural killer cells and CD8-positive cells kill most donor myoblasts immediately after transplantation [38,39]. A recent analysis of immune cell infiltration after MT shows that only neutrophils infiltrated the donor cell pockets during the early hours after transplantation [40]. The neutrophils were nearly undetectable 2 days after transplantation [40]. Macrophages were not detected until 6 hours after transplantation [40]. CD8-positive lymphocytes and natural killer cells began to infiltrate the area of donor cells 6 days after transplantation [40]. Finally, some studies have demonstrated that complement also plays a role in this early cell death [41,42]. The early stage of the host immune response remains difficult to control. Most current treatments are designed to minimize or eliminate the later immune response.

Later immune response

The success of long-term MT is most limited by the later immune response. The later immune response involves cytolytic T lymphocytes killing the donor cells by a mechanism that involves major histocompatibility complex class I on the donor cells. Although this immune response is difficult to avoid, there are ways to reduce the severity of the immune rejection.

Suppressing the host immune reaction

Immunosuppressants are used commonly for preventing immune rejection after MT. The use of cyclophosphamide for this purpose has generated negative results because its antiproliferative properties likely killed the transplanted myoblasts [43]. The use of cyclosporine A has improved the result of MT in mice, but the results of some studies involving cyclosporine A indicate side effects on the transplanted myoblasts, including inhibition of fusion and differentiation [44–48]. Sirolimus also has improved the outcome of MT in mice [49]. The use of tacrolimus during MT produced the best results in mice, however, and is efficient in monkeys [50–55]. Researchers have observed abundant hybrid myofibers and no lymphocyte infiltration for up to 1 year after MT in primates [55]. Tacrolimus is widely used in clinical organ transplantation, but its administration is associated with long-term adverse effects. Camirand and colleagues [56] recently tested the combined use of tacrolimus and mycophenolate mofetil because these agents' toxicities do not overlap and their combined use reduces the single-drug toxicities. Further study is required to ensure that mycophenolate mofetil does not inhibit myoblast fusion, however [56].

Inducement of immune tolerance

Ideally, there would be a way to enable the host to tolerate the transplanted cells while preserving its immunity against other pathogens and cancer. Our recent findings indicate that a clone of muscle-derived stem cells (MDSCs) can differentiate into T and B lymphocytes after transplantation into lethally irradiated animals [27]. This finding supports the possible use of MDSCs to induce immune tolerance by transplanting MDSCs into marrow-ablated mice before muscle cell transplantation. It is expected that the transplanted MDSCs should differentiate into T and B lymphocytes and facilitate host tolerance of the subsequently transplanted muscle cells.

It also seems to be possible to induce host immune tolerance by reducing the immunogenicity of donor cells. Researchers have used this approach in in vitro studies by genetically modifying myoblasts to express human lymphocyte antigen-G, a nonclassic major histocompatibility complex class I molecule that is a key mediator of maternal tolerance to a fetus [57]. The results of the study indicate that the presence of even a few human lymphocyte antigen-G–positive cells within a population of human lymphocyte antigen-G–negative muscle cells had significant inhibitory effects on alloreactive lysis [57].

Challenge 2: cell survival

Cell sources available for transplantation

Researchers have investigated many tissues as potential sources of donor cells for transplantation. Studies have shown that stem cells elicit better muscle regeneration than do myoblasts. The discovery of these cells has enabled scientists to begin to surmount some of the problems associated with traditional MT. The following section describes and compares different populations of cells currently used in muscle cell transplantation.

Embryonic stem cells

Embryonic stem (ES) cells are pluripotent cells derived from the inner cell mass of blastocyst-stage embryos. Their importance to modern biology and medicine is based largely on two unique characteristics that distinguish them from all other organ-specific stem cells identified to date. First, it is possible to culture ES cells and expand them indefinitely as pure populations of undifferentiated cells for extended periods of time while preserving the cells' normal karyotype. Second, ES cells are pluripotent: they possess the capacity to become every type of cell in the body. The ability of mouse ES cells to contribute to all tissues of adult mice, including the germline, after injection into host blastocysts demonstrates the pluripotent nature of these cells.

In addition to their developmental potential in vivo, ES cells display a remarkable ability to form differentiated cell types in culture. Studies during the past 20 years have led to the development of appropriate culture conditions and protocols for the generation of a broad spectrum of lineages. The ability to induce ES cells to differentiate toward multiple lineages opens exciting new opportunities to model embryonic development in vitro and study the events that regulate the earliest stages of lineage induction and specification. Comparable studies are difficult in the mouse embryo and impossible in the human embryo. In addition to providing a model of early development, the ES cell differentiation system is widely viewed as a novel and unlimited source of cells and tissues for transplantation for the treatment of various diseases. The isolation of human ES cells in 1998 dramatically elevated scientists' interest in the therapeutic applications of ES cells and moved this possibility one step closer to reality [58].

ES cells are believed to have a high therapeutic potential for the treatment of various diseases, including skeletal muscle diseases. The successful generation of skeletal muscle in vivo requires selective induction, however (ie, co-cultivation of skeletal muscle cells with ES cells). Experiments performed with ES cells mixed with a preparation from mouse muscle enriched for myogenic stem and precursor cells and injected into *mdx* mice led to the occasional formation of normal vascularized skeletal muscle by the transplanted ES cells [59]. These results, although promising, require additional investigation and validation.

Cells obtained from postnatal tissue

Skeletal muscle
Satellite cells are located between the sarcolemma and basement membrane of muscle fibers. There is evidence that satellite cells are derived from the dorsal aorta [60]. Generally, satellite cells are identifiable on the basis of their expression of M-cadherin, c-met, the receptor for hepatocyte growth factor, myocyte nuclear factor, and Pax7, a paired box transcription factor [61–63]. Research also has shown that quiescent satellite cells on single mouse muscle fibers express the myogenic regulatory factor Myf 5 and CD34, which is also present in activated hematopoietic stem cells. Some research suggests that CD34 may be downregulated in cells in a quiescent state that are ready for subsequent activation [64]. Study results indicate that all satellite cells may not be equivalent [65,66]. More recently, Collins and colleagues [67] reported that satellite cells in a single myofiber can give rise to more than 100 new myofibers after transplantation into muscle. This finding strongly indicates that satellite cells are a powerful tool for repairing skeletal muscle.

Dynamics of satellite cells. In animals, satellite cells proliferate and fuse with the growing muscle fiber; some also self-renew to form new satellite cells. Despite this replenishment of the satellite cell pool during muscle growth, the number of satellite cells declines with age [68]. Satellite cells are activated by injury. Some research has indicated that hepatocyte growth factor can activate quiescent satellite cells [69]. Like muscle precursor cells, activated satellite cells express myogenic regulatory factors during skeletal muscle development. They proliferate and then fuse to form myotubes, which mature into myofibers.

Several reports have shown that satellite cells are a heterogeneous population. After injury, some proliferate before undergoing differentiation, whereas some satellite cells that only fuse with damaged muscle fibers are believed to be more committed precursor cells [66]. A small population of stem cell–like muscle precursor cells in mouse muscle survives high doses of radiation [70]. Neither normal nor myopathic *mdx* mouse muscle exposed to radiation retains the ability to regenerate; however, when such irradiated muscles are damaged extensively by snake venom, widespread regeneration occurs. The number of radiation-resistant muscle precursor cells that are activated in response to extreme trauma is greatly reduced in *mdx* muscle compared with normal muscle; these radiation-resistant cells may represent a quiescent satellite or stem cell subpopulation [70].

Growth factors also play key roles in the chemotaxis, proliferation, and differentiation of satellite cells. Crushed muscle fibers produce many factors that are mitogenic for muscle precursor cells, including basic fibroblast growth factor, platelet-derived growth factor-BB, transferrin, and hepatocyte growth factor [71]. Macrophages also produce growth factors that are mitogenic for muscle precursor cells, including platelet-derived growth factor, transforming growth factor-β, basic fibroblast growth factor, and leukemia inhibitory factor. Growth factors, such as hepatocyte growth factor, basic fibroblast growth factor, insulin-like growth factor 1, and transforming growth factor-β, also promote chemotaxis of satellite cells in tissue culture [72,73]. Satellite cells near the injury site are induced to replicate and migrate, but satellite cells also enter the injury site from elsewhere within the muscle [60,62].

Cells other than satellite cells also may give rise to muscle. One hypothesis was that skeletal muscle regeneration occurred by dedifferentiation of mature muscle fibers, but limited evidence supports this idea. The newt, which has no satellite cells, is capable of regeneration after injury by dedifferentiation and regeneration of mature urodele muscle fibers triggered by a thrombin-activated serum-derived factor [74]. Researchers have induced mammalian myotubes to dedifferentiate in vitro by administering a microtubule-binding purine analog, myoseverin [75], forcing expression of Msx 1 [76], or applying newt regeneration extract [77].

Researchers also have begun to identify and characterize multipotent stem cells isolated from mouse skeletal muscles called MDSCs [25–27,

37,78–81]. These cells seem to be precursors to satellite cells [25–27,37, 78–81] and exhibit a high proliferative capacity [25–27,37,78–81]. Some of the properties of MDSCs also may facilitate their systemic delivery through the circulatory system [25,27,82,83]. The intramuscular injection of normal MDSCs into *mdx* mice produced tenfold more dystrophin-positive myofibers than did the injection of myoblasts derived from satellite cells [26]; however, other researchers who performed follow-up experiments did not observe an improvement in muscle function after injection of MDSCs [84]. Researchers have hypothesized that MDSCs may exhibit immune-privileged behavior that enables them to avoid immune rejection [26]. Recent evidence has suggested that MDSCs may differ from satellite cells and that cells with hematopoietic potential are not transdifferentiated muscle cells but rather bone marrow–derived cells that reside in the skeletal muscle [63,85–87]. The results of other studies indicate that MDSCs are muscle derived [25–27,37,78–82,88–90]. Identifying the source of these cells requires additional investigation.

Cells of nonmuscular sources

Although satellite cells or MDSCs are the most obvious sources of donor cells for transplantation to treat skeletal muscle diseases, the results of some recent studies suggest that they are not the only sources of myoblasts in skeletal muscle. Other potential sources include bone marrow–derived cells [91,92] and vascular-associated cells [93,94]. These other sources of myogenic cells can assist in muscle regeneration if necessary.

Bone marrow–derived cells. Researchers have focused on the isolation of bone marrow cells not only to identify an alternative source of myogenic cells but also to develop a systemic treatment for DMD based on the use of a bone marrow transfusion that enables the transfer of a therapeutic quantity of myogenic precursors from the blood to the myofibers. Previous evidence in mice indicated that nonmuscular cells play little role in muscle regeneration [83,95–97]. Researchers' hopes were bolstered somewhat by the observation of dystrophin expression in some myofibers after intravenous infusion of normal hematopoietic cells in *mdx* mice and some participation of donor cells in muscle regeneration after bone marrow transplantation in normal mice, however [98,99]. Subsequent observations revealed the efficiency of bone marrow transplantation to induce the expression of donor dystrophin in a dystrophin-deficient mouse to be negligible: only 0.25% of the myofibers expressed dystrophin during each mouse's lifespan [100]. A recent analysis of a patient who has DMD who received a bone marrow transplantation at the age of 1 year to treat an X-linked severe combined immunodeficiency showed that 13 years later less than 1% of the child's myofibers contained donor nuclei [101]. A recent study concluded that the rare bone marrow cells that fused with myofibers were not hematopoietic in origin, because the level of dystrophin expression in the injected *mdx* mice did not correlate with the degree of bone marrow reconstitution [102]. Although some bone marrow cells in mice expressed proteins specific to the skeletal muscle, transplantation of a fraction enriched with ten times the amount of cells did not increase the low percentage of dystrophin-positive myofibers compared with a normal bone marrow transfusion in *mdx* mice [103].

Researchers also have identified a special population of cells referred to as side population (SP) cells. SP cells were first isolated from the bone marrow of mice via staining with the vital DNA dye Hoechst 33,342 and subsequent analysis and purification by fluorescence-activated cell sorting [104]. Bone marrow–derived SP cells appear dull (or Hoechst low) because of Hoechst dye efflux mediated by the ABCG2/*brcp1* transporter [105,106]. SP cells also have been identified in several other tissues, including skeletal muscle [60,62,66,98,107,108]. Muscle SP cells exhibit a limited ability to differentiate into muscle in vitro [85], whereas muscle main population cells are enriched for committed myogenic precursors and are able to form myotubes. Despite their limited in vitro myogenic potential, muscle SP cells exhibit hematopoietic and myogenic potential in vivo and can give rise to satellite cells [85,98]. In Pax7 knockout mice, a mutant that lacks satellite cells, muscle SP cells are present at higher percentages than in normal mice, which suggests that muscle SP cells differ from satellite cells and might be a population of satellite cell precursors. Because these precursor cells do not differentiate into satellite cells in *Pax7* mice, the SP cells accumulate [63]. Recent findings indicate that Pax7 only directs postnatal satellite cell renewal and propagation, however, not their specification [109]. These findings raised questions about the role that Pax7 plays in satellite cell development.

The multipotent nature of skeletal muscle–derived SP cells is demonstrated by their myogenic and hematopoietic potential in vivo. Whether SP cells originate from the bone marrow is unclear, however. To study the long-term contribution of the hematopoietic system to muscle SP cells, Rivier and colleagues [110] isolated whole bone marrow cells from Ly5.1 male subjects or from e-GFP transgenic male mice and transplanted them into lethally irradiated Ly5.2 female subjects. Long-term cell trafficking of donor bone marrow cells to muscle SP cells was monitored 17 times during the 34-week study. Fluorescence-activated cell sorting analyses were used to detect Ly5.1 and GFP + donor cells, whose donor origin was confirmed by fluorescence in situ hybridization for the Y chromosome. Although the researchers observed cells of donor origin in the muscle, donor bone marrow cells had contributed little to the muscle SP. Attempts to increase cell trafficking by damaging the muscle confirmed that more than 90% of the SP cells present in the muscle were of host origin. These results demonstrated that the bone marrow does not replenish the fraction of muscle SP cells and suggested a nonhematopoietic origin of this cell population.

Together these results indicate that the use of a patient's own bone marrow–derived stem cells to treat a myopathy is possible, but successful outcomes have been rare in experimental animals. The identification, isolation, and propagation of such stem cells and creation of a suitable niche in vivo for their proliferation and differentiation into the desired tissue continue to pose major obstacles.

Fibroblasts. Some research indicates that fibroblasts can differentiate into myoblasts if genetically modified to contain *MyoD1*, a master regulator gene for myogenesis [111]. This finding suggests that fibroblasts might be an additional cell source for muscle cell transplantation. Goldring and colleagues [112] reported that normal murine dermal fibroblasts implanted into the muscles of *mdx* mice participated in new myofiber formation and restored the expression of dystrophin. They found that the lectin galectin-1 is involved in the conversion of dermal fibroblasts into a myogenic lineage. Their study confirmed the presence of galectin-1 in the medium used for conversion. They also found that exposure of clones of dermal fibroblasts to this lectin resulted in 100% conversion of the cells. Galectin-1 did not, however, induce myogenic conversion of murine muscle-derived fibroblasts.

Mesenchymal stem cells. The adherent cell fraction isolated from bone marrow, stromal cells that form the supporting structures of bone marrow, can differentiate in vitro into a mesodermal phenotype (such as skeletal muscle) and are known as mesenchymal stem cells [113]. When exposed to specific conditions in mice, these cells undergo preferential differentiation into skeletal muscle [114]. After intramuscular implantation in mice, mesenchymal stem cells isolated from the synovial membrane of adult humans can fuse with myofibers and remain as satellite cells [115]. Some research also suggests that mesenchymal stem cells can participate in muscle regeneration after intravenous injection in the same model [115]. These mesenchymal stem cells derived from the synovial membrane are believed to be similar to those derived from the bone marrow [115]. The possible use of these cells for autotransplantation in ex vivo gene therapy is of interest, but determining their actual usefulness for clinical applications requires further studies, including studies in a nonhuman primate model. The development of efficient methods to achieve a permanent genetic correction in a patient's own cells also would be necessary.

Vascular endothelial cells. The true origin of these various populations of postnatal muscle stem cells remains unknown. Their stem cell characteristics often are determined by their expression of stem cell markers, including Sca-1 and CD34, and their unique behavior after implantation in skeletal muscle, including long-term proliferation, self-renewing ability, and multipotent differentiation [26]. Although Sca-1–positive cells are present within the basal lamina of muscle fibers, the true origin of these cells is still unclear

[25,26]. Because we have reported that a low percentage of the MDSCs express endothelial markers in vitro and, importantly, spontaneously differentiate into endothelial cells after intramuscular implantation in dystrophic *mdx* skeletal muscle, we suspect that a potential relationship exists between MDSCs and endothelial cells [26]. Other studies have demonstrated the isolation of myogenic-endothelial progenitor cells from the aortae of mouse embryos and postnatal mice that coexpress myogenic and endothelial markers [93,94,116]. After intra-arterial delivery, these myogenic-endothelial progenitor cells can regenerate skeletal muscle efficiently [94]. We recently identified a population of cells that coexpress myogenic and endothelial markers within human skeletal muscle [117]. We also have shown that it is possible to isolate these cells by cell sorting and expand them in vitro. More importantly, these human cells that coexpress myogenic and endothelial markers seem to regenerate skeletal muscle fibers more effectively than do human cells that express myogenic markers only [117]. We believe that these human myogenic endothelial cells may constitute a cell population in transit between myogenic and endothelial lineage and, as such, may be a good source of progenitor or stem cells for use in muscle regeneration and repair applications designed to treat muscle injuries or disease (eg, DMD).

Challenge 3: limited dissemination

Methods for cell delivery

Efficient procedures for delivering donor cells to target tissues are crucial to achieving beneficial outcomes. The delivery method is particularly important when trying to treat myopathies because these diseases affect tissue that accounts for almost half of the body mass and represents a large target. Researchers have tested two methods of cell delivery in skeletal muscle: local and systemic.

Local injection

Intramuscular injection is the most frequent method of delivering donor cells to skeletal muscle. It ensures that sufficient numbers of donor cells reach the muscle, and it produces tissue damage, which facilitates the uptake of the donor myoblasts by regenerating myofibers. Donor myoblasts delivered by intramuscular injection fuse mainly with the myofibers in the area of injection, however, and do not spread significantly from the site of implantation [118–120]. Each myoblast injection in a primate results in only a narrow track of hybrid myofibers [50]. In monkeys, this localized fusion of donor myoblasts is compensated for by performing multiple injections in close proximity to one another. The generation of 50% hybrid fibers in monkeys required an interinjection distance of 1 mm and 3×10^7 myoblasts per cm^3 of muscle [50]. The number of injections could be reduced if the injected cells would spread to cover a larger area of a given muscle, behavior that could be achieved by increasing the diffusion of donor cells into the tissue or producing more muscle regeneration around the injection trajectory [118,121].

Improvement of transplantation by increasing the intramuscular migration of donor cells

To improve the spread of donor cells in the host, enzymes that degrade the extracellular matrix are needed. The migratory capacity of the C_2C_{12} myoblast cell line was attributed to the secretion of metalloproteinases [119]. Pretreatment of muscles with collagenase and metalloproteinases doubles the donor myoblast migration [120]. Myoblast transfection with a metalloproteinase gene also increased the number of hybrid myofibers after a single intramuscular injection [122]. The urokinase plasminogen activator is important for the migration of C_2C_{12} cells in vivo and increased the intramuscular migration of primary cultured myoblasts stimulated with basic fibroblast growth factor (from 300–700 μm) [118]. Tumor necrosis factor-α is another chemotactic factor that influences the migration of C_2C_{12} myoblasts [123].

Improvement of transplantation by increasing local regeneration while inactivating host satellite cells

Inducing muscle regeneration during MT increases the uptake of the donor myoblasts into hybrid myofibers, and inhibiting the participation of host satellite cells further promotes donor myoblast incorporation [8]. The intramuscular injection of myotoxins from snake venom has aided transplantation outcomes in mouse and some monkey experiments [51–53,124]. Local anesthetic agents also have been used for mouse experiments [125,126]. The most frequent method of inhibiting the participation of host satellite cells is local radiation at high doses [8,51,124,127,128] and pretreatment of the muscle with myotoxic agents [129,130].

Systemic delivery of donor cells through blood circulation

Delivering donor cells through the bloodstream would be ideal. Myogenic cells would be distributed to all skeletal muscles, including those not appropriate for local injections, such as the diaphragm and heart. Intravenous and intraperitoneal injections of myoblasts have proven unsuccessful, however, even after extensive muscle injury [5]. Intra-arterial injection of a myoblast cell line resulted in fusion of donor cells with the myofibers in those muscles irrigated by the arteries, but only after mechanical injury of the muscle [131]. The systemic delivery of hematopoietic stem cells, unfractionated bone marrow, and putative MDSCs also produced fusion of donor cells with host myofibers, mainly after muscle injury [25,27,82,98,99]. MDSCs spontaneously fused with host myofibers after intra-arterial injection, but only in some of the muscles irrigated by the arteries [82]. Some cells became attached to the microvasculature of the target muscles, but myofiber damage without vessel damage did not improve donor cell fusion with the myofibers [82]. These observations showed that myogenic cells delivered by the bloodstream fuse with myofibers mainly at the sites at which an injury creates a physical route from the vessels to the regenerating myofibers. The intravenous route also seems to be less efficient than the intra-arterial route. In conclusion, if muscles must be injured for intra-arterial injection to result in donor cell incorporation with host myofibers, systemic delivery has no advantage over local injections.

Challenge 4: microenvironment

Although it is important to select the best cells for transplantation, it is equally important to understand the local environment into which the cells will be transplanted. We have found that muscle-derived cells transplanted into injured skeletal muscle and exposed to transforming growth factor-β1, which is secreted by the muscle after injury, differentiate into fibrotic cells, a key event in muscle fibrogenesis [132,133]. Similarly, we have observed that MDSCs influenced by bone morphogenetic proteins, nerve growth factor, and vascular endothelial growth factor differentiate into osteogenic, neurogenic, and vascular/endothelial lineages, respectively [78]. We believe that the local environment poses additional challenges to researchers who attempt to use these cells as the basis for cell therapy to improve muscle regeneration and repair.

Future directions

Our experiences and those of others have highlighted many challenges associated with the use of cell transplantation to improve muscle regeneration and repair. It is clear that identification of the best cell type (eg, myoblasts, MDSCs, other postnatal stem cells, or ES cells) and protocol to expand them in vitro are major determinants in the success of this type of research. Researchers also must continue their efforts to better characterize the microenvironment into which cells are to be transplanted. In particular, stem cells stimulated by various cytokines and growth factors released by injured or diseased skeletal muscle might differentiate into lineages other than the myogenic lineage. It is also important to eliminate the need for sustained immunosuppression, perhaps through the use of autologous cell transplantation or induction of immune tolerance. Researchers also must find ways to increase the migration of donor cells after injection into injured or diseased muscle because the restoration of function within the dystrophic muscle requires the expression of dystrophin along the entire length of each muscle fiber. Perhaps systemic delivery of the cells will facilitate the uniform distribution of the cells within the dystrophic muscle. Fig. 1 represents the current challenges that face cell transplantation for muscle applications.

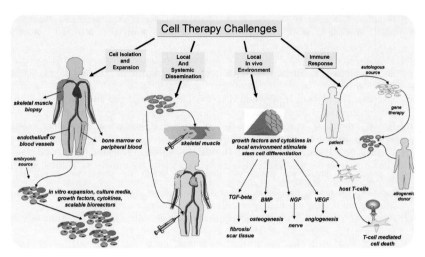

Fig. 1. Cell therapy for muscle regeneration faces several challenges, including cell isolation and expansion, effective delivery, functioning within the in vivo environment, and avoiding the immune response. The optimal cell population must be identified. Expansion without loss of cell phenotype also is necessary. Cells need to be delivered either locally to the injured site or systemically to reach several organs. Once transplanted, the cells also respond to the microenvironment, which includes biochemical stimuli that may prompt differentiation to various lineages. The donor cells also can potentially illicit an immune response that could hinder their in vivo survival and function. These challenges represent the focus of intense investigation in the field of stem cell biology and cell therapy. BMP, bone morphogenetic protein; NGF, nerve growth factor; TGF, transforming growth factor; VEGF, vascular endothelial growth factor.

Acknowledgments

The authors wish to thank R. Sauder for his outstanding editorial assistance with the manuscript.

References

[1] Hoffman EP, Brown RH Jr, Kunkel LM. Dystrophin: the protein product of the Duchenne muscular dystrophy locus. Cell 1987;51(6):919–28.

[2] Arahata K, Ishiura S, Ishiguro T, et al. Immunostaining of skeletal and cardiac muscle surface membrane with antibody against Duchenne muscular dystrophy peptide. Nature 1988; 333(6176):861–3.

[3] Bonilla E, Samitt CE, Miranda AF, et al. Duchenne muscular dystrophy: deficiency of dystrophin at the muscle cell surface. Cell 1988;54(4):447–52.

[4] Koenig M, Hoffman EP, Bertelson CJ, et al. Complete cloning of the Duchenne muscular dystrophy (DMD) cDNA and preliminary genomic organization of the DMD gene in normal and affected individuals. Cell 1987;50(3):509–17.

[5] Partridge TA. Invited review: myoblast transfer: a possible therapy for inherited myopathies? Muscle Nerve 1991;14(3):197–212.

[6] Hagiwara Y, Mizuno Y, Takemitsu M, et al. Dystrophin-positive muscle fibers following C2 myoblast transplantation into mdx nude mice. Acta Neuropathol (Berl) 1995;90(6): 592–600.

[7] Huard J, Bouchard JP, Roy R, et al. Myoblast transplantation produced dystrophin-positive muscle fibres in a 16-year-old patient with Duchenne muscular dystrophy. Clin Sci (Lond) 1991;81(2):287–8.

[8] Morgan JE, Hoffman EP, Partridge TA. Normal myogenic cells from newborn mice restore normal histology to degenerating muscles of the mdx mouse. J Cell Biol 1990;111(6 Pt 1): 2437–49.

[9] Partridge TA, Morgan JE, Coulton GR, et al. Conversion of mdx myofibres from dystrophin-negative to -positive by injection of normal myoblasts. Nature 1989;337(6203):176–9.

[10] Huard J, Bouchard JP, Roy R, et al. Human myoblast transplantation: preliminary results of 4 cases. Muscle Nerve 1992;15(5):550–60.

[11] Huard J, Roy R, Bouchard JP, et al. Human myoblast transplantation between immuno-histocompatible donors and recipients produces immune reactions. Transplant Proc 1992;24(6):3049–51.

[12] Law PK. Pioneering development of myoblast transfer therapy. In: Angelini C, editor. Muscular dystrophy research. New York: Elsevier Science; 1991. p. 109–16.

[13] Karpati G, Acsadi G. The potential for gene therapy in Duchenne muscular dystrophy and other genetic muscle diseases. Muscle Nerve 1993;16(11):1141–53.

[14] Gussoni E, Pavlath GK, Lanctot AM, et al. Normal dystrophin transcripts detected in Duchenne muscular dystrophy patients after myoblast transplantation. Nature 1992; 356(6368):435–8.

[15] Gussoni E, Blau HM, Kunkel LM. The fate of individual myoblasts after transplantation into muscles of DMD patients. Nat Med 1997;3(9):970–7.

[16] Tremblay JP, Malouin F, Roy R, et al. Results of a triple blind clinical study of myoblast transplantations without immunosuppressive treatment in young boys with Duchenne muscular dystrophy. Cell Transplant 1993;2(2):99–112.

[17] Mendell JR, Kissel JT, Amato AA, et al. Myoblast transfer in the treatment of Duchenne's muscular dystrophy. N Engl J Med 1995;333(13):832–8.

[18] Huard J, Roy R, Guerette B, et al. Human myoblast transplantation in immunodeficient and immunosuppressed mice: evidence of rejection. Muscle Nerve 1994;17(2):224–34.

[19] Beauchamp JR, Morgan JE, Pagel CN, et al. Quantitative studies of efficacy of myoblast transplantation. Muscle Nerve 1994;18(Suppl):261.

[20] Fan Y, Maley M, Beilharz M, et al. Rapid death of injected myoblasts in myoblast transfer therapy. Muscle Nerve 1996;19(7):853–60.

[21] Guerette B, Asselin I, Skuk D, et al. Control of inflammatory damage by anti-LFA-1: increase success of myoblast transplantation. Cell Transplant 1997;6(2):101–7.

[22] Guerette B, Skuk D, Celestin F, et al. Prevention by anti-LFA-1 of acute myoblast death following transplantation. J Immunol 1997;159(5):2522–31.

[23] Tremblay JP. Myoblast transplantation: a brief review of the problems and of some solutions. Basic Appl Myol 1997;7:221–30.

[24] Merly F, Huard C, Asselin I, et al. Anti-inflammatory effect of transforming growth factor-beta1 in myoblast transplantation. Transplantation 1998;65(6):793–9.

[25] Lee JY, Qu-Petersen Z, Cao B, et al. Clonal isolation of muscle-derived cells capable of enhancing muscle regeneration and bone healing. J Cell Biol 2000;150(5):1085–100.

[26] Qu-Petersen Z, Deasy B, Jankowski R, et al. Identification of a novel population of muscle stem cells in mice: potential for muscle regeneration. J Cell Biol 2002;157(5): 851–64.

[27] Cao B, Zheng B, Jankowski RJ, et al. Muscle stem cells differentiate into haematopoietic lineages but retain myogenic potential. Nat Cell Biol 2003;5(7):640–6.

[28] Bailey P, Holowacz T, Lassar AB. The origin of skeletal muscle stem cells in the embryo and the adult. Curr Opin Cell Biol 2001;13(6):679–89.

[29] Goldring K, Partridge T, Watt D. Muscle stem cells. J Pathol 2002;197(4):457–67.

[30] Seale P, Asakura A, Rudnicki MA. The potential of muscle stem cells. Dev Cell 2001;1(3): 333–42.

[31] Wada MR, Inagawa-Ogashiwa M, Shimizu S, et al. Generation of different fates from multipotent muscle stem cells. Development 2002;129(12):2987–95.

[32] Vilquin JT, Kinoshita I, Roy B, et al. Partial laminin alpha2 chain restoration in alpha2
chain-deficient dy/dy mouse by primary muscle cell culture transplantation. J Cell Biol
1996;133(1):185–97.

[33] Leriche-Guerin K, Anderson LV, Wrogemann K, et al. Dysferlin expression after normal
myoblast transplantation in SCID and in SJL mice. Neuromuscul Disord 2002;12(2):
167–73.

[34] Yao SN, Kurachi K. Implanted myoblasts not only fuse with myofibers but also survive as
muscle precursor cells. J Cell Sci 1993;105(Pt 4):957–63.

[35] Gross JG, Morgan JE. Muscle precursor cells injected into irradiated mdx mouse muscle
persist after serial injury. Muscle Nerve 1999;22(2):174–85.

[36] Heslop L, Beauchamp JR, Tajbakhsh S, et al. Transplanted primary neonatal myoblasts
can give rise to functional satellite cells as identified using the Myf5nlacZl + mouse.
Gene Ther 2001;8(10):778–83.

[37] Qu Z, Balkir L, van Deutekom JC, et al. Development of approaches to improve cell survival in myoblast transfer therapy. J Cell Biol 1998;142(5):1257–67.

[38] Hodgetts SI, Beilharz MW, Scalzo AA, et al. Why do cultured transplanted myoblasts die
in vivo? DNA quantification shows enhanced survival of donor male myoblasts in host
mice depleted of CD4 + and CD8 + cells or Nk1.1 + cells. Cell Transplant 2000;9(4):
489–502.

[39] Hodgetts SI, Spencer MJ, Grounds MD. A role for natural killer cells in the rapid death of
cultured donor myoblasts after transplantation. Transplantation 2003;75(6):863–71.

[40] Skuk D, Caron N, Goulet M, et al. Dynamics of the early immune cellular reactions after
myogenic cell transplantation. Cell Transplant 2002;11(7):671–81.

[41] Hodgetts SI, Grounds MD. Complement and myoblast transfer therapy: donor myoblast
survival is enhanced following depletion of host complement C3 using cobra venom factor,
but not in the absence of C5. Immunol Cell Biol 2001;79(3):231–9.

[42] Skuk D, Tremblay JP. Complement deposition and cell death after myoblast transplantation. Cell Transplant 1998;7(5):427–34.

[43] Vilquin JT, Kinoshita I, Roy R, et al. Cyclophosphamide immunosuppression does not per-
mit successful myoblast allotransplantation in mouse. Neuromuscul Disord 1995;5(6):
511–7.

[44] Wernig A, Irintchev A, Lange G. Functional effects of myoblast implantation into histo-
incompatible mice with or without immunosuppression. J Physiol 1995;484(Pt 2):493–504.

[45] Pavlath GK, Rando TA, Blau HM. Transient immunosuppressive treatment leads to long-
term retention of allogeneic myoblasts in hybrid myofibers. J Cell Biol 1994;127(6 Pt 2):
1923–32.

[46] Irintchev A, Zweyer M, Wernig A. Cellular and molecular reactions in mouse muscles after
myoblast implantation. J Neurocytol 1995;24(4):319–31.

[47] Hardiman O, Sklar RM, Brown RH Jr. Direct effects of cyclosporin A and cyclophosphamide on differentiation of normal human myoblasts in culture. Neurology 1993;43(7):
1432–4.

[48] Hong F, Lee J, Song JW, et al. Cyclosporin A blocks muscle differentiation by inducing oxidative stress and inhibiting the peptidyl-prolyl-cis-trans isomerase activity of cyclophilin
A: cyclophilin A protects myoblasts from cyclosporin A-induced cytotoxicity. FASEB J
2002;16(12):1633–5.

[49] Vilquin JT, Asselin I, Guerette B, et al. Myoblast allotransplantation in mice: degree of success varies depending on the efficacy of various immunosuppressive treatments. Transplant
Proc 1994;26(6):3372–3.

[50] Skuk D, Goulet M, Roy B, et al. Efficacy of myoblast transplantation in nonhuman primates following simple intramuscular cell injections: toward defining strategies applicable
to humans. Exp Neurol 2002;175(1):112–26.

[51] Kinoshita I, Vilquin JT, Guerette B, et al. Very efficient myoblast allotransplantation in mice under FK506 immunosuppression. Muscle Nerve 1994;17(12):1407–15.

[52] Vilquin JT, Wagner E, Kinoshita I, et al. Successful histocompatible myoblast transplantation in dystrophin-deficient mdx mouse despite the production of antibodies against dystrophin. J Cell Biol 1995;131(4):975–88.

[53] Skuk D, Roy B, Goulet M, et al. Successful myoblast transplantation in primates depends on appropriate cell delivery and induction of regeneration in the host muscle. Exp Neurol 1999;155(1):22–30.

[54] Kinoshita I, Roy R, Dugre FJ, et al. Myoblast transplantation in monkeys: control of immune response by FK506. J Neuropathol Exp Neurol 1996;55(6):687–97.

[55] Skuk D, Goulet M, Roy B, et al. Myoblast transplantation in whole muscle of nonhuman primates. J Neuropathol Exp Neurol 2000;59(3):197–206.

[56] Camirand G, Caron NJ, Asselin I, et al. Combined immunosuppression of mycophenolate mofetil and FK506 for myoblast transplantation in mdx mice. Transplantation 2001;72(1): 38–44.

[57] Wiendl H, Mitsdoerffer M, Hofmeister V, et al. The non-classical MHC molecule HLA-G protects human muscle cells from immune-mediated lysis: implications for myoblast transplantation and gene therapy. Brain 2003;126(Pt 1):176–85.

[58] Keller G. Embryonic stem cell differentiation: emergence of a new era in biology and medicine. Genes Dev 2005;19(10):1129–55.

[59] Bhagavati S, Xu W. Generation of skeletal muscle from transplanted embryonic stem cells in dystrophic mice. Biochem Biophys Res Commun 2005;333(2):644–9.

[60] Seale P, Rudnicki MA. A new look at the origin, function, and "stem-cell" status of muscle satellite cells. Dev Biol 2000;218(2):115–24.

[61] Cornelison DD, Wold BJ. Single-cell analysis of regulatory gene expression in quiescent and activated mouse skeletal muscle satellite cells. Dev Biol 1997;191(2):270–83.

[62] Hawke TJ, Garry DJ. Myogenic satellite cells: physiology to molecular biology. J Appl Physiol 2001;91(2):534–51.

[63] Seale P, Sabourin LA, Girgis-Gabardo A, et al. Pax7 is required for the specification of myogenic satellite cells. Cell 2000;102(6):777–86.

[64] Sato T, Laver JH, Ogawa M. Reversible expression of CD34 by murine hematopoietic stem cells. Blood 1999;94(8):2548–54.

[65] Beauchamp JR, Heslop L, Yu DS, et al. Expression of CD34 and Myf5 defines the majority of quiescent adult skeletal muscle satellite cells. J Cell Biol 2000;151(6):1221–34.

[66] Zammit P, Beauchamp J. The skeletal muscle satellite cell: stem cell or son of stem cell? Differentiation 2001;68(4–5):193–204.

[67] Collins CA, Olsen I, Zammit PS, et al. Stem cell function, self-renewal, and behavioral heterogeneity of cells from the adult muscle satellite cell niche. Cell 2005;122(2):289–301.

[68] Bischoff R. The satellite cell and muscle regeneration. In: Engel AG, Franzini-Armstrong C, editors. Myology: basic and clinical. 2nd edition. New York: McGraw-Hill; 1994. p. 97–118.

[69] Tatsumi R, Anderson JE, Nevoret CJ, et al. HGF/SF is present in normal adult skeletal muscle and is capable of activating satellite cells. Dev Biol 1998;194(1):114–28.

[70] Heslop L, Morgan JE, Partridge TA. Evidence for a myogenic stem cell that is exhausted in dystrophic muscle. J Cell Sci 2000;113(Pt 12):2299–308.

[71] Chen G, Quinn LS. Partial characterization of skeletal myoblast mitogens in mouse crushed muscle extract. J Cell Physiol 1992;153(3):563–74.

[72] Bischoff R. Chemotaxis of skeletal muscle satellite cells. Dev Dyn 1997;208(4):505–15.

[73] Sheehan SM, Allen RE. Skeletal muscle satellite cell proliferation in response to members of the fibroblast growth factor family and hepatocyte growth factor. J Cell Physiol 1999; 181(3):499–506.

[74] Brockes JP, Kumar A. Plasticity and reprogramming of differentiated cells in amphibian regeneration. Nat Rev Mol Cell Biol 2002;3(8):566–74.

[75] Rosania GR, Chang YT, Perez O, et al. Myoseverin: a microtubule-binding molecule with novel cellular effects. Nat Biotechnol 2000;18(3):304–8.

[76] Odelberg SJ, Kollhoff A, Keating MT. Dedifferentiation of mammalian myotubes induced by msx1. Cell 2000;103(7):1099–109.

[77] McGann CJ, Odelberg SJ, Keating MT. Mammalian myotube dedifferentiation induced by newt regeneration extract. Proc Natl Acad Sci U S A 2001;98(24):13699–704.

[78] Deasy BM, Huard J. Gene therapy and tissue engineering based on muscle-derived stem cells. Curr Opin Mol Ther 2002;4(4):382–9.

[79] Deasy BM, Jankowski RJ, Huard J. Muscle-derived stem cells: characterization and potential for cell-mediated therapy. Blood Cells Mol Dis 2001;27(5):924–33.

[80] Jankowski RJ, Deasy BM, Huard J. Muscle-derived stem cells. Gene Ther 2002;9(10): 642–7.

[81] Peng H, Huard J. Muscle-derived stem cells for musculoskeletal tissue regeneration and repair. Transpl Immunol 2004;12(3–4):311–9.

[82] Torrente Y, Tremblay JP, Pisati F, et al. Intraarterial injection of muscle-derived CD34(+)Sca-1(+) stem cells restores dystrophin in mdx mice. J Cell Biol 2001;152(2): 335–48.

[83] Grounds MD. Skeletal muscle precursors do not arise from bone marrow cells. Cell Tissue Res 1983;234(3):713–22.

[84] Mueller GM, O'Day T, Watchko JF, et al. Effect of injecting primary myoblasts versus putative muscle-derived stem cells on mass and force generation in mdx mice. Hum Gene Ther 2002;13(9):1081–90.

[85] Asakura A, Seale P, Girgis-Gabardo A, et al. Myogenic specification of side population cells in skeletal muscle. J Cell Biol 2002;159(1):123–34.

[86] Issarachai S, Priestley GV, Nakamoto B, et al. Bone marrow-derived CD45 + and CD45- cells reside in skeletal muscle. Blood Cells Mol Dis 2002;29(1):69–72.

[87] Issarachai S, Priestley GV, Nakamoto B, et al. Cells with hematopoietic potential residing in muscle are itinerant bone marrow-derived cells. Exp Hematol 2002;30(4):366–73.

[88] Howell JC, Yoder MC, Srour EF. Hematopoietic potential of murine skeletal muscle-derived CD45(-)Sca-1(+)c-kit(-) cells. Exp Hematol 2002;30(8):915–24.

[89] Mahmud N, Weiss P, Li F, et al. Primate skeletal muscle contains cells capable of sustaining in vitro hematopoiesis. Exp Hematol 2002;30(8):925–36.

[90] Dell'Agnola C, Rabascio C, Mancuso P, et al. In vitro and in vivo hematopoietic potential of human stem cells residing in muscle tissue. Exp Hematol 2002;30(8):905–14.

[91] Lapidos KA, Chen YE, Earley JU, et al. Transplanted hematopoietic stem cells demonstrate impaired sarcoglycan expression after engraftment into cardiac and skeletal muscle. J Clin Invest 2004;114(11):1577–85.

[92] LaBarge MA, Blau HM. Biological progression from adult bone marrow to mononucleate muscle stem cell to multinucleate muscle fiber in response to injury. Cell 2002;111(4): 589–601.

[93] Tamaki T, Akatsuka A, Ando K, et al. Identification of myogenic-endothelial progenitor cells in the interstitial spaces of skeletal muscle. J Cell Biol 2002;157(4):571–7.

[94] Sampaolesi M, Torrente Y, Innocenzi A, et al. Cell therapy of alpha-sarcoglycan null dystrophic mice through intra-arterial delivery of mesoangioblasts. Science 2003;301(5632): 487–92.

[95] Robertson TA, Grounds MD, Papadimitriou JM. Elucidation of aspects of murine skeletal muscle regeneration using local and whole body irradiation. J Anat 1992;181(Pt 2):265–76.

[96] Rosenblatt JD, Parry DJ. Gamma irradiation prevents compensatory hypertrophy of overloaded mouse extensor digitorum longus muscle. J Appl Physiol 1992;73(6):2538–43.

[97] Schultz E, Jaryszak DL, Gibson MC, et al. Absence of exogenous satellite cell contribution to regeneration of frozen skeletal muscle. J Muscle Res Cell Motil 1986;7(4):361–7.

[98] Gussoni E, Soneoka Y, Strickland CD, et al. Dystrophin expression in the mdx mouse restored by stem cell transplantation. Nature 1999;401(6751):390–4.

[99] Ferrari G, Cusella-De Angelis G, Coletta M, et al. Muscle regeneration by bone marrow-derived myogenic progenitors. Science 1998;279(5356):1528–30.

[100] Ferrari G, Stornaiuolo A, Mavilio F. Failure to correct murine muscular dystrophy. Nature 2001;411(6841):1014–5.

[101] Gussoni E, Bennett RR, Muskiewicz KR, et al. Long-term persistence of donor nuclei in a Duchenne muscular dystrophy patient receiving bone marrow transplantation. J Clin Invest 2002;110(6):807–14.

[102] Kapsa RM, Quigley AF, Vadolas J, et al. Targeted gene correction in the mdx mouse using short DNA fragments: towards application with bone marrow-derived cells for autologous remodeling of dystrophic muscle. Gene Ther 2002;9(11):695–9.

[103] Corti S, Strazzer S, Del Bo R, et al. A subpopulation of murine bone marrow cells fully differentiates along the myogenic pathway and participates in muscle repair in the mdx dystrophic mouse. Exp Cell Res 2002;277(1):74–85.

[104] Goodell MA, Brose K, Paradis G, et al. Isolation and functional properties of murine hematopoietic stem cells that are replicating in vivo. J Exp Med 1996;183(4):1797–806.

[105] Zhou S, Morris JJ, Barnes Y, et al. Bcrp1 gene expression is required for normal numbers of side population stem cells in mice, and confers relative protection to mitoxantrone in hematopoietic cells in vivo. Proc Natl Acad Sci U S A 2002;99(19):12339–44.

[106] Zhou S, Schuetz JD, Bunting KD, et al. The ABC transporter Bcrp1/ABCG2 is expressed in a wide variety of stem cells and is a molecular determinant of the side-population phenotype. Nat Med 2001;7(9):1028–34.

[107] Asakura A, Rudnicki MA. Side population cells from diverse adult tissues are capable of in vitro hematopoietic differentiation. Exp Hematol 2002;30(11):1339–45.

[108] Tamaki T, Akatsuka A, Okada Y, et al. Growth and differentiation potential of main- and side-population cells derived from murine skeletal muscle. Exp Cell Res 2003;291(1):83–90.

[109] Oustanina S, Hause G, Braun T. Pax7 directs postnatal renewal and propagation of myogenic satellite cells but not their specification. EMBO J 2004;23(16):3430–9.

[110] Rivier F, Alkan O, Flint AF, et al. Role of bone marrow cell trafficking in replenishing skeletal muscle SP and MP cell populations. J Cell Sci 2004;117(Pt 10):1979–88.

[111] Huard C, Moisset PA, Dicaire A, et al. Transplantation of dermal fibroblasts expressing MyoD1 in mouse muscles. Biochem Biophys Res Commun 1998;248(3):648–54.

[112] Goldring K, Jones GE, Thiagarajah R, et al. The effect of galectin-1 on the differentiation of fibroblasts and myoblasts in vitro. J Cell Sci 2002;115(Pt 2):355–66.

[113] Grigoriadis AE, Heersche JN, Aubin JE. Differentiation of muscle, fat, cartilage, and bone from progenitor cells present in a bone-derived clonal cell population: effect of dexamethasone. J Cell Biol 1988;106(6):2139–51.

[114] Wakitani S, Saito T, Caplan AI. Myogenic cells derived from rat bone marrow mesenchymal stem cells exposed to 5-azacytidine. Muscle Nerve 1995;18(12):1417–26.

[115] De Bari C, Dell'Accio F, Vandenabeele F, et al. Skeletal muscle repair by adult human mesenchymal stem cells from synovial membrane. J Cell Biol 2003;160(6):909–18.

[116] Ordahl CP. Myogenic shape-shifters. J Cell Biol 1999;147(4):695–8.

[117] Tavian M, Zheng B, Oberlin E, et al. The vascular wall as a source of stem cells. Ann NY Acad Sci 2005;1044:41–50.

[118] El Fahime E, Mills P, Lafreniere JF, et al. The urokinase plasminogen activator: an interesting way to improve myoblast migration following their transplantation. Exp Cell Res 2002;280(2):169–78.

[119] El Fahime E, Torrente Y, Caron NJ, et al. In vivo migration of transplanted myoblasts requires matrix metalloproteinase activity. Exp Cell Res 2000;258(2):279–87.

[120] Torrente Y, El Fahime E, Caron NJ, et al. Intramuscular migration of myoblasts transplanted after muscle pretreatment with metalloproteinases. Cell Transplant 2000;9(4):539–49.

[121] Lafreniere JF, Mills P, Tremblay JP, et al. Growth factors improve the in vivo migration of human skeletal myoblasts by modulating their endogenous proteolytic activity. Transplantation 2004;77(11):1741–7.

[122] Caron NJ, Asselin I, Morel G, et al. Increased myogenic potential and fusion of matrilysin-expressing myoblasts transplanted in mice. Cell Transplant 1999;8(5):465–76.

[123] Torrente Y, El Fahime E, Caron NJ, et al. Tumor necrosis factor-alpha (TNF-alpha) stimulates chemotactic response in mouse myogenic cells. Cell Transplant 2003;12(1):91–100.

[124] Huard J, Verreault S, Roy R, et al. High efficiency of muscle regeneration after human myoblast clone transplantation in SCID mice. J Clin Invest 1994;93(2):586–99.

[125] Cantini M, Massimino ML, Catani C, et al. Gene transfer into satellite cell from regenerating muscle: bupivacaine allows beta-Gal transfection and expression in vitro and in vivo. In Vitro Cell Dev Biol Anim 1994;30A(2):131–3.

[126] Pin CL, Merrifield PA. Developmental potential of rat L6 myoblasts in vivo following injection into regenerating muscles. Dev Biol 1997;188(1):147–66.

[127] Alameddine HS, Louboutin JP, Dehaupas M, et al. Functional recovery induced by satellite cell grafts in irreversibly injured muscles. Cell Transplant 1994;3(1):3–14.

[128] Wernig A, Zweyer M, Irintchev A. Function of skeletal muscle tissue formed after myoblast transplantation into irradiated mouse muscles. J Physiol 2000;522(Pt 2):333–45.

[129] van Deutekom JC, Floyd SS, Booth DK, et al. Implications of maturation for viral gene delivery to skeletal muscle. Neuromuscul Disord 1998;8(3–4):135–48.

[130] van Deutekom JC, Hoffman EP, Huard J. Muscle maturation: implications for gene therapy. Mol Med Today 1998;4(5):214–20.

[131] Neumeyer AM, DiGregorio DM, Brown RH Jr. Arterial delivery of myoblasts to skeletal muscle. Neurology 1992;42(12):2258–62.

[132] Li Y, Foster W, Deasy BM, et al. Transforming growth factor-beta1 induces the differentiation of myogenic cells into fibrotic cells in injured skeletal muscle: a key event in muscle fibrogenesis. Am J Pathol 2004;164(3):1007–19.

[133] Li Y, Huard J. Differentiation of muscle-derived cells into myofibroblasts in injured skeletal muscle. Am J Pathol 2002;161(3):895–907.

PHYSICAL MEDICINE
AND REHABILITATION
CLINICS OF
NORTH AMERICA

ELSEVIER
SAUNDERS

Phys Med Rehabil Clin N Am
16 (2005) 909–924

Amyotrophic Lateral Sclerosis Microgenomics

John Ravits, MD, FAAN[a,b,*], Patrick Laurie, BS[a],
Brad Stone, PhD[a]

[a]Benaroya Research Institute at Vrigina Mason, 1201 Ninth Avenue,
Seattle, WA 98101, USA
[b]Section of Neurology, Virginia Mason Medical Center,
1100 Ninth Avenue, Seattle, WA 98101, USA

Amyotrophic lateral sclerosis (ALS) is a degenerative disease of the central nervous system (CNS) characterized by progressive weakness from degeneration of motor neurons [1]. The main clinical features of weakness are focal onset at any region of the neuraxis, a mix of upper and lower motor neuron dysfunction, and contiguous spread over time [2] (Fig. 1). Onset is insidious, and progression is essentially linear. Death occurs in 90% of patients within 3 to 5 years. The age at onset is usually over 25 years. The incidence of ALS is about 2 to 3 per 100,000, and the prevalence is 6 to 10 per 100,000 (Box 1). In the United States, 5000 deaths occur per year and in the world, 100,000. Ninety to 95% of ALS is sporadic (SALS) and 5% to 10% is familial (FALS). Of the 5% to 10% of ALS that is FALS, 20% are caused by mutations in the gene encoding superoxide dismutase 1 (SOD1) at chromosome 21q22.1, and the remaining 80% are caused by unknown mutations. Approximately 100 SOD1 mutations have been identified, and nearly all are single missense dominant mutations causing toxic gain of function [3].

This article was supported by grants from the Moyer Foundation, Seattle, Washington, and the Juniper Foundation, Seattle, Washington.
* Corresponding author. Benaroya Research Institute at Vrigina Mason, 1201 Ninth Avenue, Seattle, WA 98101.
E-mail address: jravits@benaroyaresearch.org (J. Ravits).

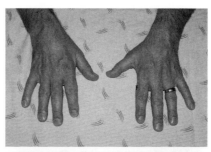

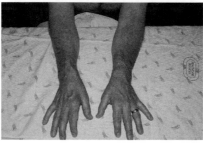

Fig. 1. Focality of ALS. Fifty-year-old man within 6 months of clinical onset sporadic ALS has weakness clinically confined to the right hand, but neurophysiologic abnormalities are also present in the right forearm and in the left hand. The pathologic center of disease, therefore, is the right C8–T1 anterior horn spinal level, and disease propagation is outward from this center. Focality is virtually invariable in ALS, but the specific vertical level in the neuraxis where it begins is highly variable.

Amyotrophic lateral sclerosis neuropathology

The major neuropathologic finding in SALS is degeneration and loss of motor neurons [4]. Three morphologic stages representing the time course of motor neuron degeneration can be seen concurrently: chromatolysis, somatodendritic attrition, and apoptosis [5]. Chromatolysis is characterized by dispersion of Nissl substance without nuclear condensation. Somato-dendritic attrition is characterized by homogenous cytoplasm, nuclear condensation, and preservation of the nucleolus. Apoptosis is characterized

---

Box 1. Amyotrophic lateral sclerosis

- Incidence: 2–3 per 100,000 (same as multiple sclerosis).
- Prevalence: 6–10 per 100,000;
- ~25,000 patients in US;
- ~500,000 patients worldwide.
- Death Counts:
- >5,000 per year in United States;
- >100,000 per year in world

by neuronal contraction (to approximately one fifth its normal size) with an extremely condensed nucleus and cytoplasm. Apoptotic bodies usually in macrophages can be seen [6]. Intracytoplasmic inclusions are seen only in a minority of neurons, and include Bunina bodies and skein-like inclusions, which may represent two different steps of the cascade leading to neuronal degeneration [7–9]. Other neuropathologic findings in ALS include axonal loss in the descending motor tracts, anterior roots, and nerve; denervated muscle; and subtle involvement of the frontal lobes, hippocampal area, substantia nigra, and dorsal columns [4,8]. SOD1 FALS differs from SALS because of intracytoplasmic hyaline conglomerates and prominent degeneration of spinocerebellar tracts and posterior columns and sometimes of Clarke's columns [9]. Because intracytoplasmic hyaline conglomerates are not seen in SALS, pathologic cascades leading to neuronal degeneration may be different [9]. Exact neuropathologic distinctions between of SOD1-FALS, non-SOD1-FALS, and SALS are unclear because the best descriptions of FALS predated discovery of SOD1 mutation [10]. Motor neuron degeneration in both SALS and FALS begins focally and spreads to contiguous regions in the neuraxis until the neurons controlling respiration are affected, at which time death arrests the degenerative process. Around the disease center, numbers of motor neurons and spectrum of motor neuron degeneration vary for any individual patient, in large part determined by the site of onset and rate of progression [11].

Mechanisms of motor neuron degeneration and apoptosis

The mechanisms for neuronal degeneration, for the select motor neuron vulnerability, and for the linear and contiguous propagation through the motor system that characterize ALS are unknown (Box 2). Current hypotheses include oxidative stress, neuroexcitatory toxicity, mitochondrial dysfunction, intermediate neurofilament disorganization, failure of intracellular mineral homeostasis involving zinc, copper, or calcium, disrupted axonal transport, abnormal protein aggregation or folding, and neuroinflammation [1,12–16]. Evidence is mounting that motor neuron death at least in SOD1 transgenic mouse models of FALS is nonautonomous [17–21]. Whatever upstream molecular mechanisms occur, evidence favors apoptosis as the final common pathway of cell death in ALS (reviewed in [22] and [23]).

Box 2. Mechanisms

- Unknown—many hypotheses.
- Neuronal death may be noncell autonomous.
- Final common pathway appears to be apoptosis.

RNA quality

Individual messenger RNA (mRNA) transcripts have intrinsic decay rates ranging from minutes to days. RNA can be routinely recovered from postmortem nervous systems for up to 36 hours [24–26]. The major factors that compromise it postmortem are agonal state, postmortem interval, tissue pH, and time in storage [24,27,28]. RNA may be isolated from formalin-fixed, paraffin-embedded (FFPE) tissues [29–34]. RNA is best isolated from frozen tissues, but it is degraded by repeated thawing and refreezing due to RNases released from lysosomes by membrane disruption from rapid freezing. Quantitative and qualitative assessments of RNA have been difficult. Traditional techniques to assess RNA are spectrophotometry, agarose gel electrophoresis, fluorometry, and RT-PCR including ratios of 5' to 3' amplicons within housekeeping genes. All have problems with sensitivity, accuracy, quantification, and technical difficulty. Recently, microelectrophoresis, a chip-based technology that uses microfluidics, has become available ("Lab-on-a-chip" Agilent 2100 Bioanalyzer, Agilent Technologies, Palo Alto, California). When compared with traditional gel electrophoresis, it requires miniscule sample size (1 μL), miniscule RNA concentrations (250 pg/μL), is quantitative, digital, fast, automated, and reproducible. RNA can be objectively and quantitatively assessed by way of electropherograms, digital gels, and a variety of metrics such as RNA integrity numbers (RINs). We used it to evaluate RNA in our ALS nervous system tissue bank specifically designed for RNA preservation and delivery to downstream technologies and established it is on a par with that obtained in a controlled laboratory setting [11] (Box 3). The explanation for this is that the agonal state is hypercarbic respiratory failure that is without significant acidemia or hypoxemia that would degrade RNA. We have also tested RNA quality at each step of histologic processing and found that it is slightly and predictably decreased but sufficiently maintained for molecular investigation.

Difficulties and opportunities for amyotrophic lateral sclerosis investigation

Difficulties in detecting pathogenic factors in ALS include (Box 4): (1) severe reduction of the targets of investigation, motor neurons, due to

---

Box 3. RNA in amyotrophic lateral sclerosis

- Death is by chronic hypercarbic respiratory failure, which is without acidemia or hypoxemia—this allows RNA integrity to remain high, on par with a controlled laboratory settings.
- Death is predictable, which provides opportunity for tissue acquisition specifically designed for RNA preservation and delivery to downstream technologies.

Box 4. Difficulties for amyotrophic lateral sclerosis research

- Disappearance of targets of investigation, the motor neurons.
- Inaccessible location of motor neurons within CNS.
- Topographic variation of pathology along neuraxis.
- Small ratio of pathogenic signal to nonpathogenic noise.
- Difficult cell isolation.
- Biochemical compromise of tissue by necrolysis and tissue processing.

---

elimination by the disease; (2) the remote and inaccessible location of the diseased cells in the CNS; (3) variation of regional topography of pathology along the neuraxis; (4) infinitesimal signal-to-noise ratio of pathogenic to nonpathogenic factors; (5) technical challenges of cell isolation; and (6) biochemical compromise caused by necrolysis and by tissue processing.

The fact that fundamentally ALS is a focal disease that begins at variable vertical levels of the neuraxis and propagates in contiguous manner outward from this center to summate over time and space until it is seemingly diffuse can be exploited for molecular research (Box 5). When motor neuron degeneration propagates to the respiratory system and death ensues, there are the two unique consequences discussed above [11]: (1) further degeneration is arrested and a spectrum of degeneration exists radially away from the disease center; and (2) RNA is preserved. Thus, the postmortem ALS nervous system is neither burnt out by the degeneration if one knows where to look vertically nor degraded biochemically by necrolysis if tissue is optimally acquired. This is unlike other neurodegenerative disease where the degenerative process itself is not directly fatal and degeneration continues to advance to end stages until the patients succumb to unpredictable

---

Box 5. Opportunities for amyotrophic lateral sclerosis research

- Disease has focal onset and contiguous progression—motor neuron degeneration summates in space and time.
- A spectrum of motor neuron degeneration representing the full time course of degeneration exist radially away from the disease center in each nervous system.
- Involvement of respiratory system arrests degenerative process at a point in time.
- RNA is preserved during death by hypercarbic respiratory failure.

---

supervening medical complications allowed but not directly caused by the degeneration. The possibilities for genomics in ALS are even greater than previously appreciated for postmortem tissue [24,27,28,34,35]. When delivered to new biotechnologies that bridge histology and molecular biology, a new and direct route of molecular investigation is possible [36,37].

Laser-based tissue microdissection

Tissue microdissection is a computer-assisted microscopic technique that applies laser technology to histologic sections to microdissect tissue for molecular analysis and thus frees the latter from its traditional reliance on bulk tissue [38–42]. A number of commercial systems with differing approaches to microdissection are available (reviewed in [43]). Microdissection can be an essential technology for investigation of heterogeneous tissues with complex architecture such as the nervous system, and for diseases with selective vulnerability of single-cell populations such as motor neurons in ALS. Motor neurons are large 40 to 120 μm-diameter neurons located in the prefrontal gyrus of the cerebral cortex (giant cells of Betz); brainstem motor nuclei of cranial nerves 5, 7, 9, 10, 11, and 12; and spinal cord anterior horns [44]. They are easily microdissected from any CNS region, especially from the spinal anterior horns. Applied to ALS (Fig. 2), microdissection (Box 6): (1) isolates that miniscule portion of the nervous system that is pathologic, and separates it from the majority of tissue that is not pathologic; (2) ensures sampling is selective, thus overcoming sampling error posed by the regional nature of pathology; (3) pools samples of the degenerating neuronal population to obtain sufficient quantities for investigation; (4) standardizes and quantifies input to molecular investigation; and (5) allows investigation of different cellular compartments coexisting in the same specific tissues.

RNA amplification

Amplification technologies make nucleic acids accessible to investigation by exploiting their ability for high-fidelity duplication to make millions and billions of exact or complementary copies of original sequences. There are two main ways to amplify RNA: exponential amplification based on the polymerase chain reaction (PCR) and linear amplification based on in vitro transcription (IVT). Exponential amplifications, PCR, and its variations, involve repeated cycles of duplication using a set of target-specific oligonucleotide primers and a thermostable DNA polymerase. The primers select the borders of the DNA sequence to be amplified, called the amplicon. For PCR of RNA, reverse transcription must first produce complementary DNA (cDNA), which then is amplified by PCR (hence, reverse-transcriptase PCR, or RT-PCR). Twenty-five cycles of amplification can produce 33 million copies of the original sequence, and 30 cycles can produce one billion

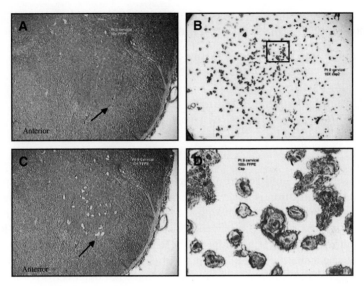

Fig. 2. LCM of spinal cord motor neurons in SALS. (*A*) Transverse section showing one side of cervical cord before LCM; arrow points to anterior horn cells (×12.5). (*B*) LCM cap at low power; the cap is full of hundreds of motor neurons that have been microdissected from contiguous histological sections; the cap will fit into a microtube containing RNA extraction buffer for RNA isolation (×12.5). (*C*) After LCM; the small white blanks are where motor neurons have been removed (×12.5). (*D*) LCM cap at high power; the motor neurons are from the region outlined in top right figure (×200). (SALS, FFPE tissue used on a Pixcell IIe Laser Capture Microdissection System with stained with HistoGene LCM Frozen Section Staining Kit; Arcturus Bioscience, Mountain View, California.)

copies. Because of its dependence on target-specific oligonucleotide primers to define the specific DNA sequence to be amplified, only one or a few sequences can be amplified concurrently.

Linear amplification uses IVT rather than DNA duplication as the basis of RNA amplification [45,46] (Box 7). Here, again, reverse transcription must first produce cDNA by priming off the 3′ poly-A tail, which is unique to mRNA in general but not specific to individual mRNA transcripts. Then, through a sequence of primers, promoters, enzymes, and thermal cycles that promote IVT from cDNA, antisense mRNA (aRNA) is made. One round of IVT amplification can produce thousands of antisense copies of original

---

Box 6. Tissue microdissection

- Bridges histology and molecular biology.
- Isolates and collects degenerating neurons.
- Pools samples to have sufficient and standardized quantity.

Box 7. Linear amplification by in vitro transcription

- Isolates mRNA, which is only 1–3% of total RNA.
- Nonselective—isolates *all* mRNA 3′ ends, not specific sequences like PCR.
- Amplifies sequences by up to a few 1000-fold per round.
- Can incorporate labels for microarray.

---

mRNA sequences, and two rounds can produce millions. Even though the degree of amplification is less with linear amplification than exponential amplification, it has four main advantages: (1) it separates mRNA, which is only 1% to 3% of total RNA (largely comprised of transfer and ribosomal RNA) from non-mRNA; (2) it amplifies *all* mRNA contained in total RNA and does not select specific target oligonucleotide sequences such as PCR has to; (3) all mRNA is commensurately amplified, and what bias occurs is consistent between samples and generally has little effect on array comparisons [47]; and (4) fluorescent or radiolabeled nucleotides can be incorporated so that the resulting aRNA can be used as probes in microarray studies.

Microarray and microgenomics

DNA microarray technology allows the simultaneous determination of expression of thousands of genes in a single substrate and allows high throughput profiling (Box 8). The basis of this technology is hybridization between two complementary strands of nucleic acid. Genes of interest are represented by oligonucleotide sequences, which are immobilized at specific X- and Y-coordinant addresses on a solid substrate. The sample or test RNA is labeled with fluorescent or radioactive tags and hybridized to the array. A detected signal correlates with gene expression. Two major DNA array platforms exist: spotted (or cDNA arrays), and manufactured (or

---

Box 8. Microarray and genomics

- Microarray performs simultaneous high throughput gene expression profiling.
- Quantitative, self-validating, digital, and objective.
- Allows exploration and discovery of genome (*genomics*) and is hypothesis generating.
- Does not distinguish primary from secondary pathologic changes in gene expression.

---

short oligonucleotide arrays). Oligonucleotide microarray chips now contain the whole genome. The technology generates huge quantities of data, and a new subfield of bioinformatics has developed to mine the data [48]. Rather than traditional hypothesis-driven (or hypothesis limited) investigation, such investigations are *exploratory or discovery driven*—they generate data and that can be mined to develop new hypotheses [49,50].

Genomic study at the cellular level is referred to as *microgenomics* [51,52] (Box 9). To date, most of the work has been in oncology and is already achieving clinical applications [53]. Given the complexity and heterogeneity of the nervous system, microgenomics offers new promise for neurodegenerative diseases (Fig. 3): (1) it provides high throughput gene expression profiling of degenerating cell lines; (2) profiles the relevant neuronal population of the complex and heterogeneous nervous system to improve the pathologic-to-nonpathologic signal-to-noise ratio; (3) allows separate and parallel profiling of different cellular compartments coexisting in the same specific tissues, such as neurons and surrounding glia, to better understand their interaction; (4) allows molecular investigation to bear directly on sporadic human disease; (5) allows profiling of time course of gene expression to define early events; (6) may be applied to transgenic disease models; and (7) may be applied to other neurodegenerative disease characterized by select neuronal degeneration such as Parkinson's disease.

Despite the power of microarray technology, there are problems and cautions. (1) Expression profiling is dependent upon the quality of the input, underscoring the critical importance of upstream tissue processing discussed above. (2) Expression profiling may not be complete, and only represent 75% of a cell's expressed genes, thus giving rise to false negatives (mistakenly thinking that a gene that is expressed is not) [54,55]. (3) The genes identified represent the summation of the genes in the profiled tissues—an important caution when profiling cells at various stages of degeneration. (4) As with all such research, microgenomic discoveries do not differentiate changes that are pathogenic from those that are secondary. (5) Even if primary gene expression changes can be defined, the initial causative factors initiating such expression remain to be defined. (6) The relationship between

---

Box 9. Microgenomics (cell-specific genomics)

- Genomics at the cellular level.
- Profiles specific relevant neuronal and glial compartments of architecturally complex and heterogeneous CNS.
- Allows molecular investigation to bear directly on sporadic human disease.
- May be used in transgenic disease models or in other neurodegenerative disease.

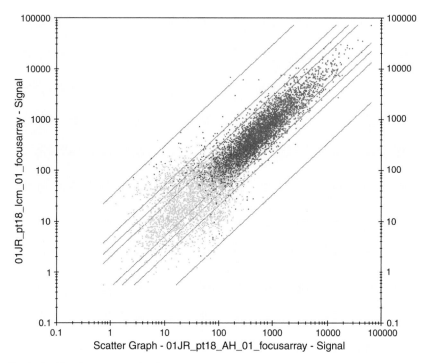

Fig. 3. Profile of gene expression in ALS motor neurons compared with surrounding anterior horn. Scatterplot displays gene expression of motor neurons on the ordinate and the gene expression of the surrounding anterior horn after motor neuron removal on the abscissa. Gene expression is performed by oligonucleotide microarray of amplified mRNA from the respective compartments isolated by laser microdissection. From bioinformatics, uniquely expressed or nonexpressed genes can be discovered. (Studies performed on a GeneChip Human Genome Focus Array and Affymetrix Microarray System; Affymetrix, Santa Clara, California).

genomics and proteomics is unknown—what happens at the gene level may or may not accurately reflect what is happening at the protein level [56]. Technical issues in evaluating this are significant and changing [57]. Despite these problems and cautions, the prospect of profiling gene expression of motor neurons is a new frontier in ALS research, and may identify areas for therapeutic intervention.

Therapeutic implications: RNAi and molecular Trojan horses

If molecular mechanisms of degeneration could be discovered, a variety of methods of gene replacement, gene knock-down, and gene regulation are imaginable. Recent technologies called RNA interference (RNAi), for example, are emerging for gene knock-down using antisense nucleic acid sequences to inhibit posttranscriptional gene expression [58–61] (Box 10). RNAi works through generation of small 21 to 23 nucleotide antisense

---

Box 10. RNA Inhibitors (RNAi)

- Antisense RNA oligonucleotide sequences.
- Delivered as small inhibitor RNA (siRNA) or short hairpin RNA (shRNA).
- Knock-down specified gene expression at post transcriptional level.

RNA, called small inhibitory RNA (siRNA) and short hairpin RNA (shRNA). These oligonucleotides use endogenous multiprotein complexes called RNA-induced silencing complex (RISC) to guide cleavage of the mRNA in the cytoplasm. It has the following advantages: effective, effective in low concentrations, may evade host interferon defenses, can be generated by multiple pathways, tissue-specific expression, nontoxic, and reasonably long lived. It has the following disadvantages: cannot target nuclear RNA or introns, no option for improving if target is refractory, and off-target effects are possible. It has greater promise than older methods such as oligonucleotides and ribozymes, all facing greater problems of efficient delivery, adequate stability, target-specificity, and target sequence selection.

Delivering gene therapy to the nervous system is a major challenge. One barrier that protects the nervous system is the blood–brain barrier (BBB), which divides the vascular and nervous system compartments. A new technology called molecular Trojan horses exploits the BBB by employing its transcytosis systems to deliver therapeutic cargo to neurons [62]. More than 100 billion capillaries that stretch for approximately 300 miles and extend to virtually every neuron perfuse the brain. Molecular Trojan horses are liposome nanocontainers that can contain genes or gene modulators such RNAi (Box 11). They are mounted on peptides that fit into receptor-mediated transcytosis systems to carry the cargo across the BBB. The liposome nanocontainers are conjugated with polyethyleneglycol to stabilize them in blood.

Box 11. Molecular Trojan horses

- Cargo genes or gene modulators packaged in liposomal nanocontainers that are stable in blood and nonimmunogenic.
- Nanocontainers are mounted on peptides with affinity for receptor-ediated transcytosis systems, which cargo them across the BBB.
- Gene or gene modulators could have specific promoters to achieve neuronal specificity.

The peptides immunogenicity can be circumvented with genetic engineering. Both the pegylation and genetic engineering are Federal Drug Administration approved. Because this therapeutic route does not disrupt the BBB, brain regulation is not altered. Because it does not entail viral vectors, other cellular functions are not impacted, immune defenses are not invoked, and mutagenesis does not occur. Also, because they are not directly injected by intracerebral, intraventricular, or intrathecal routes, delivery is noninvasive and widespread.

Review of relevant amyotrophic lateral sclerosis literature

A number of investigations have employed either tissue microdissection or microarray technologies to ALS, but only one has combined them and only one has validated this approach. Two investigations have applied tissue microdissection [63,64]. Heath et al [63] used laser capture microdissection (LCM) to isolate neurons from non-ALS postmortem spinal cords for RT-PCR assessment of mRNA levels for a subtype of glutamate receptor—they established uniqueness in the motor neuron profile, possible important for its select vulnerability. Mawrin et al [64] used laser pressure capturing to isolate neurons from postmortem nervous systems to look for mitochondrial DNA damage as an indicator of oxidative stress—they found no significant difference between ALS and controls.

Six investigations have applied microarrays or other methods of high-throughput gene expression profiling—three to human postmortem tissue and three to the G93A-SOD1 transgenic mice (reviewed in [65]) [66–71]. Malaspina et al [66] used high-density cDNA filters with a gene discovery array of 18,400 expressed sequence tags to profile gene expression in frozen anterior gray matter from postmortem lumbar spinal cords—they found differentially expressed genes in SALS involving antioxidant function, neuroinflammation, lipid metabolism, protease inhibition, and protection against apoptosis. Ishigaki et al [67] used molecular indexing combined with custom-spotted cDNA microarrays to profile gene expression in frozen anterior gray matter from postmortem lumbar spinal cords—they observed differentially expressed genes in SALS associated with the ubiquitin–proteasome system, oxidative toxicity, transcription, neuronal differentiation, and inflammation; they made no comment about apoptosis. Dangond et al [68] used oligonucleotide microarrays containing ~6800 genes to profile gene expression in postmortem lumbar gray matter in frozen spinal cords obtained from local or national tissue banks—they identified alterations in genes involved in mitochondrial function, oxidative stress, excitotoxicity, apoptosis, cytoskeletal architecture, RNA transcription and translation, proteasomal function, and growth and signaling; FALS and SALS had different gene expression profiles. Olsen et al [69] used murine oligonucleotide microarray of 6500 genes to profile gene expression at 30, 60, 90, and 120 days in G93A–SOD1 transgenic mice bulk spinal cords and found emergence of glial activation coincidental with clinical weakness and then activation of genes involved in metal ion regulation. Yoshihara et al [70] used cDNA microarrays containing 1081 genes to profile gene expression at 4, 11, 14, and 17 weeks in G93A–SOD1 transgenic mice bulk lumbar spinal cords—they observed upregulation of genes related to inflammation and apoptosis at 11 weeks, still the presymptomatic stage. Hensley et al [71] used multiprobe ribonuclease protection assays to profile 36 genes involved with cytokines and apoptosis at 80 and 120 days G93A–SOD1 transgenic mice frozen bulk thoracic and lumbar spinal cords, and found cytokine expression probably precedes protein oxidation and apoptosis and macrophages but not lymphocytes contribute to cytokine expression.

Jiang et al [72] used laser pressure catapulting to isolate motor neurons from postmortem frozen lumbar spinal cords of SALS patients to provide cell-specific cDNA microarrays containing 4845 genes; they found 3% of genes were downregulated, and these were associated with cytoskeleton and axonal transport, transcription, and cell surface antigens and receptors; 1% of genes were unregulated, and these included promoters for cell death pathways. Ravits et al [11] has performed extensive evaluation of motor neuron topography and RNA quality to show that if the nervous system in ALS is optimally acquired and processed upfront for downstream technologies, microgenomics will yield high-quality molecular exploration at the cellular level.

References

[1] Rowland LP, Shneider NA. Amyotrophic lateral sclerosis. N Engl J Med 2001;344: 1688–700.
[2] Brooks BR. The role of axonal transport in neurodegenerative disease spread: a meta-analysis of experimental and clinical poliomyelitis compares with amyotrophic lateral sclerosis. Can J Neurol Sci 1991;18:435–8.
[3] Figlewicz DA, Orrell RW. The genetics of motor neuron disease. Amyotroph Lateral Scler Other Motor Neuron Disord 2003;4:225–31.
[4] Ince PG, Lowe J, Shaw PJ. Amyotrophic lateral sclerosis: current issues in classification, pathogenesis, and molecular pathology. Neuropathol Appl Neurobiol 1998;24:104–17.
[5] Martin LJ. Neuronal death in amyotrophic lateral sclerosis is apoptosis: possible contribution of a programmed cell death mechanism. J Neuropathol Exp Neurol 1999;58: 459–71.
[6] Troost D, Aten J, Morsink F, et al. Apoptosis in amyotrophic lateral sclerosis is not restricted to motor neurons. Bcl-2 expression is increased in unaffected post-central gyrus. Neuropathol Appl Neurobiol 1995;21:498–504.
[7] Van Welsem ME, Hogenhuis JA, Meininger V, et al. The relationship between Bunina bodies, skein-like inclusions and neuronal loss in amyotrophic lateral sclerosis. Acta Neuropathol (Berl) 2002;103:583–9.
[8] Piao Y-S, Wakabayashi K, Kakita A, et al. Neuropathology with clinical correlations of sporadic amyotrophic lateral sclerosis: 102 autopsy cases examined between 1962–2000. Brain Pathol 2003;12:10–22.
[9] Ince PG, Tomkins J, Slade JY, et al. Amyotrophic lateral sclerosis associated with genetic abnormalities in the gene encoding Cu/Zn superoxide dismutase: molecular pathology of

five new cases, and comparison with previous reports and 73 sporadic cases of ALS. J Neuropathol Exp Neurol 1998;57:895–904.

[10] Hirano A, Kurland LT, Sayre GP. Familial amyotrophic lateral sclerosis. A subgroup
characterized by posterior and spinocerebellar tract involvement and hyaline inclusions
in the anterior horn cells. Arch Neurol 1967;16:232–43.

[11] Ravits J, Laurie P, Stone B: The implications of focality in amyotrophic lateral sclerosis for
microgenomics. In preparation.

[12] Cleveland DW, Rothstein JD. From Charcot to Lou Gehrig: deciphering selective motor
neuron death in ALS. Nat Rev Neurosci 2001;2:806–19.

[13] Cluskey S, Ramsden DB. Mechanisms of neurodegeneration in amyotrophic lateral sclerosis. J Clini Pathol: Mol Pathol 2001;54:386–92.

[14] Buuijn LI, Miller TM, Cleveland DW. Unraveling the mechanisms involved in motor neuron
degeneration in ALS. Annu Rev Neurosci 2004;27:723–49.

[15] Strong MJ. The basic aspects of therapeutics in amyotrophic lateral sclerosis. Pharmacol
Ther 2003;98:379–414.

[16] Weydt P, Moller T. Neuroinflammation in the pathogenesis of amyotrophic lateral sclerosis.
Neuroreport 2005;16:527–31.

[17] Rothstein JD. Excitotoxicity hypothesis. Neurology 1996;47(suppl 2):S19–25.

[18] Appel SH, Simpson EP. Activated microglia: the silent executioner in neurodegenerative disease? Curr Neurol Neurosci Rep 2001;1:303–5.

[19] Hall ED, Oostveen JA, Gurney ME. Relationship of microglial and astrocytic activation
to disease onset and progression in a transgenic model of familial ALS. Glia 1998;23:
249–56.

[20] Elliott JL. Cytokine upregulation in a murine model of familial amyotrophic lateral sclerosis.
Brain Res Mol Brain Res 2001;95:172–8.

[21] Kawamata T, Akiyama H, Yamada T, et al. Immunologic reactions in amyotrophic lateral
sclerosis brain and spinal cord tissue. Am J Pathol 1992;140:691–707.

[22] Sathasivam S, Ince PG, Shaw PJ. Apoptosis in amyotrophic lateral sclerosis: a review of the
evidence. Neuropathol Appl Neurobiol 2001;27(4):257–74.

[23] Guégan C, Przedborski S. Programmed cell death in amyotrophic lateral sclerosis. J Clin
Invest 2003;111:153–61.

[24] Hynd MR, Lewhol JM, Scott HL, et al. Biochemical and molecular studies using human
autopsy brain tissue. J Neurochem 2003;85:543–62.

[25] Johnson SA, Forgan DG, Finch CE. Extensive post-mortem stability of RNA from rat and
human brain. J Neurosci Res 1986;16:267–80.

[26] Ross BM, Knowler JT, McCulloch J. On the stability of messenger RNA and ribosomal
RNA in the brains of control human subjects and patients with Alzheimer's disease. J Neruochem 1992;58:1810–9.

[27] Bahn S, Augood SJ, Ryan M, et al. Gene expression profiling in the post-mortem human
brain—no cause for dismay. J Chem Neuroanal 2001;22:79–94.

[28] Ginsberg SD, Che S. RNA amplification in brain tissues. Neruochem Res 2002;27:981–92.

[29] Rupp GM, Locker J. Purification and analysis of RNA from paraffin-embedded tissues. Biotechniques 1988;6:56–60.

[30] Ben-Ezra J, Johnson DA, Rossi J, et al. Effect of fixation on the amplification of nucleic acids
from paraffin-embedded material by the polymerase chain reaction. J Histochem Cytochem
1991;39:351–4.

[31] Foss RD, Buha-Thakurta N, Conran R, et al. Effects of fixative and fixation time on the
extraction and polymerase chain reaction amplification of RNA from paraffin-embedded
tissue. Comparison of two housekeeping gene mRNA controls. Diagn Mol Pathol 1994;
3:148–55.

[32] Dakhama A, Macek V, Hogg JC, et al. Amplification of human β-actin gene by the reverse
transcriptase-polymerase chain reaction: implications for assessment of RNA from formalin-
fixed, paraffin-embedded material. J Histochem Cytochem 1996;44:1205–7.

[33] Coombs NJ, Gough AC, Primrose JN. Optimization of DNA and RNA extraction from archival formalin-fixed tissue. Nucleic Acids Res 1999;27(16):i–iii.

[34] Masuda N, Ohnishi T, Kawamoto S, et al. Analysis of chemical modification of RNA from formalin-fixed samples and optimization of molecular biology applications for such samples. Nucleic Acids Res 1999;27:4436–43.

[35] Van Deerlin VMD, Ginsberg SD, Lee VM-Y, et al. The use of fixed human postmortem brain tissue to study mRNA expression in neurodegenerative diseases: applications of microdissection and mRNA amplification. In: Geshwind DH, Gregg JP, editors. Microarrays for the neurosciences: an essential guide. Cambridge (MA): A Bradford Book; 2002. p. 201–36.

[36] Wilson KE, Ryan MM, Prime JE, et al. Functional genomics and proteomics: application in neurosciences. J Neurol Neurosurg Psychol 2004;75:529–38.

[37] Van Deerlin VM, Gill LH, Nelson PT. Optimizing gene expression analysis in archival brain tissue. Neurochem Res 2002;27:993–1003.

[38] Emmert-Buck MR, Bonner RF, Smith PD, et al. Laser capture microdissection. Science 1996;274:998–1001.

[39] Bonner RF, Emmert-Buck M, Cole K, et al. Laser capture microdissection: molecular analysis of tissue. Science 1997;278:1481–3.

[40] Simone NL, Bonner RF, Gillespie JW, et al. Laser-capture microdissection: opening the microscopic frontier to molecular analysis. Trends Genet 1998;14:272–6.

[41] Suarez-Quian CA, Goldstein SR, Pohida T, et al. Laser-capture microdissection of single cells from complex tissues. Biotechniques 1999;26:328–35.

[42] Hergenhahn M, Kenzelmann M, Gröne H-J. Laser-controlled microdissection of tissues opens a window of new opportunities. Pathol Res Pract 2003;199:419–23.

[43] Eltoum IA, Siegal GP, Frost AR. Microdissection of histological sections: past, present, and future. Adv Anat Pathol 2002;9:316–22.

[44] Lissek AM. The pyramidal tract: its status in medicine. Springfield (IL): Charles C Thomas; 1954.

[45] Ginsberg SD, Che S. RNA amplification in brain tissues. Neurochem Res 2002;27:981–92.

[46] Kelz MB, Dent GW, Therlanos S, et al. Single-cell antisense RNA amplification and microarray analysis as a tool for studying neurological degeneration and restoration. Sci Aging Knowledge Environ 2002;1:1–10.

[47] Li J, Schwartz SM, Bumgarner RE. RNA amplification, fidelity and reproducibility of expression profiling. C R Biol 2003;326:1021–30.

[48] Speed T, editor. Statistical analysis of gene expression microarray data. Boca Raton (FL): Chapman & Hall/CRC Press LLC; 2003.

[49] Brown PO, Botstein D. Exploring the new world of the genome with DNA microarrays. Nat Genet 1999;21(1 Suppl):33–7.

[50] Goodman L. Hypothesis-limited research. Genome Res 1999;9:673–4.

[51] Nisenbaum LK. The ultimate chip shot: can microarray technology deliver for neuroscience? Genes Brain Behav 2002;1:27–34.

[52] Mills JC, Roth KA, Cagan RL, et al. DNA microarrays and beyond: completing the journey from tissue to cell. Nat Cell Biol 2001;3:E175–8.

[53] Liu ET, Karuturi KR. Microarrays and clinical investigations. N Engl J Med 2004;350:1595–6.

[54] Kacharmina JE, Crino PB, Eberwine J. Preparation of cDNA from single cells and subcellular regions. Methods Enzymol 1999;303:3–18.

[55] Crino PB, Trojanowski JQ, Dichter MA, et al. Embryonic neuronal markers in tuberous sclerosis: single-cell molecular pathology. Proc Natl Acad Sci USA 1996;93:14152–7.

[56] Humphery-Smith I, Cordwell SJ, Blackstock WP. Proteome research: complementarity and limitations with respect to the RNA and DNA worlds. Electrophoresis 1997;18:1217–42.

[57] Greenbaum D, Colangelo C, Williams K, et al. Comparing protein abundance and mRNA expression levels on a genomic scale. Genome Biol 2003;4:117–24.

[58] Scherer LJ, Rossi JJ. Approaches for the sequence-specific knockdown of mRNA. Nat Bio-
     technol 2003;21:1457–65.
[59] Dorsett Y, Tuschl T. siRNASs: applications in functional genomics and potential as thera-
     peutics. Nat Rev 2004;3:318–29.
[60] Dykxhoorn DM, Novina CD, Sharp PA. Killing the messenger: short RNAs that silence
     gene expression. Nat Rev 2004;4:457–67.
[61] Stevenson M. Therapeutic potential of RNA interference. N Engl J Med 2004;351:1772–7.
[62] Schlachetzki F, Zhang Y, Boado RJ, et al. Gene therapy of the brain, the transvascular ap-
     proach. Neurology 2004;62:1275–81.
[63] Heath PR, Tomkins J, Ince PG, et al. Quantitative assessment of AMPA receptor mRNA in
     human spinal motor neurons isolated by laser capture microdissection. Neuroreport 2002;
     13(14):1753–7.
[64] Mawrin C, Kirches E, Dietzmann K. Single-cell analysis of mtDNA in amyotrophic lateral
     sclerosis: towards the characterization of individual neurons in neurodegenerative disorders.
     Pathol Res Pract 2003;199:415–8.
[65] Malaspina A, de Belleroche J. Spinal cord molecular profiling provides a better under-
     standing of amyotrophic lateral sclerosis pathogenesis. Brain Res Brain Res Rev 2004;
     45:213–29.
[66] Malaspina A, Kaushik N, de Belleroche J. Differential expression of 14 genes in amyotrophic
     lateral sclerosis spinal cord detected using gridded cDNA arrays. J Neurochem 2001;77:
     132–45.
[67] Ishigaki S, Niwa J, Ando Y, et al. Differentially expressed genes in sporadic amyotrophic
     lateral sclerosis spinal cords—screening by molecular indexing and subsequent cDNA
     microarray analysis. FEBS Lett 2002;531:354–8.
[68] Dangond F, Hwang D, Camelo S, et al. Molecular signature of late-stage human ALS re-
     vealed by expression profiling of postmortem spinal cord gray matter. Physiol Genomics
     2004;16:229–39.
[69] Olsen MK, Roberds SL, Ellerbrock BR, et al. Disease mechanisms revealed by transcription
     profiling in SOD1–G93A transgenic mouse spinal cord. Ann Neurol 2001;50:730–40.
[70] Yoshihara T, Ishigaki S, Yamamoto M, et al. Differential expression of inflammation- and
     apoptosis-related genes in spinal cords of a mutant SOD1 transgenic mouse model of familial
     amyotrophic lateral sclerosis. J Neurochem 2002;80:158–67.
[71] Hensley K, Floyd RA, Gordon B, et al. Temporal patterns of cytokine and apoptosis-related
     gene expression in spinal cords of the G93A–SOD1 mouse model of amyotrophic lateral
     sclerosis. J Neurochem 2002;82:365–74.
[72] Jiang Y-M, Yamamoto M, Koyayashi Y, et al. Gene expression profile of spinal motor neu-
     rons in sporadic amyotrophic lateral sclerosis. Ann Neurol 2005;57:236–51.

ELSEVIER
SAUNDERS

Phys Med Rehabil Clin N Am
16 (2005) 925–949

PHYSICAL MEDICINE
AND REHABILITATION
CLINICS OF
NORTH AMERICA

Redox Mechanisms of Muscle Dysfunction in Inflammatory Disease

Michael B. Reid, PhD[a],*, Francisco H. Andrade, PhD[a],
C. William Balke, MD, FACP[b], Karyn A. Esser, PhD[a]

[a]Department of Physiology, University of Kentucky Medical Center, 800 Rose Street,
MS-509, Lexington, KY 40536-0298, USA
[b]College of Medicine, University of Kentucky Medical Center, 800 Rose Street, MN-150,
Lexington, KY 40536-0298, USA

Oxidative stress in muscle pathology

Free radicals first were detected in skeletal muscle by Commoner et al [1] in 1952 using the emerging technology of electron paramagnetic resonance spectroscopy. The pathophysiologic importance of this finding was largely unappreciated until the mid-1980s, when scattered reports began to link muscle disease with oxidative stress [2–6]. In the ensuing 2 decades, an increasing number of publications has made it clear that oxidative stress is a fundamental part of inflammatory disease and is linked inextricably to muscle dysfunction under pathologic conditions. Oxidative stress has been linked to loss of muscle performance in widely diverse pathologies that include heart failure [7,8], cancer [9,10], muscular dystrophy [11–13], chronic obstructive pulmonary disease [14], rheumatoid arthritis [15], obstructive sleep apnea [16–18], rhabdomyolysis [19], renal insufficiency [20], and AIDS [21]. The prevalence of this association and the disparate nature of the underlying diseases raise obvious questions about the factors that induce oxidative stress in muscle and the mechanisms whereby oxidative stress compromise muscle function.

Biology of reactive oxygen species

Oxidative stress is defined as an increase in the cellular steady-state concentration of reactive oxygen species (ROS). More precisely, this increase in the

This work was supported by grants HL59878 (M.B. Reid), EY12998 and DC06410 (F.H. Andrade), HL071865 and HL68733 (C.W. Balke), and AR43349 and AR45617 (K.A. Esser).
* Corresponding author.
E-mail address: michael.reid@uky.edu (M.B. Reid).

doi:10.1016/j.pmr.2005.08.016

cellular steady-state concentration of ROS represents the alteration of the baseline ratio of oxidant and antioxidant factors, which may involve the incomplete reduction of molecular oxygen [22] or a decreased antioxidant capacity [23]. ROS include superoxide anions, hydroxyl radicals, hydrogen peroxide (H_2O_2), and, as a consequence of superoxide anion scavenging, peroxynitrite. These reactive molecules are cytotoxic via a variety of mechanisms, including lipid peroxidation, DNA damage and mutagenesis, depletion of intracellular ATP, disruption of intracellular calcium homeostasis, protein oxidation and apoptosis, and tissue necrosis. ROS are generated by several intracellular signaling pathways, including the xanthine-hypoxanthine system [24], mitochondrial respiratory enzymes, lipoxygenase, certain P-450 enzymes, nitric oxide synthase, and membrane-bound NADPH oxidase [25,26]. Among the endogenous antioxidant systems, superoxide dismutase dismutes superoxide anions to form H_2O_2, which is dehydrated by catalase to H_2O.

Focus of current review

A comprehensive review of ROS involvement in muscle pathophysiology is beyond the scope of this article. Rather, the authors illustrate the importance of ROS biology and the primary mechanisms of ROS action by focusing on a subset of selected topics. These topics are intentionally diverse, highlighting the range of research in this field, but have specific criteria in common. First, this article addresses muscle-derived ROS as intracellular modulators of contractile function and muscle mass. These actions are most clearly evident in diseases of remote tissues in which humoral mediators stimulate ROS production without local invasion of inflammatory cells or overt tissue damage. This criterion excludes the primary muscle pathologies (eg, muscular dystrophy, rhabdomyolysis, and muscle injury), although the mechanisms discussed are likely to pertain in these diseases. Second, data from skeletal and cardiac muscle are compared. This comparison illustrates cellular responses and signaling pathways that are robust, common to both types of striated muscle. It also highlights intriguing differences that warrant further investigation. Third, each topic in this article is an application of the experimental model shown in Fig. 1. This model proposes that diseases of remote tissues act via specific mediators to stimulate ROS production by muscle cells. Muscle-derived ROS may cause loss of muscle function via two parallel and independent mechanisms. ROS may oxidize regulatory proteins of the myofilament lattice or sarcoplasmic reticulum directly, altering contraction, or may activate redox-sensitive signaling pathways to modify gene expression and muscle mass.

Role of reactive oxygen species in cachexia

One of the best-recognized associations between oxidative stress and muscle dysfunction is in the clinical condition of cachexia. Cachexia is a debilitating loss of respiratory and limb muscle mass that occurs in inflammatory

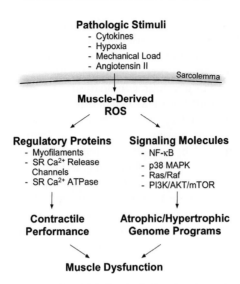

Fig. 1. General mechanisms of ROS-induced dysfunction in striated muscle. Pathway delineates pathologic stimuli that increase ROS production by striated muscle in inflammatory disease and illustrates two parallel mechanisms by which ROS may cause muscle dysfunction; see text for details. mTOR, mammalian target of rapamycin; PI3K, phosphatidylinositol 3-kinase; SR, sarcoplasmic reticulum. (*Adapted from* Reid MB, Li Y-P. Cytokines and oxidative signalling in skeletal muscle. Acta Physiol Scand 2001;171:225–32; with permission.)

diseases, including chronic obstructive pulmonary disease [14], congestive heart failure [7,8], cancer [9,10], AIDS [21], and rheumatoid arthritis [15]. The resulting weakness makes patients more susceptible to the complications of disease and may contribute directly to premature death [27]. Cachexia is caused in part by persistent elevation of circulating cytokines [27–31]. These polypeptide molecules are produced by macrophages and monocytes and promote antitumor and immune responses. With chronic inflammation, cytokines enter the circulation to exert systemic effects that include progressive loss of adipose tissue, loss of muscle protein, and a shift to negative nitrogen balance. This catabolic syndrome is thought to be mediated by five different cytokines—tumor necrosis factor (TNF)-α, interleukin (IL)-1α, IL-1β, interferon (IFN)-γ, and IL-6 [27,32]—each known to promote protein loss. Despite the pathophysiologic importance of these cytokines, their mechanisms of action on skeletal muscle remain poorly understood.

Oxidative stress is strongly implicated in the catabolic process. Biochemical markers of oxidant activity are elevated in the circulation and muscle of cachectic patients [33–38]. Direct exposure of muscle to ROS stimulates procatabolic signaling [39–44], increases protein degradation [45–47], and inhibits myosin expression [48,49]. There is growing evidence that cytokine actions and oxidative stress are closely related. Muscle-derived ROS seem to function as intracellular signaling molecules that alter muscle gene expression, promoting cytokine-induced catabolism [48,50].

Animal studies indicate that systemic elevation of catabolic cytokine levels can affect synthesis and degradation of muscle proteins [29,32,51–54]. The predominant response of differentiated muscle cells to direct cytokine exposure is increased protein breakdown [41]. This response seems to reflect a generalized increase in ubiquitin conjugation [41,55,56]. As reviewed elsewhere [57,58], the ubiquitin/proteasome pathway degrades the bulk of all intracellular proteins during muscle atrophy. Pathway activity depends on coordinated interactions among several enzyme families. First, ubiquitin monomers are activated by the ubiquitin-activating enzyme (E1 protein), an ATP-dependent step in which ubiquitin is linked to E1 via a high-energy thiolester bond. Only one E1 protein has been identified in mammalian cells, an abundant 110-kD protein that is essential for cell survival. Second, the activated ubiquitin is transferred to a ubiquitin-conjugating enzyme (E2 protein) that functions as a carrier protein. Third, activated ubiquitin is transferred to ubiquitin ligase (E3 protein), which catalyzes the formation of polyubiquitin chains on the substrate protein, marking it for degradation by the 26S-proteasome complex. This enzyme complex is a major cell constituent, composing 1% of total cell protein. Proteasomal degradation of a ubiquitin-conjugated protein involves recognition, unfolding, and degradation of the protein to small peptides (3–25 residues), an ATP-dependent process. The specificity of protein degradation via the ubiquitin/proteasome pathway is conferred by E2 and E3 proteins that recognize selected substrates based on structural determinants.

General activity of the ubiquitin/proteasome pathway is increased during muscle catabolism, a response mediated at the transcriptional level [59]. Pathway components that are upregulated include ubiquitin [60,61], subunits of the proteasome complex [62–65], and muscle-specific E2 and E3 proteins [55,56,66–68]. Current evidence indicates the E2 and E3 proteins are rate-limiting. Availability of E2 and E3 proteins determines overall activity of the ubiquitin-conjugating pathway [55,69]. More importantly, selective inhibition of individual E proteins has been shown to prevent net protein loss in animal and cell culture models of atrophy [70,71].

Integrating the available data, it seems that a subset of catabolic cytokines may act via ROS-sensitive signaling events to upregulate specific E2 and E3 proteins selectively. This action would provide a robust mechanism for coordinated upregulation of complementary gene products, increasing ubiquitin conjugation and favoring protein loss. A proposed model of these interactions is depicted in Fig. 2, which includes putative stimuli, proposed pathways, and target genes. The rationale for this model and the data on which it is based are detailed in the following sections.

Catabolic cytokines and ROS-dependent signaling

Among cytokines that are most likely to stimulate muscle catabolism, the cellular mechanisms of TNF-α action are best understood. TNF-α acts

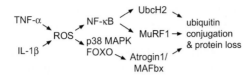

Fig. 2. ROS-dependent signaling events that mediate ubiquitin conjugation and protein loss in cytokine-stimulated muscle. Pathway illustrates ROS-dependent mechanisms by which cytokines increase E2/E3 mRNA and ubiquitin conjugating activity; see text for details.

directly on differentiated muscle to stimulate intracellular oxidant activity [72], activate nuclear factor–κB (NF-κB) and the mitogen-activated protein kinases (MAPKs) [41,56], increase ubiquitin conjugation [55,56], and cause net loss of muscle protein [41]. These features make TNF-α the prototype for cytokines in this category. In human disease, TNF-α is never elevated in isolation, however. Circulating levels of other catabolic cytokines—IL-1α, IL-1β, IFN-γ, and IL-6—also are elevated in chronic inflammatory disease [27–31]. Each of these cytokines induces muscle catabolism in vivo, but their mechanisms of action in skeletal muscle are largely unstudied. Available data suggest that a subset of these cytokines uses ROS-dependent signaling.

The two isoforms of IL-1 are most strongly implicated. Among organs, IL-1α and IL-1β exhibit different patterns of constitutive expression [73], but have considerable overlap and redundancy in their biologic activities [74]. Rodent studies indicate that muscle catabolism can be caused by IL-1 stimulation [75,76], and that an IL-1 receptor antagonist prevents the decrement in muscle protein synthesis that occurs in sepsis [77]. IL-1β does not increase ubiquitin mRNA in rat muscle in vivo [61], but it does activate NF-κB and p38 MAPK in cultured myoblasts [78] and is reported to increase mRNA levels for several muscle-specific E3 proteins [71]. Data from nonmuscle cell types provide further support: ROS function as second messengers for IL-1 in some systems [79]. NF-κB may be activated by IL-1-stimulated ROS signaling [79]. IL-1 also increases activity of the MAPKs, including p38 MAPK [80]. These responses are cell type specific [74] and have not been evaluated systematically in muscle.

There is less evidence to support IFN-γ or IL-6 involvement. Neither IFN-γ nor IL-6 is known to stimulate ROS production in muscle or to regulate transcription via p38 MAPK and NF-κB signaling. IFN-γ and IL-6 seem to increase muscle catabolism by separate mechanisms. Both alter muscle metabolism [81,82], stimulate cathepsin expression [80,83–85], and function as coactivators with TNF-α to inhibit muscle differentiation and growth [86–88]. IL-6 can stimulate ubiquitin conjugation, but this is caused by upregulation of E3α [89], a ubiquitin ligase that does not respond to ROS stimulation [44]. IL-6 seems to act primarily by altering the balance of growth factor–related signaling to produce a more catabolic profile [90], rather than stimulating catabolism directly [91].

ROS/NF-κB signaling regulates UbcH2/E2-20 and Muscle RING Finger 1

More recent studies [41,55,88,92–96] have identified NF-κB as a redox-sensitive transcription factor that promotes muscle atrophy. In differentiated muscle, NF-κB signaling seems to be essential for protein loss stimulated by disuse [96], denervation [93], tumor implantation [88], and catabolic cyto-kines [92]. Much is known about NF-κB regulation. As reviewed elsewhere [97], the canonical pathway involves a family of five proteins—p65, p50, p52, Rel B, and c-Rel. These reside in the cytosol as inactive heterodimers or homodimers that complex with the inhibitor protein I-κB. Cytokine stimu-lation triggers rapid degradation of I-κB via the ubiquitin-proteasome path-way, activating NF-κB. The active NF-κB dimer undergoes nuclear translocation and DNA binding to activate transcription of target genes. An alternative mechanism regulates NF-κB activity during disuse atrophy; this alternative pathway does not seem to mediate cachexia or cytokine-stimulated losses; see review by Jackman and Kandarian [98].

Direct exposure to either TNF-α [94,95] or H_2O_2 simulates activation and nuclear translocation of NF-κB in skeletal muscle cells [41,50,92,99,100]. The response to TNF-α is rapid and dose-dependent, it seems to be mediated by mitochondrial-derived ROS [50], and it involves phosphorylation and protea-somal degradation of the NF-κB-inhibitory protein, I-κB [41]. In immature myoblasts, this pathway inhibits MyoD expression and slows growth and dif-ferentiation [88,94,95]. In differentiated muscle, NF-κB signaling is essential for the increase in ubiquitin conjugation and loss of muscle protein stimulated by TNF-α [92]. This catabolic response seems to depend on NF-κB-dependent upregulation of cytokine-responsive E-proteins. TNF-α/NF-κB signal-ing stimulates expression of UbcH2/E2-20k, an E2 protein that increases ubiquitin-conjugating activity in muscle [55]. Muscle RING Finger 1 (MuRF1) is another likely target of ROS-activated NF-κB. MuRF1 is an E3 protein upregulated in at least 10 different experimental models of muscle atrophy, including mechanical unloading [96,101], tumor implantation [93], denervation [93], and sepsis [102]. Importantly, mice deficient in MuRF1 are resistant to denervation and glucocorticoid-induced atrophy [93]. NF-κB signaling is essential for MuRF1 upregulation in animal models of muscle wasting [93], but the upstream events that activate NF-κB/MuRF1 signaling are largely undefined. Cytokine effects on MuRF1 expression have not been reported.

ROS/p38 MAPK signaling regulates atrogin1/MAFbx

Among elements of the ubiquitin-proteasome system, the component induced most dramatically during muscle atrophy is atrogin1/MAFbx, a ubiquitin ligase. Atrogin1/MAFbx mRNA is increased in experimental atrophy induced by tumor implantation [70], sepsis [102], denervation [71], food restriction [70], unloading [71,101,103], immobilization [71], and renal failure [70]. Of particular interest, mice deficient in atrogin1/MAFbx are resistant to muscle atrophy [71]. Skeletal muscle upregulates atrogin1/MAFbx mRNA in response to either TNF-α [56] or H_2O_2 [44] stimulation.

Understanding of the signaling events that regulate this response is limited. Atrogin1/MAFbx expression is regulated by the Forkhead box O (FOXO) transcription factors [68], but FOXO signaling is not known to be redox sensitive [104]. NF-κB does not seem to regulate this response either; selective NF-κB activation has no effect on atrogin1/MAFbx mRNA [93]. Data suggest that signaling via p38 MAPK (also known as protein kinase B) promotes muscle atrophy [105–108] and atrogin1/MAFbx expression [93]. Inhibition of p38 MAPK blocks atrogin1/MAFbx upregulation and prevents the increase in ubiquitin conjugation stimulated by TNF-α [93]. It also has been established that TNF-α increases ROS activity [72], and that ROS activate p38 MAPK [93]. In combination, these observations suggest that TNF-α acts via ROS/p38 MAPK signaling to stimulate atrogin1MAFbx expression.

Reactive oxygen species effects on growth and repair of striated muscle

In many models of skeletal muscle atrophy, a decrease in the rate of protein synthesis precedes any increase in protein degradation rate [109–112]. ROS likely modulate anabolic mechanisms in striated muscle—both protein synthesis and myogenic responses of progenitor cells—but this biology remains poorly defined. This section outlines known effects of ROS on cardiac and skeletal muscle myocytes. Data on angiotensin II (Ang II), a known effector of ROS production and skeletal muscle size, are provided as a novel example of biologic relevance.

Angiotensin II treatment as a model for ROS regulation of skeletal muscle size

Ang II is a peptide hormone that binds to a G-protein-coupled receptor and can stimulate signaling through the Ras/Raf/MAPK pathways [113,114]. Nishida et al [115] provided the first solid evidence that ROS production promotes G-protein dissociation and activation. These findings were crucial for acceptance that the associated changes in ROS are partly the downstream mechanism of action of Ang II binding. Although Ang II has had a relatively long and established connection to cardiac hypertrophy, there are only limited and conflicting reports with Ang II and skeletal muscle size.

In studies of skeletal muscle hypertrophy, Gordon et al [116] suggested that tissue expression of Ang II positively contributes to skeletal muscle growth. In these studies, rats underwent bilateral synergist ablation, a commonly used surgical procedure to produce mechanical overload of the muscle and induce skeletal muscle hypertrophy. The model involves the surgical removal of the gastrocnemius muscle in the hind limb, and the remaining plantaris and soleus muscles take on the increased functional load and grow to compensate for the loss in synergistic muscle mass. After synergist ablation, the rats were treated with an angiotensin-converting enzyme inhibitor, enalapril maleate, to inhibit Ang II formation or perfused with an Ang II type 1 receptor antagonist, losartan potassium. Under these conditions, the hypertrophy of the soleus and plantaris muscles was decreased from about 70% to 95% at 28 days after ablation. These results indicated that Ang II signaling is a necessary component of the normal growth response of skeletal muscle to functional overload. More recent studies from Gordon's laboratory suggest that Ang II and potentially ROS play an important role in regulating the activity of satellite cell proliferation and fusion during the skeletal muscle hypertrophy in response to mechanical overload [117].

In contrast, studies in which Ang II is infused (500 ng/kg/min) in either rats or mice resulted in a significant reduction in skeletal muscle mass and body weight by 7 days [118,119]. Associated with the decline in muscle mass, the investigators detected a decrease in circulating levels of insulin-like growth factor I, which is a well-known anabolic factor for skeletal muscle mass. The investigators link the effects of Ang II to decreased insulin-like growth factor I levels because transgenic mice overexpressing insulin-like growth factor I in skeletal muscle do not exhibit the same loss in muscle mass in response to Ang II infusion. The Ang II effect also was associated with diminished signaling through the PI3 kinase/Akt/mTOR pathway. This finding was highlighted as this pathway is known to lie downstream of insulin-like growth factor I signaling, and it has been shown several times to be necessary for skeletal muscle hypertrophy [120–123].

At this time, there are not enough data to make any firm conclusions about the role of Ang II or ROS in skeletal muscle size because the models used for the studies cited were quite different. Gordon et al studied loss of Ang II function in a skeletal muscle experiencing increased mechanical loading, whereas the studies from Delafontaine's laboratory determined the impact of "overexpression" of Ang II on skeletal muscle size. The fact that Gordon did not detect any alteration in the skeletal muscle at rest with either angiotensin-converting enzyme inhibition or Ang II type 1 receptor blocking indicates that low levels of Ang II are not necessary for maintaining resting muscle size, but that Ang II is necessary, in part, for hypertrophy in response to mechanical overload. The results from Delafontaine's laboratory indicate that increasing the circulating levels of Ang II results in loss of muscle mass. It is most likely that the differences between the cellular response to Ang II are dose dependent in skeletal muscle. As is suggested by several studies of ROS signaling, smaller amounts may be associated more with growth/survival responses, whereas higher levels and prolonged exposure to ROS likely lead to atrophy/apoptotic responses [124–126].

Cellular mechanisms of ROS effects on growth and repair

Several studies in recent years suggested that ROS play a role in cardiac hypertrophy [127–134]. In cardiac cells, ROS levels have been implicated in communicating the growth signal from numerous extracellular stimuli, including mechanical strain, Ang II, norepinephrine, endothelin-1, cytokines (eg, IL-1β and TNF-α), and mitogens. The peptides, hormones, and growth factors bind to their specific cell-surface receptors, and these couple with multiple signal transduction cascades that link receptor activation to the regulation of hypertrophic growth. These signal cascades include tyrosine kinases (growth factor receptors, src, focal adhesion kinase), MAPKs (ERK1/2, p38, JNK, ERK5), protein kinase C (PKC), calcineurin, and PI3-kinase/Akt [128,129,131,134–138]. It is now clear that ROS are capable of directly activating nearly all of these signaling cascades. Specifically, studies using H_2O_2 in cardiac myocytes have shown the activation of src, PKC, and p38, ERK1/2, and JNK MAPKs, and a study by Tu et al [138] showed that signaling through PI3-kinase is required for H_2O_2-induced hypertrophy in the heart.

Activation and signaling through these pathways also are seen in models of skeletal muscle hypertrophy. H_2O_2 exposure activates p38, ERK1/2, and JNK MAPKs in skeletal muscle [56] and, at low concentrations, can activate cell growth [139], which requires signaling through the PI3-kinase/Akt/mTOR pathway in vivo and in vitro [140]. At higher concentrations, H_2O_2 has deleterious effects. Brief exposure can decrease the viability and life span of human satellite cells, arresting the cells in a nonproliferative state [141]. Similarly, oxidative stress induced by either H_2O_2 or bleomycin causes growth arrest, chromosomal aberrations, and apoptosis in L6C5 rat myoblasts [139].

Skeletal muscle and heart differ distinctly in their phenotypic response to cytokines, particularly TNF-α. In the heart, TNF-α acts to induce hypertrophy and likely plays a role in the progression of hypertrophy to a functional pathology. In skeletal muscle, TNF-α effects seem to be pleiotropic and differentiation-dependent. Preceding sections of this article describe the association of TNF-α with muscle catabolism and atrophy in differentiated muscle. In injured muscle, muscle-derived TNF-α seems to play an essential role in the repair process [142], however, exerting autocrine/paracrine effects as an endogenous myogenic factor to stimulate early differentiation of satellite cells [143] and myoblasts [99]. In all striated muscle cell types, the downstream targets of TNF-α function include increased ROS levels and NF-κB activation [41,130,136,144,145]. Identification of the downstream molecules responsible for the divergent responses of cardiac myocytes, mature skeletal muscle, and undifferentiated skeletal muscle cells is perplexing, but with the increase in chronic inflammation in the US population, the answer to this specificity is of great biomedical importance.

Data from cardiac muscle suggest ROS signaling also modulates the response to mechanical strain. Similar to skeletal muscle, cardiac cells hypertrophy in response to mechanical overload or stretch [146]. Aikawa et al [127] was the first to report increased ROS in response to mechanical strain. These studies showed that mechanical strain induced ROS-mediated increases in protein synthesis and hypertrophy of heart cells. The mechanism of the increased ROS levels in response to mechanical strain have been linked primarily to the paracrine actions of Ang II and endothelin I [126]. Yamamoto et al [147] showed, however, that the antioxidants N-acetyl-L-cysteine, catalase, and 1,2-dihydroxybenzene-3,5-disulfonate, but not blocking of the Ang II type 1 receptor, significantly inhibited cardiac growth. It is unclear what all the sources for ROS signaling in cardiac muscle are in response to mechanical signaling.

Sleep-disordered breathing, oxidative stress, and cardiac dysfunction

Oxidative stress contributes to cardiac dysfunction in a variety of pathologic states. Among these, sleep-disordered breathing (SDB) is a more recently recognized condition that illustrates a novel mechanism of ROS induction. SDB describes a variety of disorders of respiration, all of which are characterized by periods of hypoxia during sleep, including central sleep apnea, Cheyne-Stokes respiration, obesity-related hypoventilation and hypoxemia, and obstructive sleep apnea (OSA). As a group, these disorders are highly prevalent in the United States, and more than 12 million individuals have been diagnosed with some form of SDB [148,149]. In addition to its pulmonary manifestations, SDB is associated with considerable cardiovascular morbidity and mortality, with an increased risk for hypertension, coronary artery disease, myocardial infarction, and stroke [150–153]. The most compelling data for the association of SDB and hypertension comes from the Wisconsin Sleep Cohort Study. This prospective study showed an independent association of SDB and the development of hypertension, which was attenuated with the treatment of SDB [151]. With respect to coronary artery disease, the large prospective Sleep Heart Health Study [152] convincingly showed that even mild-to-modest levels of SDB conferred a significantly increased risk for cardiovascular disease [154]. The clear association of SDB with two major cardiac diseases shown in these two landmark prospective trials has been supported by many other retrospective and cross-sectional studies. The mechanisms responsible for the generation and exacerbation of cardiovascular comorbidities in SDB are considerably less clear, however.

Obstructive sleep apnea and chronic intermittent hypoxia

OSA is the most common of the SDB syndromes. OSA is characterized by intermittent partial or complete airway obstruction during sleep and is manifested clinically by sleep fragmentation, daytime somnolence, and a variety of neurocognitive deficits. Similar to all SDB disorders, OSA is associated with increased cardiovascular morbidity and mortality, and it is an independent risk factor for cardiovascular diseases, including hypertension; atherosclerotic vascular disease, particularly coronary artery disease and myocardial infarction; congestive heart failure; and strokes [154–159]. The three major components of OSA that are associated with cardiovascular disease are wide variations in intrathoracic pressure, postapneic arousals, and chronic intermittent hypoxia (CIH) [155]. In principle, CIH may represent the mechanistic link between OSA and OSA-related cardiovascular disease to the extent that CIH precipitates a form of oxidative stress that leads to tissue injury. Oxidative stress has been strongly implicated as an important component of cardiovascular disease, including atherosclerosis and ischemia-reperfusion injury [25]. In support of this hypothesis, CIH has been associated with hypertension and increased sympathetic tone in animal models [160–165]. Relatively little information is available regarding the consequences of CIH-mediated oxidative stress on cardiac function.

Oxidative stress in intermittent hypoxia

ROS can be produced in cell culture conditions with short periods of hypoxia [166] and in neural tissue exposed to CIH [167]. Oxidative stress [16–18] and decreased cellular antioxidant capacity have been shown in patients with OSA. Clinical studies are inherently limited in their ability to identify the mechanisms responsible for oxidative stress, however, owing to a variety of confounding influences, including comorbidities, postapneic arousals, and mechanical arousals. In addition, markers for oxidative stress in clinical studies were determined from peripheral blood and as such were incapable of providing any insight on the relationship between oxidative stress and myocardial dysfunction.

Studies [168] in a validated rodent model of CIH [161–165] provide new evidence that a CIH-mediated increase in the ratio of oxidant-to-antioxidant components underlies the increased incidence of myocardial dysfunction associated with OSA. Rats exposed to CIH mimicking that seen in patients with OSA developed significant hypertension within 2 weeks and significant cardiac hypertrophy, left ventricular dilation, decreased contractility, increased lipid peroxide levels, and decreased myocardial superoxide dismutase levels within 5 weeks. This model, which uniquely isolates the CIH component of OSA, shows that the development of hypertension and myocardial dysfunction is time-dependent and is associated with an increase in ROS coupled with a decrease in antioxidant activity. In addition, this study showed a correlation between the severity of cardiac dysfunction and the degree of myocardial oxidative stress. Because association does not prove causation, however, additional studies are required to confirm a causal relationship between oxidative stress and myocardial dysfunction.

Physiologic mechanisms of cardiac dysfunction

With regard to the mechanistic links between CIH and myocardial dysfunction, CIH resembles the classic model of myocardial ischemia-reperfusion injury [169,170]. The reintroduction of molecular oxygen after ischemia provides excess ROS that are capable of damaging cell components, such as lipids, DNA, and proteins, and initiating apoptosis. Several investigators have documented ischemia-generated ROS. Hypoxia per se or CIH-mediated reoxygenation could be capable of generating ROS. Alternatively, because tissue blood flow is intermittently disrupted during ischemia-reperfusion injury and not during CIH, the generalization between CIH and ischemia-reperfusion may be limited because the continued perfusion characteristic of CIH could allow for washout of potentially toxic metabolites.

Skeletal muscle dysfunction in heart failure: a role for reactive oxygen species?

Contractile dysfunction without atrophy

Muscle weakness and fatigue can accompany inflammatory disease in the absence of cachexia or overt muscle wasting [171–173]. Such symptoms commonly affect patients with congestive heart failure [174]. In this patient population, exercise intolerance is not related to ventricular function, and increased fatigability is evident even when the exercise affects small muscle groups that require limited increases in cardiac output [174,175]. It follows that decreased endurance in heart failure may be explained at least partly by adaptive changes in skeletal muscle, such as fiber type shifts, reduced oxidative capacity, or loss of contractile proteins [176]. Some of these alterations are likely due to cytokines and chemokines, inflammatory mediators that can induce muscle wasting, but that also may alter functional properties directly [176,177].

ROS as modulators of contraction

Cytokines can exert their effects on skeletal muscle by increasing the production of muscle-derived ROS and activating redox-sensitive signaling pathways [178]. This activity is consistent with the association between exercise intolerance and oxidative stress in patients with heart failure [179]. ROS can influence multiple determinants of contractile function: Voltage-gated ion channels, calcium release channels, myofilaments, and calcium ATPase are known to be redox sensitive. Oxidants increase twitch forces and prolong the time to peak tension and half-relaxation time. In contrast, antioxidants shorten time to peak tension and half-relaxation time and decrease twitch and submaximal tetanic forces [180].

Intracellular targets of ROS action

Oxidative stress induces cellular changes known collectively as a *stress response,* which typically includes loss of calcium homeostasis. Although calcium release channels in the sarcoplasmic reticulum open when reactive protein thiol groups are oxidized [181,182], the sensitivity of contractile function to changes in cellular ROS levels is not dependent on altered calcium kinetics. Brief exposures to high concentrations of H_2O_2, an oxidant, and dithiothreitol (DTT), a reducing agent, do not change tetanic free cytosolic calcium ($[Ca^{++}]_i$), but increase and decrease force. Prolonged exposures to H_2O_2 decrease force, without altering tetanic $[Ca^{++}]_i$. This late-phase effect of H_2O_2 can be completely reversed with DTT. Even longer exposures to H_2O_2 are needed to alter calcium reuptake by the sarcoplamic reticulum and increase tetanic $[Ca^{++}]_i$ [183]. The divergent results obtained with H_2O_2 and DTT and the time dependence of the H_2O_2 effects strongly suggest that the cellular targets of these reagents have optimal redox states [183]. In other words, the function of certain determinants of contractile activity depends on the redox state of their component proteins. Calcium release and reuptake seem to be fairly insensitive to redox modulation because fibers have to be exposed to high oxidant concentrations or for prolonged periods before sarcoplasmic reticulum function is affected. Likewise, in heart failure models, abnormal calcium handling by skeletal myocytes does not explain contractile dysfunction [184]. There is a significant increase in resting $[Ca^{++}]_i$ during fatigue, however [184]; this may be more relevant for the chronic changes in skeletal muscle structure and metabolism in response to heart failure.

Myofibrillar calcium sensitivity seems to be exquisitely susceptible to variations of the cellular redox balance [183,185,186]. Similarly the cytokine TNF-α has been shown to compromise contractile function by decreasing myofibrillar calcium sensitivity [187]. Redox effects on myofibrillar calcium sensitivity require an intact sarcolemma; this suggests the existence of transducing steps that sense increased cellular oxidant loads and induce the resultant changes in contractile function [188,189]. ROS are small, reactive, and diffusible molecules generated and metabolized rapidly in response to various stimuli. These characteristics make ROS ideal second messengers. In heart failure, pathologic fluctuations in cellular ROS levels can alter multiple cellular processes by interacting with free thiol residues, disulfide bonds, and metal centers that are crucial for the function of redox-sensitive receptors and enzymes [190,191]. The specificity of such signals is determined by the fact that relatively few proteins have cysteine residues that are susceptible to oxidation at normal intracellular pH. The list includes key signaling molecules, such as PKC, protein tyrosine phosphatases, and protein disulfide isomerase. Conditions of ROS dysregulation, such as heart failure, may be amenable to therapy with antioxidant compounds. Data supporting this concept in heart failure were reported recently. TNF-α was shown to increase ROS production in skeletal muscle and induce contractile dysfunction that was partially reversible on administration of the antioxidant N-acetyl cysteine [72].

Integrating divergence: a model of redox homeostasis in muscle

The preceding sections describe two general mechanisms by which muscle-derived oxidants cause muscle dysfunction: loss of contractile regulation and maladaptation of muscle mass. In both cases, the mechanisms are incompletely understood, and the published findings contain apparent paradoxes. ROS increase contractile force in resting muscle [180,192–194], but decrease force during fatiguing exercise [194–197]. Antioxidants inhibit contraction in the resting state [180,192,198–200], but oppose the loss of force during fatigue [198,201–205]. ROS also have divergent effects on striated muscle mass, stimulating atrophy in skeletal muscle [65,104,178] and hypertrophy in cardiac muscle [127–134]. Even within a single cell type, ROS can have diametrically opposed actions, stimulating skeletal muscle myoblast growth at low levels [139] and causing growth arrest or cell death at higher levels [139,206].

To help integrate these seemingly disparate data, the authors have developed the experimental model shown in Fig. 3. This model proposes that ROS are physiologic modulators of muscle function, that ROS are ubiquitous components of the cellular milieu, that ROS levels are relatively low under basal conditions (Fig. 3, point A), and that changes in ROS levels alter muscle function. In this model, ROS effects on function are biphasic. Function is maximized at some "optimal" ROS level (Fig. 3, point B) and is maintained largely across the range of ROS levels encountered under physiologic conditions. Function is compromised, however, when ROS levels fall outside the physiologic range because of either excess ROS accumulation (Fig. 3, point C) or ROS depletion (Fig. 3, point D).

This logic is applied most clearly to contractile function. It is consistent with reports that force is increased by low-intensity ROS exposure (Fig. 3, points A–B) and is depressed by intense stimulation (Fig. 3, points A–C) or by exposing resting muscle to antioxidants (Fig. 3, points A–D). Andrade

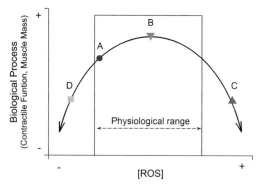

Fig. 3. Proposed relationship between ROS levels and muscle function. Curve depicts theoretical changes in contractile function or muscle mass as a function of ROS levels ([ROS]). *A*, basal state; *B*, optimal ROS level; *C*, excess ROS; *D*, ROS deficiency; see text for further details. (*Data from* Reid MB, Khawli FA, Moody MR. Reactive oxygen in skeletal muscle: III. contractility of unfatigued muscle. J Appl Physiol 1993;75:1081–7; and Andrade FH, Reid MB, Allen DG, Westerblad H. Effect of hydrogen peroxide and dithiothreitol on contractile function of single skeletal muscle fibres from mouse. J Physiol 1998;509:565–75.)

et al [183] tested this model using intact single fibers from mouse limb muscle. Within a given fiber, H_2O_2 exposure first increased and then decreased force. This force decrement was reversed by exposing the fiber to DTT, a reducing agent that opposes sulfhydryl oxidation. DTT had the opposite effect under basal conditions; force was depressed. These data supported the proposed model and suggested that ROS effects on force reflect changes in myofilament calcium sensitivity.

ROS regulation of muscle mass has not been studied systematically, but may conform to a similar model. Low-level ROS exposure stimulates growth in a variety of cell types, including skeletal muscle myoblasts and cardiac myocytes (Fig. 3, points A–B). More intense ROS stimulation triggers responses that oppose muscle growth, including ubiquitin conjugation, protein loss, cell cycle arrest, and cell death (Fig. 3, points A–C). Many of these latter responses can be blunted by pretreating muscle preparations with exogenous antioxidants. Little is known about antioxidant effects on muscle mass under basal conditions (Fig. 3, points A–D), which limits overall evaluation of the model. Hypothesis-driven experiments are needed to define better the role of muscle-derived ROS in regulating striated muscle mass.

Summary

Oxidative stress is a major component of the pathology that affects striated muscle in a wide variety of inflammatory diseases. Under these conditions, muscle-derived ROS exceed the local buffering capacity of tissue antioxidants; this perturbs the regulation of contractile function and gene expression, leading to loss of function via two parallel and largely independent mechanisms. The underlying biology can be illustrated using four different pathologic settings.

First, in cachexia, elevated levels of circulating cytokines (notably TNF-α and IL-1B) act via receptor-mediated mechanisms to stimulate ROS production within muscle fibers. The resulting increase in ROS levels activates redox-sensitive signal transduction pathways that involve NF-κB and p38 MAPK as essential elements. These signaling events increase mRNA levels for muscle-specific E2 and E3 proteins, elevating the general rate of ubiquitin conjugation. This elevation results in loss of structural proteins and overt muscle atrophy. Second, ROS modulate growth and repair of skeletal and cardiac muscles in response to humoral mediators, including Ang II. Studies of cellular mechanisms indicate that growth-related pathways, particularly the Ras/Raf and PI3K/Akt/mTOR pathways, are redox sensitive and can be activated by ROS that function as second messengers. Third, studies have identified intermittent hypoxia as a novel stimulus for oxidative stress in the clinical setting of SDB. This is a persistent problem in individuals with chronic sleep apnea. It can lead to hypertension, cardiac hypertrophy, and decrements in cardiac function via mechanisms that remain poorly understood. New experimental approaches are being used to dissociate the components of this pathology and identify the physiologic mechanisms of oxidant effects on the heart. Fourth, heart failure provides a clinical example of ROS-mediated contractile dysfunction that can develop in skeletal muscle without overt atrophy or injury. Loss of function seems to reflect redox modulation of regulatory proteins within muscle fibers, components of either the myofilament lattice (myosin heavy chains, troponin C, actin) or the sarcoplasmic reticulum complex (ryanodine-sensitive calcium release channel, calcium-dependent ATPase). In these and other inflammatory pathologies, muscle-derived ROS and the antioxidant interventions used to study ROS actions can have complex, apparently divergent effects. The authors approach the problem in the context of redox homeostasis, viewing muscle-derived ROS as physiologic components of the cellular milieu and inflammatory mediators as perturbing stimuli. This context provides a useful model for interpreting existing data and for identifying new directions of experimental research.

Acknowledgments

The authors thank Dr. Jennifer Moylan for assistance with graphics.

References

[1] Commoner B, Townsend J, Pake GE. Free radicals in biological materials. Nature 1954; 174:689–91.
[2] Amemiya T. Differences in muscular changes in rats with vitamin E and with selenium deficiency. Int J Vitam Nutr Res 1987;57:139–43.
[3] Murphy ME, Kehrer JP. Free radicals: a potential pathogenic mechanism in inherited muscular dystrophy. Life Sci 1986;39:2271–8.
[4] Murphy ME, Kehrer JP. Activities of antioxidant enzymes in muscle, liver and lung of chickens with inherited muscular dystrophy. Biochem Biophys Res Commun 1986;134: 550–6.
[5] Hunter MI, Mohamed JB. Plasma antioxidants and lipid peroxidation products in Duchenne muscular dystrophy. Clin Chim Acta 1986;155:123–31.
[6] Steiss JE. Effect of disulfiram in experimentally induced vitamin E deficiency myopathy in lambs. Am J Vet Res 1985;46:2141–4.
[7] Stassijns G, Lysens R, Decramer M. Peripheral and respiratory muscles in chronic heart failure. Eur Respir J 1996;9:2161–7.
[8] Harrington D, Coats AJ. Skeletal muscle abnormalities and evidence for their role in symptom generation in chronic heart failure. Eur Heart J 1997;18:1865–72.
[9] Morrison SD. Cancer cachexia. In: Liotta AL, editor. Influence of tumor development on the host. Amsterdam: Kluwer Academic Publishers; 1989. p. 176–213.
[10] Tisdale MJ. Protein loss in cancer cachexia. Science 2000;289:2293–4.
[11] Haycock JW, MacNeil S, Jones P, Harris JB, Mantle D. Oxidative damage to muscle protein in Duchenne muscular dystrophy. Neuroreport 1996;8:357–61.
[12] Murphy ME, Kehrer JP. Oxidative stress and muscular dystrophy. Chem Biol Interact 1989;69:101–73.

[13] Ragusa RJ, Chow CK, Porter JD. Oxidative stress as a potential pathogenic mechanism in an animal model of Duchenne muscular dystrophy. Neuromuscul Disord 1997;7:379–86.

[14] Heunks LM, Dekhuizen PN. Respiratory muscle function and free radicals: from cell to COPD. Thorax 2000;55:704–16.

[15] Vreugdenhil G, Lowenberg B, VanEijk HG, Swaak JG. Tumor necrosis factor alpha is associated with disease activity and the degree of anemia in patients with rheumatoid arthritis. Eur J Clin Invest 1992;22:488–93.

[16] Lavie L. Obstructive sleep apnoea syndrome—an oxidative stress disorder. Sleep Med Rev 2003;7:35–51.

[17] Schultz R, Mahmoudi S, Sibelius U, et al. Enhanced release of superoxide from polymorphonuclear neutrophils in obstructive sleep apnea. Am J Respir Crit Care Med 2000;162: 566–70.

[18] Barcelo A, Barbe A. Oxidative stress and sleep apnea-hypopnea syndrome. Arch Bronconeumol 2005;41:393–9.

[19] Reeder BJ, Sharpe MA, Kay AD, Kerr M, Moore K, Wilson MT. Toxicity of myoglobin and haemoglobin: oxidative stress in patients with rhabdomyolysis and subarachnoid haemorrhage. Biochem Soc Trans 2002;30:745–8.

[20] Lim PS, Cheng YM. Large-scale mitochondrial DNA deletions in skeletal muscle of patients with end-stage renal disease. Free Radic Biol Med 2000;29:454–63.

[21] Roubenoff R. Tumor necrosis factor and AIDS. Am J Clin Nutr 1995;61:161–2.

[22] Kehrer JP, Lund LG. Cellular reducing equivalents and oxidative stress. Free Radic Biol Med 1998;17:65–75.

[23] Christou IK, Moulas AN, Pastaka C, Gouroulianis KI. Antioxidant capacity in obstructive sleep apnea patients. Sleep Med 2003;4:225–8.

[24] McCord JM. Oxygen derived free radicals in postischemic tissue injury. N Engl J Med 1985; 312:159–63.

[25] Griendling KK, Sorescu D, Ushio-Fukai M. NAD(P)H oxidase: role in cardiovascular biology and disease. Circ Res 2000;86:1236–46.

[26] Ronson RS, Nakamura M, Vinten-Johnson J. The cardiovascular effects and implication of peroxynitrite. Cardiovasc Res 2000;44:47–59.

[27] Chamberlain JS. Cachexia in cancer—zeroing in on myosin. N Engl J Med 2004;351: 2124–5.

[28] Elborn JS, Cordon SM, Western PJ, Macdonald IA, Shales DJ. Tumour necrosis factoralpha, resting energy expenditure and cachexia in cystic fibrosis. Clin Sci 1993;85:563–8.

[29] Argiles JM, Garcia-Martinez C, Llovera M, Lopez-Soriano FJ. The role of cytokines in muscle wasting: its relation with cancer cachexia. Med Res Rev 1992;12:637–52.

[30] Anker SD, Rauchaus M. Insights into the pathogenesis of chronic heart failure: immune activation and cachexia. Curr Opin Cardiol 1999;14:211–6.

[31] Hasselgren PO, Fischer JE. Muscle cachexia: current concepts of intracellular mechanisms and molecular regulation. Ann Surg 2001;233:9–17.

[32] Argiles JM, Lopez-Soriano FJ. Catabolic proinflammatory cytokines. Curr Opin Clin Nutr Metab Care 1998;1:245–51.

[33] Llesuy S, Evelson P, Gonzalez-Flecha B, et al. Oxidative stress in muscle and liver of rats with septic syndrome. Free Radic Biol Med 1994;16:445–51.

[34] MacNee W. Oxidants/antioxidants and COPD. Chest 2000;117(Suppl 1):303S–17S.

[35] Romero-Alvira D, Roche E. The keys of oxidative stress in acquired immune deficiency syndrome apoptosis. Med Hypotheses 1998;51:169–73.

[36] Ray G, Batra S, Shukla NK, et al. Lipid peroxidation, free radical production and antioxidant status in breast cancer. Breast Cancer Res Treat 2000;59:163–70.

[37] Kojda G, Harrison D. Interactions between NO and reactive oxygen species: pathophysiological importance in atherosclerosis, hypertension, diabetes and heart failure. Cardiovasc Res 1999;43:562–71.

[38] Chien KR. Stress pathways and heart failure. Cell 1999;98:555–8.

[39] Tidball JG. Inflammatory cell response to acute muscle injury. Med Sci Sports Exerc 1995; 27:1022–32.

[40] Kumamoto T, Ueyama H, Sugihara R, Kominami E, Goll DE, Tsuda T. Calpain and cathepsins in the skeletal muscle of inflammatory myopathies. Eur Neurol 1997;37:176–81.

[41] Li Y-P, Schwartz RJ, Waddell ID, Holloway BR, Reid MB. Skeletal muscle myocytes undergo protein loss and reactive oxygen-mediated NF-κB activation in response to tumor necrosis factor α. FASEB J 1998;12:871–80.

[42] Goossens V, De Vos K, Vercammen D, et al. Redox regulation of TNF signaling. Biofactors 1999;10:145–56.

[43] Li Y-P, Reid MB. TNF-alpha and H₂O₂ stimulate ubiquitin conjugation of proteins in skeletal muscle myotubes [abstract]. FASEB J 2001;15:A1080.

[44] Li Y-P, Chen Y, Li AS, Reid MB. Hydrogen peroxide stimulates ubiquitin-conjugating activity and expression of genes for specific E2 and E3 proteins in skeletal muscle myotubes. Am J Physiol Cell Physiol 2003;285:C806–12.

[45] Shanely RA, Zergeroglu MA, Lennon SL, et al. Mechanical ventilation-induced diaphragmatic atrophy is associated with oxidative injury and increased proteolytic activity. Am J Respir Crit Care Med 2002;15:1369–74.

[46] Nakashima K, Nonaka I, Masaki S. Myofibrillar proteolysis in chick myotubes during oxidative stress. J Nutr Sci Vitaminol (Tokyo) 2004;50:45–9.

[47] Betters JL, Criswell DS, Shanely RA, et al. Trolox impairs mechanical ventilation-induced diaphragmatic dysfunctiona and proteolysis. Am J Respir Crit Care Med 2004;170: 1179–84.

[48] Buck M, Chojkier M. Muscle wasting and dedifferentiation induced by oxidative stress in a murine model of cachexia is prevented by inhibitors of nitric oxide synthesis and antioxidants. EMBO J 1996;15:1753–65.

[49] Aragno M, Mastracola R, Catalano MG, Grignardello E, Danni O, Boccuzzi G. Oxidative stress impairs skeletal muscle repair in diabetic rats. Diabetes 2004;53:1082–8.

[50] Li Y-P, Atkins CM, Sweatt JD, Reid MB. Mitochondria mediate tumor necrosis factor-α/ NF-κB signaling in skeletal muscle myotubes. Antiox Redox Signal 1999;1:97–104.

[51] Williams G, Brown T, Becker M, Prager M, Giroir BP. Cytokine-induced expression of nitric oxide synthase in C2C12 skeletal muscle myocytes. Am J Physiol 1994;267:R1020–5.

[52] Chang HR, Bistrian B. The role of cytokines in the catabolic consequences of infection and injury. J Parenter Enteral Nutr 1998;22:156–66.

[53] Berry C, Clark AL. Catabolism in chronic heart failure. Eur Heart J 2000;21:521–32.

[54] Tracey KJ, Cerami A. Tumor necrosis factor, other cytokines and disease. Annu Rev Cell Biol 1993;9:343.

[55] Li Y-P, Lecker SH, Chen Y, Waddell ID, Goldberg AL, Reid MB. TNF-α increases ubiquitin-conjugating activity in skeletal muscle by up-regulating UbcH2/E2–20k. FASEB J 2003;17:1048–57.

[56] Li Y-P, Chen Y, John J, et al. TNF-α acts via p38 MAPK to stimulate expression of the ubiquitin ligase atrogin1/MAFbx in skeletal muscle. FASEB J 2005;19:362–70.

[57] Lecker SH, Solomon V, Mitch WE, Goldberg AL. Muscle protein breakdown and the critical role of the ubiquitin-proteasome pathway in normal and disease states. J Nutr 1999; 129:227S–37S.

[58] Wilkinson KD. Ubiquitin-dependent signaling: the role of ubiquitination in the response of cells to their environment. J Nutr 1999;129:1933–6.

[59] Hershko A, Ciechanover A. The ubiquitin system. Annu Rev Biochem 1998;67:425–79.

[60] Garcia-Martinez C, Llovera M, Agell N, Lopez-Soriano FJ, Argiles JM. Ubiquitin gene expression in skeletal muscle is increased by tumour necrosis factor-alpha. Biochem Biophys Res Commun 1994;201:682–6.

[61] Garcia-Martinez C, Llovera M, Agell N, Lopez-Soriano FJ, Argiles JM. Ubiquitin gene expession in skeletal muscle is increased during sepsis: involvement of TNF-alpha but not IL-1. Biochem Biophys Res Commun 1995;217:839–44.

[62] Llovera M, Garcia-Martinez C, Agell N, et al. Ubiquitin and proteasome gene expression is increased in skeletal muscle of slim AIDS patients. Int J Mol Med 1998;2:69–73.

[63] Williams A, Sun X, Fischer JE, Hasselgren PO. The expression of genes in the ubiquitin-proteasome proteolytic pathway is increased in skeletal muscle from patients with cancer. Surgery 1999;126:744–9.

[64] Kumamoto T, Fujimoto S, Ito T, Horinouchi H, Ueyama H, Tsuda T. Proteasome expression in the skeletal muscles of patients with muscular dystrophy. Acta Neuropathol (Berl) 2000;100:595–602.

[65] Gomes-Marcondes MCC, Tisdale MJ. Induction of protein catabolism and the ubiquitin-proteasome pathway by mild oxidative stress. Cancer Lett 2002;180:69–74.

[66] Lecker SH, Solomon V, Price SR, Kwon YT, Mitch WE, Goldberg AL. Ubiquitin conjugation by the N-end rule pathway and mRNAs for its components increase in muscles of diabetic rats. J Clin Invest 1999;104:1411–20.

[67] Dehoux MJ, van Beneden RP, Fernandez-Celemin L, Lause PL, Thissen JP. Induction of MAFbx and MuRF ubiquitin ligase mRNAs in skeletal muscle after LPS injection. FEBS Lett 2003;544:214–7.

[68] Sandri M, Sandri C, Cilbert A, et al. Foxo transcription factors induce the atrophy-related ubiquitin ligase atrogin-1 and cause skeletal muscle atrophy. Cell 2004;117:399–412.

[69] Solomon V, Lecker SH, Goldberg AL. The N-end rule pathway catalyzes a major fraction of the protein degradation in skeletal muscle. J Biol Chem 1998;273:25216–22.

[70] Gomes MD, Lecker SH, Jagoe RT, Navon A, Goldberg AL. Atrogin-1, a muscle-specific F-box protein highly expressed during muscle atrophy. Proc Natl Acad Sci U S A 2001;98:14440–5.

[71] Bodine SC, Latres E, Baumhueter S, et al. Identification of ubiquitin ligases required for skeletal muscle atrophy. Science 2001;294:1704–8.

[72] Li X, Moody MR, Engel D, et al. Cardiac-specific overexpression of TNF-α causes oxidative stress and contractile dysfunction in mouse diaphragm. Circulation 2000;102:1690–6.

[73] Hacham M, Argov S, White RM, Segal S, Apte RN. Different patterns of interleukin-1alpha and interleukin-1beta expression in organs of normal young and old mice. Eur Cytokine Netw 2002;13:55–65.

[74] Dunne A, O'Neill LA. The interleukin-1 receptor/Toll-like receptor superfamily: signal transduction during inflammation and host defense. Sci STKE 2003;171:re3.

[75] Kumar S, Kishimoto H, Chua HL, et al. Interleukin-1alpha promotes tumor growth and cachexia in MCF-7 xenograft model of breast cancer. Am J Pathol 2003;163:2531–41.

[76] Zamir O, Hasselgren PO, von Allmen D, Fischer JE. The effect of interleukin-1 alpha and the glucocorticoid receptor blocker RU 38486 on total and myofibrillar protein breakdown in skeletal muscle. J Surg Res 1991;50:579–83.

[77] Cooney R, Owens E, Jurasinski C, Gray K, Vannice J, Vary T. Interleukin-1 receptor antagonist prevents sepsis-induced inhbition of protein sythesis. Am J Physiol 1994;267:E636–41.

[78] Luo G, Hershko DD, Robb BW, Wray CJ, Hasselgren PO. IL-1beta stimulates IL-6 production in cultured skeletal muscle cells through activation of MAP kinase signaling pathway and NF-kappa B. Am J Physiol Regul Integr Comp Physiol 2003;284:R1249–54.

[79] Brigelius-Flohe R, Banning A, Kny M, Bol G-F. Redox events in interleukin-1 signaling. Arch Biochem Biophys 2004;423:66–73.

[80] Fujishiro M, Gotoh Y, Katagire H, et al. MKK3/6 and p38 MAPK pathway activation is not necessary for insulin-induced glucose uptake but regulates glucose transporter expression. J Biol Chem 2001;276:19800–6.

[81] Petersen EW, Carey AL, Sacchetti M, et al. Acute IL-6 treatment increases fatty acid turnover in elderly humans in vivo and in tissue culture in vivo. Am J Physiol Endocrinol Metab 2005;288:155–62.

[82] Khanna S, Roy S, Packer L, Sen CK. Cytokine-induced glucose uptake in skeletal muscle: redox regulation and the role of alpha-lipoic acid. Am J Physiol 1999;276:R1327–33.

[83] Tsujinaka T, Kishibuchi M, Yano M, et al. Involvement of interleukin-6 in activation of lysosomal cathepsin and atrophy of muscle fibers induced by intramuscular injection of turpentine oil in mice. J Biochem (Tokyo) 1997;122:595–600.

[84] Fujita J, Tsujinaka T, Yano M, et al. Anti-interleukin-6 receptor antibody prevents muscle atrophy in colon-26 adenocarcinoma-bearing mice with modulation of lysosomal and ATP-ubiquitin-dependent proteolytic pathways. Int J Cancer 1996;68:637–43.

[85] Gallardo E, de Andres I, Illa I. Cathepsins are upregulated by IFN-gamma/STAT1 in human muscle culture: a possible active factor in dermatomyositis. J Neuropathol Exp Neurol 2001;60:847–55.

[86] Alvarez B, Quinn LS, Busquets S, Quiles MT, Lopez-Soriano FJ, Argiles JM. Tumor necrosis factor-alpha exerts interleukin-6-dependent and independent effects on cultured skeletal muscle cells. Biochim Biophys Acta 2002;1542:66–72.

[87] Acharyya S, Ladner KJ, Nelsen LL, et al. Cancer cachexia is regulated by selective targeting of skeletal muscle gene products. J Clin Invest 2004;114:370–8.

[88] Guttridge DC, Mayo MW, Madrid LV, Wang CY, Baldwin AS. NF-kappaB-induced loss of MyoD messenger RNA: possible role in muscle decay and cachexia. Science 2000;289: 2363–6.

[89] Kwak KS, Zhou X, Solomon V, et al. Regulation of protein catabolism by muscle-specific and cytokine-inducible ubiquitin ligase E3alpha-II during cancer cachexia. Cancer Res 2004;64:8193–8.

[90] Haddad F, Zaldivar F, Cooper DM, Adams GR. IL-6-induced skeletal muscle atrophy. J Appl Physiol 2005;98:911–7.

[91] Williams A, Wang JJ, Wang L, Sun X, Fischer JE, Hasselgren PO. Sepsis in mice stimulates muscle proteolysis in the absence of IL-6. Am J Physiol 1998;275:R1983–91.

[92] Li Y-P, Reid MB. NF-κB mediates the protein loss induced by TNF-α in differentiated skeletal muscle myotubes. Am J Physiol Regul Integr Comp Physiol 2000;279:R1165–70.

[93] Cai D, Franz JD, Tawa NE Jr, et al. IKKbeta/NF-kappaB activation causes severe muscle wasting in mice. Cell 2004;119:285–98.

[94] Guttridge DC, Albanese C, Reuther JY, Pestell RG, Baldwin ASJ. NF-kappaB controls cell growth and differentiation through transcriptional regulation of cyclin D1. Mol Cell Biol 1999;19:5785–99.

[95] Langen RCJ, Schols AMWJ, Kelders MCJM, Wouters EFM, Janssen-Heininger YMW. Inflammatory cytokines inhibit myogenic differentiation through activation of nuclear factor-kappaB. FASEB J 2001;15:1169–80.

[96] Hunter RB, Stevenson E, Koncarevic A, Mitchell-Felton H, Essig DA, Kandarian SC. Activation of an alternative NF-kappaB pathway in skeletal muscle during disuse atrophy. FASEB J 2002;16:529–38.

[97] Baeuerle PA, Baltimore D. NF-kappa B: ten years after. Cell 1996;87:13–20.

[98] Jackman RW, Kandarian SC. The molecular basis of skeletal muscle atrophy. Am J Physiol Cell Physiol 2004;287:C834–43.

[99] Li Y-P, Schwartz RJ. TNF-alpha regulates early differentiation of C2C12 myoblasts in an autocrine fashion. FASEB J 2001;15:1413–5.

[100] Sen CK, Khanna S, Resznick AZ, Roy S, Packer L. Glutathione regulation of tumor necrosis factor-α-induced NF-κB activation in skeletal muscle-derived L6 cells. Biochem Biophys Res Commun 1997;237:645–9.

[101] DeRuisseau KC, Kavazis AN, Deering MA, et al. Mechanical ventilation induces alterations of the ubiquitin-proteasome pathway in the diaphragm. J Appl Physiol 2005;98: 1314–21.

[102] Wray CJ, Mammen JM, Hershko DD, Hasselgren PO. Sepsis upregulates the gene expression of multiple ubiquitin ligases in skeletal muscle. Int J Biochem Cell Biol 2003;35: 698–705.

[103] Stevenson EJ, Giresi PG, Koncarevic A, Kandarian SC. Global analysis of gene expression patterns during disuse atrophy in rat skeletal muscle. J Physiol 2003;551:33–68.

[104] Stitt TN, Drujan D, Clarke BA, et al. The IGF-1/PI3K/Akt pathway prevents expression of muscle atrophy-induced ubiquitin ligases by inhibiting FOXO transcription factors. Mol Cell 2004;14:395–403.

[105] Childs TE, Spangenburg EE, Vyas DR, Booth FW. Temporal alterations in protein signaling cascades during recovery from muscle atrophy. Am J Physiol Cell Physiol 2003;285: C391–8.

[106] Di Giovanni S, Molon A, Broccolini A, et al. Constitutive activation of MAPK cascade in acute quadriplegic myopathy. Ann Neurol 2004;55:195–206.

[107] Koistinen HA, Chibalin AV, Zierath JR. Aberrant p38 mitogen-activated protein kinase signaling in skeletal muscle from type 2 diabetic patients. Diabetologia 2003;46:1324–8.

[108] Williamson D, Gallagher P, Harber M, Hollon C, Trappe S. Mitogen-activated protein kinase (MAPK) pathway activation: effects of age and acute exercise on human skeletal muscle. J Physiol 2003;547:977–87.

[109] Bates PC, Millward DJ. Changes in the relative rates of protein synthesis and breakdown during muscle growth and atrophy. Biochem Soc Trans 1978;6:612–4.

[110] Booth FW, Nicholson WF, Watson PA. Influence of muscle use on protein synthesis and degradation. Exerc Sport Sci Rev 1982;10:27–48.

[111] Gibson JN, Smith K, Rennie MJ. Prevention of disuse muscle atrophy by means of electrical stimulation: maintenance of protein synthesis. Lancet 1988;2:767–70.

[112] Hornberger TA, Hunter RB, Kandarian SC, Esser KA. Regulation of translation factors during hindlimb unloading and denervation of skeletal muscle in rats. Am J Physiol Cell Physiol 2001;281:C179–87.

[113] Yamazaki T, Komuro I, Yazaki Y. Role of the renin-angiotensin system in cardiac hypertrophy. Am J Cardiol 1999;83:53H–7H.

[114] Yamazaki T, Komuro I, Yazaki Y. Signalling pathways for cardiac hypertrophy. Cell Signal 1998;10:693–8.

[115] Nishida M, Maruyama Y, Tanaka R, Kontani K, Nagao T, Kurose H. G alpha(i) and G alpha(o) are target proteins of reactive oxygen species. Nature 2000;408:492–5.

[116] Gordon SE, Davis BS, Carlson CJ, Booth FW. ANG II is required for optimal overload-induced skeletal muscle hypertrophy. Am J Physiol Endocrinol Metab 2001;280:E150–9.

[117] Westerkamp CM, Gordon SE. Angiotensin converting enzyme inhibition attenuates myonuclear addition in overloaded slow-twich skeletal muscle. Am J Physiol Regul Integr Comp Physiol, in press.

[118] Brink M, Price SR, Chrast J, et al. Angiotensin II induces skeletal muscle wasting through enhanced protein degradation and down-regulates autocrine insulin-like growth factor 1. Endocrinology 2001;142:1489–96.

[119] Song YH, Godard M, Li Y, Richmond SR, Rosenthal N, Delafontaine P. Insulin-like growth factor I-mediated skeletal muscle hypertrophy is characterized by increased mTOR-p70S6K signaling without increased Akt phosphorylation. J Invest Med 2005;53: 135–42.

[120] Dardevet D, Sornet C, Vary T, Grizard J. Phosphatidylinositol 3-kinase and p70 s6 kinase participate in the regulation of protein turnover in skeletal muscle by insulin and insulin-like growth factor I. Endocrinology 1996;137:4087–94.

[121] Hornberger TA, McLoughlin TJ, Leszczynski JK, et al. Selenoprotein-deficient transgenic mice exhibit enhanced exercise-induced muscle growth. J Nutr 2003;133:3091–7.

[122] Semsarian C, Sutrave P, Richmond DR, Graham RM. Insulin-like growth factor (IGF-I) induces myotube hypertrophy associated with an increase in anaerobic glycolysis in a clonal skeletal-muscle cell model. Biochem J 1999;339:443–51.

[123] Xu Q, Wu Z. The insulin-like growth factor-phosphatidylinositol 3-kinase-Akt signaling pathway regulates myogenin expression in normal myogenic cells but not in rhabdomyosarcoma-derived RD cells. J Biol Chem 2000;275:36750–7.

[124] Aslan M, Oxben T. Oxidants in receptor tyrosine kinase signal transduction pathways. Antiox Redox Signal 2003;5:781–8.

[125] Matsuzawa A, Ichijo H. Stress-responsive protein kinases in redox-regulated apoptosis signaling. Antiox Redox Signal 2005;7:472–81.

[126] Sabri A, Hughie HH, Lucchesi PA. Regulation of hypertrophic and apoptotic signaling pathways by reactive oxygen species in cardiac myocutes. Antiox Redox Signal 2003;5: 731–40.

[127] Aikawa R, Nagai T, Tanaka M, et al. Reactive oxygen species in mechanical stress-induced cardiac hypertrophy. Biochem Biophys Res Commun 2001;289:901–7.

[128] Bianchi P, Pimentel DR, Murphy MP. A new hypertrophic mechanism of serotonin in cardiac myocytes: receptor-independent ROS generation. FASEB J 2005;19:641–3.

[129] Cheng TH, Shih NL, Chen CH, et al. Role of mitogen-activated protein kinase pathway in reactive oxygen species-mediated endothelin-1-induced beta-myosin heavy chain gene expression and cardiomyocyte hypertrophy. J Biomed Sci 2005;12:123–33.

[130] Higuchi Y, Otsu K, Nishida K, et al. Involvement of reactive oxygen species-mediated NF-kappaB activation in TNF-alpha-induced cardiomyocyte hypertrophy. J Mol Cell Cardiol 2002;34:233–40.

[131] Kashiwase K, Higuchi Y, Hirotani S, et al. CaMKII activates ASK1 and NF-kappaB to induce cardiomyocyte hypertrophy. Biochem Biophys Res Commun 2005;327:136–42.

[132] Nakamura K, Fushimi K, Kouchi H, et al. Inhibitory effects of antioxidants on neonatal rat cardiac myocyte hypertrophy induced by tumor necrosis factor-alpha and angiotensin II. Circulation 1998;98:794–9.

[133] Tsujimoto I, Hikoso S, Yamaguchi O, et al. The antioxidant edaravone attenuates pressure overload-induced left ventricular hypertrophy. Hypertension 2005;45:921–6.

[134] Yamazaki T, Komuro I, Zou Y, Yazaki Y. Hypertrophic responses of cardiomyocytes induced by endothelin-1 through the protein kinase C-dependent but Src and Ras-independent pathways. Hypertens Res 1999;22:113–9.

[135] Chen QM, Tu VC, Wu Y, Bahl JJ. Hydrogen peroxide dose dependent induction of cell death or hypertrophy in cardiomyocytes. Arch Biochem Biophys 2000;373:242–8.

[136] Hirotani S, Otsu K, Nishida K, et al. Involvement of nuclear factor-kappaB and apoptosis signal-regulating kinase 1 in G-protein-coupled receptor agonist-induced cardiomyocyte hypertrophy. Circulation 2002;105:509–12.

[137] Tu VC, Bahl JJ, Chen QM. Distinct roles of p42/p44(ERK) and p 38 MAPK in oxidant-induced AP-1 activation and cardiomyocyte hypertrophy. Cardiovasc Toxicol 2003;3: 133.

[138] Tu VC, Bahl JJ, Chen QM. Signals of oxidant-induced cardiomyocyte hypertrophy: key activation of p70 S6 kinase-1 and phosphoinositide 3-kinase. J Pharmacol Exp Ther 2002; 300:1101–10.

[139] Caporossi D, Ciafre SA, Pittaluga M, Savini I, Farache MG. Cellular responses to H(2)O(2) and bleomycin-nduced oxidative stress in L6C5 rat myoblasts. Free Radic Biol Med 2003;35:1355–64.

[140] Bolster DR, Jefferson LS, Kimball SR. Regulation of protein synthesis associated with skeletal muscle hypertrophy by insulin-, amino acid- and exercise-induced signaling. Proc Nutr Soc 2004;63:351–6.

[141] Renault V, Thornell LE, Butler-Browne G, Mouly V. Human skeletal muscle satellite cells: aging, oxidative stress and the mitotic clock. Exp Gerontol 2002;37:1229–36.

[142] Chen S-E, Gerken E, Zhang Y, et al. Role of TNF-alpha signaling in regeneration of cardiatoxin-injured muscle. Am J Physiol Cell Physiol, in press.

[143] Li Y-P. TNF-alpha is a mitogen in skeletal muscle. Am J Physiol Cell Physiol 2003;285: C370–6.

[144] Ladner KJ, Caligiuri MA, Guttridge DC. Tumor necrosis factor-regulated biphasic activation of NF-kappaB is required for cytokine-induced loss of skeletal muscle gene products. J Biol Chem 2003;278:2294–303.

[145] Zhou LZ, Johnson AP, Rando TA. NF-kappaB and AP-1 mediate transcriptional responses to oxidative stress in skeletal muscle cells. Free Radic Biol Med 2001;31:1405–16.

[146] Lammerding J, Kamm RD, Lee RT. Mechanotransduction in cardiac myocytes. Ann N Y Acad Sci 2004;1015:53–70.

[147] Yamamoto K, Dang QN, Kennedy SP, Osathanonth R, Kelly RA, Lee RT. Induction of tenascin-C in cardiac myocytes by mechanical deformation: role of reactive oxygen species. J Biol Chem 1999;274:21840–6.

[148] Young T, Patta M, Dempsey J, Skatrud J, Weber SK, Badr S. The occurance of sleep-disordered breathing among middle-aged adults. N Engl J Med 1993;328:1230–5.

[149] Young T, Peppard PE. Epidemiological evidence for the association of sleep disordered breathing with hypertension and cardiovascular disease. In: Bradley TD, Floras JS, editors. Sleep apnea: implications in cardiovascular and cerebrovascular disease. New York: Marcel Dekker; 2000. p. 261–84.

[150] He J, Kryger MH, Zorick FJ, Conway W, Roth T. Mortality and apnea index in obstructive sleep apnea: experience in 385 male patients. Chest 1988;94:9–14.

[151] Peppard PE, Young T, Palta M, Skatrud J. Prospective study of the association between sleep-disordered breathing and hypertension. N Engl J Med 2000;342:1378–84.

[152] Nieto FJ, Young TB, Lind BK, et al. Association of sleep disordered breathing, sleep apnea, and hypertension in a large community-based study. Sleep Heart Health Study. JAMA 2000;283:1829–36.

[153] Koskenvuo M, Kaprio J, Telakivi T, Partinen M, Heikkila K, Sarna S. Snoring as a risk factor for ischaemic heart disease and stroke in men. BMJ 1987;294:16–9.

[154] Shahar E, Whitney CW, Redline S, et al. Sleep-disordered breathing and cardiovascular disease: cross-sectional results of the Sleep Heart Health Study. Am J Respir Crit Care Med 2001;163:19–25.

[155] Podszuz TE, Greenberg H, Scharf SM. Influence of sleep state and sleep-disordered breathing on cardiovascular function. In: Sullivan CE, Sanders NA, editors. Sleep and breathing II. New York: Marcel Dekker; 1993. p. 257–310.

[156] Lavie P, Here P, Hoffstein V. Obstructive sleep apnoea syndrome as a risk factor for hypertension: population study. BMJ 2000;320:479–82.

[157] Grote L, Hedner J, Peter JH. Sleep-related breathing disorder is an independent factor for uncontrolled hypertension. J Hypertens 2000;18:670–85.

[158] Moore T, Rabben T, Wiklund U, Franklin KA, Eriksson P. Sleep-disordered breathing in men with coronary artery disease. Chest 1996;109:659–63.

[159] Lavie L. Sleep apnea syndrome, endothelial dysfunction, and cardiovascular morbidity. Sleep 2004;27:1053–5.

[160] Chen L, Sica AL, Scharf SM. Mechanisms of acute cardiovascular response to periodic apneas in sedated pigs. J Appl Physiol 1999;86:1236–46.

[161] Fletcher EC, Lesske J, Qian W, Miller CC III, Strauss H, Unger TI. Repetitive episodic hypoxia causes diurnal elevations of systemic blood pressure in rats. Hypertension 1992;19:555–61.

[162] Fletcher EC, Lesske J, Behm R, Miller CC III, Unger TI. Carotid chemoreceptors, systemic blood pressure, and chronic episodic hypoxia. J Appl Physiol 1992;72:1978–84.

[163] Fletcher EC, Lesske J, Culman J, Miller CC III, Unger TI. Sympathetic denervation blocks blood pressure elevation in episodic hypoxia. Hypertension 1992;20:612–9.

[164] Greenberg HE, Sica A, Batson D, Scharf SM. Chronic intermittent hypoxia increases sympathetic responsiveness to hypoxia and hypercapnea. J Appl Physiol 1999;86:305.

[165] Sica AL, Greenberg HE, Ruggiero DA, Scharf SM. Chronic intermittent hypoxia: a model of sympathetic activation in the rat. Resp Physiol 2000;121:173–84.

[166] Prabhakar NK, Kumar GK. Oxidative stress in the systemic and cellular responses to intermittent hypoxia. Biol Chem 2004;385:217–21.

[167] Row BW, Liu R, Xu W, Kneirandish L, Gozal D. Intermittent hypoxia is associated with oxidative stress and spatial learning deficits in the rat. Am J Respir Crit Care Med 2003;167:1548–53.

[168] Chen L, Einbinder E, Zhang Q, et al. Oxidative stress and left ventricular function with chronic intermittent hypoxia in rats. Am J Respir Crit Care Med, in press.
[169] Becker LB. New concepts in reactive oxygen species and cardiovascular reperfusion physiology. Cardiovasc Res 2004;61:461–70.
[170] Dhalla MS, Elmoselhi AB, Hata T, Makino N. Status of myocardial antioxidants in ischemia-reperfusion injury. Cardiovasc Res 2000;47:446–56.
[171] Budgett R. Fatigue and underperformance in athletes: the overtraining syndrome. Br J Sports Med 1998;32:107–10.
[172] Friman G, Ilback NG. Acute infection: metabolic responses, effects on performance, interaction with exercise, and myocarditis. Int J Sports Med 1998;19(Suppl 3):S172–82.
[173] Simon AM, Zittoun R. Fatigue in cancer patients. Curr Opin Oncol 1999;11:244–9.
[174] Harrington D, Coats AJ. Mechanisms of exercise intolerance in congestive heart failure. Curr Opin Cardiol 1997;12:224–32.
[175] Yamani MH, Sahgal P, Wells L, Massie BM. Exercise intolerance in chronic heart failure is not associated with impaired recovery of muscle function or submaximal exercise. J Am Coll Cardiol 1995;25:1232–8.
[176] Lunde PK, Sjaastad I, Schiotz Thorud H-M, Sejersted OM. Skeletal muscle disorders in heart failure. Acta Physiol Scand 2001;171:277–94.
[177] Blum A, Miller H. Pathophysiological role of cytokines in congestive heart failure. Annu Rev Med 2001;52:15–27.
[178] Reid MB, Li Y-P. Cytokines and oxidative signalling in skeletal muscle. Acta Physiol Scand 2001;171:225–32.
[179] Nishiyama Y, Ikeda H, Haramaki N, Yoshida M, Imaizumi T. Oxidative stress is related to exercise intolerance in patients with heart failure. Am Heart J 1998;135:115–20.
[180] Reid MB, Khawli FA, Moody MR. Reactive oxygen in skeletal muscle: III. contractility of unfatigued muscle. J Appl Physiol 1993;75:1081–7.
[181] Abramson JJ, Salama G. Sulfhydryl oxidation and Ca^{2+} release from sarcoplasmic reticulum. Mol Cell Biochem 1988;82:81–4.
[182] Favero TG, Zable AC, Abramson JJ. Hydrogen peroxide stimulates the Ca^{2+} release channel from skeletal muscle sarcoplasmic reticulum. J Biol Chem 1995;270:25557–63.
[183] Andrade FH, Reid MB, Allen DG, Westerblad H. Effect of hydrogen peroxide and dithiothreitol on contractile function of single skeletal muscle fibres from mouse. J Physiol 1998;509:565–75.
[184] Lunde PK, Dahlstedt AJ, Bruton JD, et al. Contraction and intracellular Ca^{2+} handling in isolated skeletal muscle of rats with congestive heart failure. Circ Res 2001;88:1299–305.
[185] Posterino GS, Lamb GD. Effects of reducing agents and oxidants on excitation-contraction coupling in skeletal muscle fibres of rat and toad. J Physiol 1996;496:809–25.
[186] Andrade FH, Reid MB, Westerblad H. Contractile response to low peroxide concentrations: myofibrillar calcium sensitivity as a likely target for redox modulation of skeletal muscle function. FASEB J 2001;15:309–11.
[187] Reid MB, Lannergren J, Westerblad H. Respiratory and limb muscle weakness induced by tumor nectosis factor-alpha: involvement of muscle myofilaments. Am J Respir Crit Care Med 2002;166:479–84.
[188] Callahan LA, She Z-W, Nosek TM. Superoxide, hydroxyl radical, and hydrogen peroxide effects on single-diaphragm fiber contractile apparatus. J Appl Physiol 2001;90:45–54.
[189] Plant DR, Lynch GS, Williams DA. Hydrogen peroxide modulates Ca^{2+} activation of single permeabilized fibers from fast- and slow-twitch skeletal muscles of rats. J Muscle Res Cell Motil 2000;21:747–52.
[190] Wang XT, Culotta VC, Klee CB. Superoxide dismutase protects calcineurin from inactivation. Nature 1996;383:434–7.
[191] Rouault TA, Klausner RD. Iron-sulfur clusters as biosensors of oxidants and iron. Trends Biochem Sci 1996;21:174–7.

[192] Lancaster JR. Nitric oxide in cells: this simple molecule plays Janus-faced roles in the body, acting as both messenger and destroyer. Am Sci 1992;80:248–59.

[193] Oba T, Koshita M, Yamaguchi M. H_2O_2 modulates twitch tension and increases Po of Ca^{2+} release channel in frog skeletal muscle. Am J Physiol 1996;63:460–8.

[194] Lawler JM, Cline CC, Hu Z, Coast JR. Effect of oxidant challenge on contractile function of the aging rat diaphragm. Am J Physiol 1997;272(2 Pt 1):E201–7.

[195] Nashawati E, Dimarco A, Supinski G. Effects produced by infusion of a free radical-generating solution into the diaphragm. Am Rev Respir Dis 1993;147:60–5.

[196] Barclay JK, Hansel M. Free radicals may contribute to oxidative skeletal muscle fatigue. Can J Physiol Pharmacol 1991;69:279–84.

[197] Lawler JM, Cline CC, Hu Z, Coast JR. Effect of oxidative stress and acidosis on diaphragm contractile function. Am J Physiol 1997;273(2 Pt 2):R630–6.

[198] Khawli FA, Reid MB. N-acetylcysteine depresses contractility and inhibits fatigue of diaphragm in vitro. J Appl Physiol 1994;77:317–24.

[199] Sams WM, Carroll NV, Crantz PL. Effect of dimethyl sulfoxide on isolated-innervated skeletal, smooth, and cardiac muscle. Proc Soc Exp Biol Med 1966;122:103–7.

[200] Reid MB, Moody MR. Dimethyl sulfoxide depresses skeletal muscle contractility. J Appl Physiol 1994;76:2186–90.

[201] Reid MB, Haack KE, Franchek KM, Valberg PA, Kobzik L, West MS. Reactive oxygen in skeletal muscle: I. intracellular oxidant kinetics and fatigue in vitro. J Appl Physiol 1992;73:1797–804.

[202] Shindoh C, Dimarco A, Thomas A, Manubray P, Supinski G. Effect of N-acetylcysteine on diaphragm fatigue. J Appl Physiol 1990;68:2107–13.

[203] Supinski G, Nethery D, Stofan D, Dimarco A. Effect of free radical scavengers on diaphragmatic fatigue. Am J Respir Crit Care Med 1997;155:622–9.

[204] Medved I, Brown MJ, Bjorksten AR, et al. N-acetylcysteine enhances muscle cysteine and glutathione availability and attenuates fatigue during prolonged exercise in endurance-trained individuals. J Appl Physiol 2004;97:1477–85.

[205] Travaline JM, Sudarshan S, Roy BG, Cordova F, Leyenson V, Criner GJ. Effect of N-acetylcysteine on human diaphragm strength and fatigue. Am J Respir Crit Care Med 1997;156:1567–71.

[206] Stangel M, Zettl UK, Mix E, et al. H_2O_2 and nitric oxide-mediated oxidative stress induce apoptosis in rat skeletal muscle myoblasts. J Neuropath Exp Neurol 1996;55:36–43.

PHYSICAL MEDICINE
AND REHABILITATION
CLINICS OF
NORTH AMERICA

ELSEVIER
SAUNDERS

Phys Med Rehabil Clin N Am
16 (2005) 951–965

Single Muscle Fiber Physiology in Neuromuscular Disease

Lisa S. Krivickas, MD*, Walter R. Frontera, MD, PhD

*Harvard Medical School, Spaulding Rehabilitation Hospital, 125 Nashua Street,
Boston, MA 02114, USA*

Assessment of skeletal muscle function is an integral part of clinical trials of pharmacology and other interventions in patients with neuromuscular disorders. Muscle function can be assessed on multiple levels ranging from the whole organism to the molecular level. At the level of the organism or person, timed functional tests such as a 30-m walk or rising from a chair can be used. At the level of the organ or muscle, strength and power can be measured using a variety of techniques including manual muscle testing, hand-held dynamometry, maximum voluntary isometric contraction measurement, and isokinetic testing. At the cellular level, the skinned single muscle fiber preparation may be used to measure cellular force and power production and contractile velocity. Finally, at the molecular level, the in vitro motility assay can be used to measure the translation velocity of actin filaments on myosin. This article will present a discussion of the usefulness of the cellular approach in the evaluation of patients with neuromuscular disease.

In neuromuscular disorders, cellular muscle physiology may be directly or indirectly impaired. Thus, it is important to have a tool to directly assess the degree of impairment and the effect of rehabilitation, pharmacologic, and gene therapy interventions on that impairment. In muscle diseases, muscle physiology is directly affected. The manner in which muscle physiology is affected depends on whether the muscle protein abnormality is in the extracellular matrix (laminin), sarcolemma (dystrophin, sarcoglycan, dysferlin), sarcomere (actin, myosin, tropomyosin, titin), nuclear membrane (lamin A/C, emerin), or in energy metabolism pathways (glycogenoses, mitochondrial disorders). In neuromuscular disorders where skeletal muscle is indirectly affected by pathology in the anterior horn cell, peripheral nerve, or neuromuscular junction, secondary changes in muscle physiology may occur. The

---

* Corresponding author.
  E-mail address: lkrivickas@partners.org (L.S. Krivickas).

skinned single fiber preparation directly assesses function of the sarcomeric proteins. Thus, the technique is ideally suited for study of myopathies caused by abnormalities in the sarcomeric proteins; these disorders are all relatively rare, but include Laing distal myopathy (myosin heavy chain [MyHC]), uncommon forms of limb girdle muscular dystrophy (myotilin, titin), desmin myopathy, and nemaline myopathy (actin, tropomyosin, nebulin). The skinned single-fiber preparation may also detect secondary impairment in disorders affecting regions of the motor unit outside the sarcomere. In addition, the single fiber technique has been used to study the deleterious effects of aging, malnutrition, and immobilization on skeletal muscle [1–4].

Muscle fiber contraction force is determined mainly by the number of activated actin–myosin crossbridges and the force generated by each crossbridge. Total crossbridge number may be reduced either by decreasing the number of muscle fibers (muscle atrophy) or by decreasing the number of crossbridges per fiber. The spacing or packing of myofibrils within the single muscle fiber may also determine force generation, and may be affected by neuromuscular disease [5]. Force per crossbridge can be reduced by biochemical alterations that impair the function of actin or myosin, resulting in a lower percentage of strongly bound crossbridges.

The product of force and velocity determines the power generating capability of muscle that has a direct impact on function. Thus, a decrease in either force or velocity will decrease power generation. It has been suggested that muscle fibers with a range of shortening velocities are needed for muscles to generate varying levels of power over a full range of motion in response to the demands of different activities [6]. The specific force (SF) concept is critical when designing experiments to study muscle force. Force and power production correlate directly with muscle size and must be normalized to the cross-sectional area (CSA) of either the whole muscle or the single muscle fiber, whichever entity is being studied. Clearly, in healthy individuals, larger muscles are capable of greater force production than smaller muscles. Comparisons among patients and study volunteers with varying amounts of muscle mass can only be made if strength values are adjusted for muscle size. However, when studying patients with muscular dystrophies, adjustment for muscle size alone may be inadequate because of infiltration of the muscle by fat and connective tissue. When assessing the contractile properties of muscle, we are interested in qualitative, not only quantitative, changes that occur with neuromuscular disease.

Several difficulties with in vivo measurement of whole muscle SF confound studies on the macroscopic level. These difficulties include differences in intramuscular fiber orientation or pennation, the presence of intramuscular connective tissue, differences in mechanical leverage related to joint position, the possible coactivation of antagonist muscles during strength testing, variation in motor unit recruitment patterns, central drive, and subject motivation. In addition, measurements of SF in whole muscle are complicated by the heterogeneous mix of fiber types. Many of these confounding variables are eliminated by using single muscle fibers to study contractile properties. The parameters measured using this technique are unloaded maximal shortening velocity (V_o), maximal force, and muscle fiber CSA that are then used to calculate SF, absolute power, and specific power. Muscle tissue for these studies can be obtained easily by a relatively noninvasive percutaneous needle biopsy under local anesthesia, or when an open biopsy is obtained for other reasons, such as diagnosis. Fig. 1 depicts the percutaneous needle biopsy technique using the Bergstrom biopsy needle [7,8].

Skinned single muscle fiber methodology

The methodology used for single-fiber experiments in our laboratory is described in this section. Other laboratories performing single-fiber work have slight variations in their methods. Thus, the absolute value of measurements obtained in different laboratories may not be directly comparable. Single-fiber maximal force, SF, and V_o can be assessed by performing a series of isometric contractions. Power and specific power are assessed by performing a series of isotonic contractions.

Once a biopsy specimen has been obtained, it is immediately placed in relaxing solution at 4°C. Bundles of ~50 fibers are dissected from the biopsy

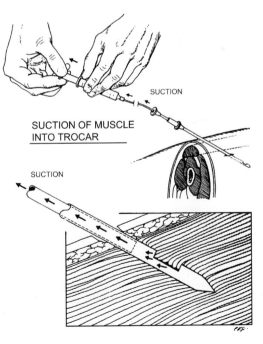

SUCTION

SUCTION OF MUSCLE
INTO TROCAR

SUCTION

Fig. 1. Technique for percutaneous needle muscle biopsy. (*From* Mubarak SJ, Chambers HG, Wenger DR. Percutaneous muscle biopsy in the diagnosis of neuromuscular disease. J Pediatr Orthop 1992;12:191–6; with permission.)

samples and then tied with surgical silk to glass capillary tubes at slightly stretched lengths. The fibers are chemically skinned for 24 hours in relaxing solution containing 50% (v/v) glycerol at 4°C and are then stored at −20°C [9]. Chemical skinning disrupts the sarcolemma and sarcoplasmic reticulum without damaging the myofilament structure. Fig. 2 depicts a chemically skinned fiber with breaks in the cell membrane. Skinning allows the fibers to be maximally and quickly activated in a controlled fashion by the addition of exogenous calcium. The disruption of the sarcoplasmic reticulum prevents accumulation of calcium within the fiber that would interfere with the ability to rapidly activate and relax the fiber.

On the day of an experiment, fibers are mounted in an experimental apparatus (Fig. 3) with one end of a fiber segment attached to a force transducer and the other to a lever arm that can be moved by a motor [10]. Using surgical silk, the fiber is tied on either end to small wire connectors that are fixed to the force transducer and lever arm. The sarcomere length, the segment width and depth, and the length of segment between the connectors are measured with an image analysis system. Fiber CSA is calculated from the width and depth. SF is calculated as maximum force (P_o) normalized to CSA and is corrected for the 20% swelling that is known to occur during skinning [10,11]. The fiber is activated by submerging it in a solution with a high calcium concentration (pCa^{++} 4.5); relaxing solution has a low calcium concentration (pCa^{++} 9.0).

Isometric contractile measurements

V_o is measured by the slack test procedure [12,13]. Fibers are activated at pCa^{++} 4.5, and once steady tension is reached, various amplitudes of slack are rapidly introduced (within 1–2 ms) at one end of the fiber. This breaks all of the attached crossbridges so that fiber force rapidly falls to zero. Because the fiber remains in a calcium solution, the crossbridges

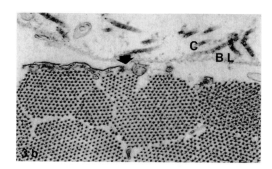

Fig. 2. A chemically skinned single muscle fiber demonstrates disruption of the sarcolemma between the arrow and the right side of the micrograph. (*From* Salviati G, Sorenson MM, Eastwood AB. Calcium accumulation by the sarcoplasmic reticulum in two populations of chemically skinned human muscle fibers. Effects of calcium and cyclic AMP. J Gen Physiol 1982;79:603–32; with permission.)

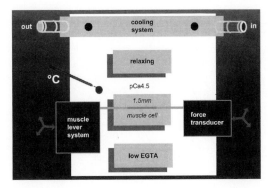

Fig. 3. Diagram of the apparatus used for single muscle fiber experiments. The apparatus on which the single fibers are mounted has three chambers that can be filled with different solutions for use in activating and relaxing the muscle fiber. A cooling system maintains the temperature of the solutions at 15°C.

then begin to reattach, and the time required to take up the imposed slack is measured from the onset of the length step to the beginning of tension re-development. After each amplitude of slack, the fiber is reextended while relaxed to minimize nonuniformity of sarcomere length. A straight line is fitted to a plot of slack length versus time, using least-squares regression, and the slope of the line divided by the segment length is recorded as V_o for that fiber. Fig. 4 depicts the steps involved in the slack test. P_o is calculated as the difference between the total tension in activating solution and the resting tension measured in the same segment while in the relaxing solution. All contractile measurements are performed at 15°C in our laboratory.

Isotonic contractile measurements

Force velocity curves are generated by performing a series of isotonic contractions of the muscle fiber after completion of the slack test [14]. The muscle fiber is placed in activating solution, and once P_o is reached, a series of three isotonic steps varying from 8% to 78% of P_o are performed. A custom software program is used to collect data from the force transducer and the lever arm as well as to control the lever arm's position so that the desired force level is maintained during each step. Fig. 5 shows the recordings from both the lever arm and the force transducer during a typical series of isotonic steps. During each step, the velocity of muscle fiber shortening (ie, rate of lever arm movement) required to maintain the desired force level is measured by determining the slope of the lever arm trace. Following the series of contractions, the fiber is allowed to relax. A total of six series of isotonic contractions is performed generating 18 pairs of relative force (%P_o) and velocity measurements. Velocity is plotted as a function of %P_o generating a hyperbolic curve, and the Hill equation [15] is fit to the data. The Hill equation states that $(P + a)(V + b) = (P_o + a)/b$, where $P =$ force,

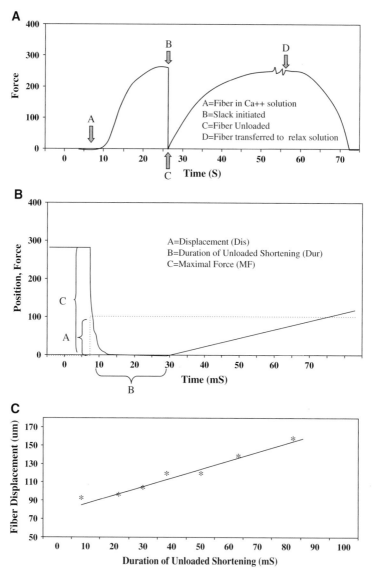

Fig. 4. (*A*) Activation of a single muscle fiber with calcium followed by introduction of a slack in fiber length, force redevelopment, and transfer to relaxing solution. (*B*) Measurement of time to take up the imposed slack (*dur*: ms), lever arm displacement (*dis*: um), and maximal force (*MF*: uN) for an individual slack. (*C*) Plot of duration versus displacement used to determine V_o. V_o is the slope of the regression line divided by fiber segment length.

V = velocity, and P_o = maximal isometric force. From the fitted curve, Hill constants a and b, having dimensions of force and velocity respectively, are derived. Fig. 6A shows a typical force velocity curve. The parameter a/P_o^{-1} describes the concavity of the curve; the lower the ratio, the more concave

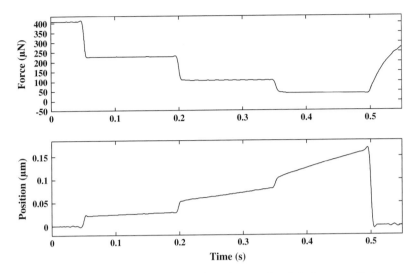

Fig. 5. Recordings from both the force transducer (*top trace*) and the lever arm (*bottom trace*) during a typical series of isotonic steps.

the curve. The force velocity curve is more concave for Type I fibers than for Type II fibers. Thus, in Type II fibers a higher percentage of peak velocity can be maintained as load is increased.

Next, the power generated during each isotonic step, calculated as force times velocity, is plotted as a function of $\%P_o$. The fitted velocity curve is multiplied by the corresponding force points to generate a fitted power curve (Fig. 6B). Peak power is defined as the peak of this curve and is reported in uN × FL s^{-1}. Peak power is then normalized for fiber CSA to yield a measure of specific power in kN m^{-1} × FL s^{-1}. The $\%P_o$ at which peak power occurs on the fitted power curve is also noted.

Myosin heavy chain composition

After mechanical measurements, each fiber is placed in sodium dodecyl sulfate sample buffer in a plastic microfuge tube and stored at $-20°$C. The MyHC composition of single fibers is determined by sodium dodecyl sulfate-polyacrylamide gel electrophoresis (SDS-PAGE) [16]. Most fibers express either MyHC I, IIa or IIx; but, some fibers, known as hybrids, express more than one MyHC isoform (eg, Type I/IIa fibers or IIax fibers). Fig. 7 shows a representative gel demonstrating the presence of hybrid fibers. Many of these hybrid fibers are thought to be undergoing transition from one MyHC isoform to another, and this appears to be more prevalent in patients with neuromuscular disorders who are experiencing either muscle regeneration or denervation and reinnervation. The MyHC isoform is the primary determinant of both V_o and power. Type II fibers have higher V_o and power measurements than Type I fibers. They also often generate greater *SF*.

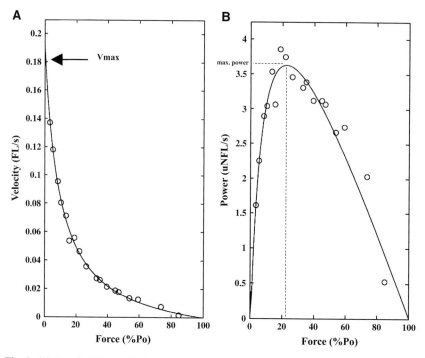

Fig. 6. (*A*) A typical force velocity curve generated from a series of isotonic single fiber contractions. (*B*) Power curve derived from force velocity curve in (*A*).

Single fiber studies in patients with neuromuscular disease

Use of the single-fiber technique to study muscle physiology and dysfunction in patients with neuromuscular disease is relatively recent, and the existing body of literature is limited. The studies that have been performed may be divided into those evaluating patients with anterior horn cell disorders (prior polio and amyotrophic lateral sclerosis [ALS]) and those

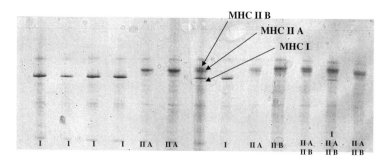

Fig. 7. SDS PAGE gel shows single muscle fibers expressing individual myosin heavy chain (MHC) isoforms as well as hybrid fibers expressing more than one MHC isoform. The middle lane with the larger labels is a control lane made from a muscle homogenate.

evaluating patients with myopathies or muscular dystrophies (such as inclusion body myositis, dermatomyositis, myotonic dystrophy, and facioscapulohumeral [FSH] dystrophy). These studies have reported data on isometric contractile properties only. Although the isotonic contractile property measurements of power are extremely relevant to muscle function in patients with neuromuscular disease, these measurements only have been reported in healthy individuals, primarily in aging studies [4,17,18]. The existing literature on single-fiber contractile properties in neuromuscular disease is summarized below.

Anterior horn cell disorders

To our knowledge, only one study has examined single muscle fiber contractile properties in patients with prior polio [19]. The tibialis anterior was biopsied in 10 patients with prior polio who had mild residual weakness in the biopsied muscle, suggesting that the muscle was chronically overused. The tibialis anterior in these patients consisted of 97% Type I fibers, whereas the tibialis anterior from control subjects consisted of 67% Type I, 27% Type IIa, and 7% Type IIx fibers. Type I fibers from the polio patients were 87% larger than those from control subjects. SF was reduced by 22% in the prior polio subjects, and V_o in the polio subjects was 86% higher than in the control subjects. The authors' interpretation of this data is that prior polio subjects have lost the diversity of V_o (both type II fibers and the slowest type I fibers) in their muscle because the chronically overused tibialis anterior is used in an all or nothing fashion during ambulation and everyday activities. In control subjects, low threshold, Type I motor units are used during casual walking and higher threshold (Type II) motor units are activated during more strenuous activity. In the weakened tibialis anterior of prior polio subjects, it is likely that all surviving motor units are needed for casual walking, so less diversity of fiber type is necessary. The hypertrophic Type I fibers function suboptimally because they produce less SF than normal-sized fibers.

Prior polio is a static or very slowly progressive anterior horn cell disorder. In contrast, ALS is a rapidly progressive anterior horn cell disease, although the rate of progression varies significantly from one patient to the next. We have studied single fiber contractile properties of the vastus lateralis muscle in six men with ALS [20]. We found that patients with ALS have a higher percentage of hybrid fibers (including Type I/IIa, Type IIa/IIx, and Type I/IIa/IIx) but do not demonstrate a distinct shift in MyHC toward either slower or faster isoforms. Patients with ALS have larger muscle fibers than control subjects, but SF is not different, suggesting that the force-generating capacity per unit of tissue (fiber quality) is well maintained in the remaining muscle fibers. The increase in size of the remaining fibers may be a mechanism to compensate for loss of motor units.

V_o is increased in Type I fibers of ALS patients, but not to the same extent as seen in prior polio. When our ALS patients were divided into those who were relatively slowly progressing and those who were more rapidly progressing, the slow progressors had very large muscle fibers, similar in size to those observed in prior polio patients. Type I fibers were 77% larger than those seen in control subjects. Some of these very large fibers generated reduced levels of SF suggesting, as in prior polio, that extreme muscle fiber hypertrophy may impair the fiber's ability to optimally generate force. Two possible explanations for this finding are that the fiber hypertrophy is produced by abnormal myofilaments with altered cross-bridge cycling or that the addition of cytoplasm without a proportional increase in myofilament number produces the hypertrophy. Slow progressors also had a higher percentage of hybrid fibers than the fast progressors (49% versus 18%). The differences in single fiber size and MyHC composition suggest that assessment of these properties in single fibers may be a useful predictor of disease progression if a biopsy is obtained early in the course of ALS.

The transgenic SOD1 G93A mouse overexpresses mutant human superoxide dismutase 1 (SOD1), which causes some cases of dominantly inherited familial ALS. This transgenic mouse is a popular model for ALS, and is widely used in preclinical drug trials. Atkin et al [21] have studied chemically skinned single muscle fibers in the SOD1 G93A mouse with methodology similar to that applied in our human study. They found markedly reduced SF in the fast fibers of symptomatic mice but no alteration in force generation in slow fibers; V_o was not measured. These findings differ somewhat from those in humans but highlight the potential utility of using single-fiber contractile property measurement to help assess the appropriateness of animal models for human neuromuscular disease. Drug trials performed in the ALS transgenic mouse model often have quite different results than those performed in humans with ALS, and it is important to understand the physiology underlying these differences.

Our findings in ALS, in conjunction with those of Larsson et al [19,20] in prior polio, suggest that anterior horn cell diseases produce single muscle fiber hypertrophy when disease is slowly progressing. This may be a compensatory mechanism for the loss of a significant number of muscle fibers in denervated motor units. However, when fibers become extremely hypertrophic, their function is impaired, and they generate reduced levels of SF. A second compensatory mechanism appears to be alteration of V_o. The increased V_o in Type I fibers may be an attempt to maintain power output despite loss of some muscle fibers and reduced SF generating capacity in other fibers.

Myopathic disorders

The myopathic disorders can be divided into two broad categories: those that are inherited, and those that are acquired. To our knowledge, myotonic muscular dystrophy type 1 (DM1) and FSH muscular dystrophy are the only hereditary myopathic disorders in which single-fiber contractile properties have been studied. The acquired disorders in which single-fiber studies have been performed include dermatomyositis, inclusion body myositis (IBM), and critical illness myopathy.

We have studied single-fiber contractile properties in the tibialis anterior of five patients with genetically confirmed DM1 [22]. Two of the subjects were symptomatic and three were asymptomatic carriers of the DM1 mutation (260–400 CTG repeats). Type I fiber size in DM1 was similar to that of control subjects, but Type IIa fibers were hypertrophic (73% larger for asymptomatic subjects and 46% larger for symptomatic subjects). Hybrid fibers were detected in the symptomatic, but not the asymptomatic, subjects. The most striking finding was that SF was reduced in all DM1 subjects, and it was reduced to a greater extent in symptomatic than in asymptomatic subjects for Type I fibers. SF in the symptomatic subjects was 64% of that in the asymptomatic subjects. V_o was reduced in Type I fibers but not Type IIa fibers when compared with healthy control subjects; no difference was seen between the symptomatic and asymptomatic DM1 subjects. Thus, force-generating capacity, and, by extrapolation, the ability to generate power, are reduced in single fibers in DM1. Furthermore, this reduction is present in the presymptomatic stages of the disease. This implies that the myotonic dystrophy protein kinase (DMPK) mutation, which causes DM1, in some way impairs the actin–myosin interaction. To date, the true function of DMPK has not been identified; one of several proposed DMPK functions is regulation of actin–myosin contractility [23].

We have studied one young man with severe infantile onset FSH dystrophy [24]. A biopsy of the vastus lateralis showed a high percentage of hybrid fibers and a shift toward a fast fiber phenotype when compared with age-matched control subjects. All fiber types were hypertrophic, with Type IIax fibers most significantly affected; these fibers were more than twice the size of fibers from control subjects. Despite the marked muscle fiber hypertrophy, SF and V_o were no different than that of the control subjects for any fiber type. Thus, in contrast to DM1, the remaining muscle fibers in FSH have normal contractile properties. This finding suggests that the mutation responsible for FSH dystrophy does not alter the function of sarcomeric proteins. FSH dystrophy is caused by a mutation in a nonprotein-encoding region of the gene for a DNA repeat sequence known as D4Z4, and the mechanism by which this mutation causes disease is unknown.

We have studied single-fiber contractile properties in adults with two forms of inflammatory myopathy: inclusion body myositis, and dermatomyositis [25]. As in patients with hereditary muscular dystrophy, we found an increased percentage of hybrid fibers (22% in dermatomyositis, 9% in IBM, and 2% in controls). Type I and IIa fibers were hypertrophic in patients with IBM, but not in those with dermatomyositis. Patients with dermatomyositis underwent biopsy within a few months of symptom onset, whereas patients with IBM underwent biopsy 1 to 5 years after the onset of muscle weakness. The hypertrophic fibers in IBM may be a marker of disease chronicity. In both diseases, SF

was no different from that of control subjects, indicating that force-generating capacity is well preserved in these disorders. V_o was increased for Type I fibers in patients with dermatomyositis, but no alterations were seen in V_o of Type IIa fibers. The increased V_o in Type I fibers in dermatomyositis may be a compensatory mechanism to help maintain muscle power output in the face of progressive loss of muscle mass and single-fiber atrophy.

Larsson et al [26] have studied single-fiber contractile properties in critical illness myopathy. The patients studied developed acute quadriplegia following treatment with a combination of neuromuscular junction blocking agents and high-dose corticosteroids in the intensive care unit setting. The muscle fibers from these patients were extremely atrophic with a CSA less than 50% that of control subjects. SF in these fibers was markedly reduced to 25% that of control fibers. Additional studies of the biopsies from these subjects revealed a general decrease in myofibrillar protein, partial or complete loss of myosin, absence of myosin messenger RNA, and a very low thick filament-to-thin filament protein ratio, indicating that actin was preserved. The very low SF is consistent with the overall loss of myosin. We have seen a similar reduction in SF, without a change in V_o, in a patient whom we studied on the day of intensive care unit admission and 10 days following admission.

Table 1 summarizes the data from single-fiber studies performed in patients with neuromuscular disease. Patients with neurogenic disorders or more chronic myopathic disorders have increased muscle fiber size; patients with acute myopathic disorders tend to develop atrophic muscle fibers. In some patients with fiber hypertrophy (postpolio and DM1), the increase in P_o is less than that in CSA such that SF is reduced. In the neurogenic disorders and dermatomyositis, V_o of some fibers is increased, possibly as a compensatory mechanism. In all of the neuromuscular disorders studied thus far, the percentage of hybrid fibers is increased.

Table 1
Summary of single fiber studies in neuromuscular disease

Disease	P_o	CSA	SF	V_o	% hybrid
Polio [19]		↑	↓	↑	
ALS [20]	↑	↑	↔	↑ (T. I) ↔ (T. IIA)	↑
DM1 [22]	↓	↔ (T. I) ↑ (T. IIA)	↓	↓ (T. I) ↔ (T. IIA)	↑
FSH [24]	↑	↑	↔	↔	↑
IBM [25]	↑	↑	↔	↔	↑
Dermatomyositis [25]	↔	↔	↔	↑ (T. I) ↔ (T. IIA)	↑
CIM [26]	↓	↓	↓		

Abbreviations: ALS, amyotrophic lateral sclerosis; CIM, critical illness myopathy; CSA, cross-sectional area; DM1, myotonic dystrophy type I; FSH, facioscapulohumeral muscular dystrophy; IBM, inclusion body myositis; P_o, maximal force; SF, specific force; V_o, maximal unloaded shortening velocity.

Future research applications

To date, the assessment of single muscle fiber contractile properties in patients with neuromuscular disease primarily has been used to characterize physiologic changes that occur in different disease processes. In slowly progressive neuropathic and myopathic disorders, we have observed single-fiber hypertrophy and an increase in the percentage of hybrid fibers. In the neuropathic disorders, the hypertrophic fibers appear to function suboptimally with a reduction in force-generating capacity; this is not generally the case for hypertrophic fibers observed in slowly progressing myopathic disorders (IBM and FSH dystrophy). In the more acute myopathic disorders (dermatomyositis and critical illness myopathy), we see fiber atrophy. In myopathic disorders, the ability to maintain SF appears to be dependent on whether or not the sarcomeric proteins are directly (critical illness myopathy) or indirectly (possibly DM1) affected by the disease process; if the sarcomeric proteins are affected, SF is reduced. V_o may be altered in some of the diseases studied (anterior horn cell disorders, dermatomyositis) as a secondary compensatory mechanism, but this remains to be proven definitively. In other diseases, such as myotonic dystrophy, V_o may be altered because of an effect of the disease process on sarcomeric protein function.

In the future, the single-fiber technique may be applied to evaluate the direct effect of various treatments, including exercise, pharmacologic interventions, and gene therapy, on the physiology of individual muscle cells in patients with neuromuscular disease. This approach has already been applied to the study of interventions to reduce sarcopenia in healthy adults [17,18,27] and improve performance in athletes [28–31]. The single-fiber technique also may be applied to animal models of neuromuscular diseases where it might be useful for assessing how well the model mirrors the disease in humans. In addition, single muscle fiber contractile properties may be used as a functional outcome measure for preclinical studies in animal models of neuromuscular disease. This approach will be particularly useful for muscle diseases in which the sarcomeric proteins are directly affected.

In future studies, it is important to assess isotonic as well as isometric contractile properties. Because power is a function of both muscle strength and contractile speed, it may be the single most important functional parameter to measure, and it may be more sensitive than either SF or V_o to subtle changes induced by either disease or treatment of the disease.

Summary

The skinned single muscle fiber preparation allows investigators to directly assess the impact of neuromuscular disease on contractile function at the cellular level. It is complementary to other measurement techniques that assess muscle function on a larger scale. The single-fiber technique allows one to assess the impact of disease and/or treatment differentially on

Type I, IIa, IIx, and hybrid fibers, as well as on atrophic and hypertrophic fibers. With some diseases, particular muscle fiber types are preferentially affected. When applying the technique to the study of neuromuscular disease, one must recognize that in vivo muscle strength and power generation involve multiple additional steps such as central activation of motor neurons, neural transmission, neuromuscular junction transmission, and excitation–contraction coupling, which are not addressed by the single-fiber preparation. In addition, a number of mechanical processes involved in force transduction modify single muscle fiber strength and power before it is translated into in vivo whole muscle strength and power.

Thus far, single-fiber contractile properties of patients with prior polio, ALS, myotonic and FSH dystrophies, inflammatory myopathy, and critical illness myopathy have been studied. The findings from these studies have been summarized in this article, and future research applications suggested.

References

[1] Krivickas L, Suh D, Wilkins J, et al. Age- and gender-related differences in maximum shortening velocity of skeletal muscle fibers. Am J Phys Med Rehabil 2001;80:447–55.
[2] Frontera WR, Suh D, Krivickas LS, et al. Skeletal muscle fiber quality in older men and women. Am J Physiol 2000;279:C611–8.
[3] Larsson L, Li X, Berg HE, et al. Effects of removal of weight bearing function on contractility and myosin isoform composition in single human skeletal muscle cells. Eur J Appl Physiol 1996;432:320–8.
[4] Trappe S, Gallagher P, Harber M, et al. Single muscle fibre contractile properties in young and old men and women. J Physiol 2003;552:47–58.
[5] Metzger JM, Moss RL. Shortening velocity in skinned muscle fibers: influence of lattice spacing. Biophys J 1987;52:127–31.
[6] Rome LC, Funke RP, Alexander RM, et al. Why animals have different muscle fiber types. Nature 1988;335:824–7.
[7] Bergstrom J. Muscle electrolytes in man. Scand J Clin Lab Med 1962;14:511–3.
[8] Evans W, Phinney S, Young V. Suction applied to a muscle biopsy maximizes sample size. Med Sci Sports Exerc 1982;14:101–2.
[9] Larsson L, Salviati G. A technique for studies of the contractile apparatus in single human muscle fibre segments obtained by percutaneous biopsy. Acta Physiol Scand 1992;146: 485–95.
[10] Moss R. Sarcomere length-tension relations in frog skinned muscle fibers during calcium activation at short lengths. J Physiol 1979;292:177–92.
[11] Godt R, Maughan D. Swelling of skinned muscle fibers of the frog. Biophys J 1977;19: 103–16.
[12] Edman K. The velocity of unloaded shortening and its relation to sarcomere length and isometric force in vertebrate muscle fibers. J Physiol 1979;291:143–50.
[13] Larsson L, Moss R. Maximum velocity of shortening in relation to myosin isoform composition in single fibres from human skeletal muscles. J Physiol 1993;472:595–614.
[14] Widrick J, Trappe S, Costill D, et al. Force-velocity and force-power properties of single muscle fibers from elite master runners and sedentary men. Am J Physiol 1996;271: C676–83.
[15] Hill A. The head of shortening and the dynamic constants of muscle. Proc R Soc Lond B Biol Sci 1938;126:136–95.

[16] Laemmli U. Cleavage of structural proteins during the assembly of the head of bacterio-phage T4. Nature 1970;227:680–5.

[17] Trappe S, Williamson D, Godard M, et al. Effect of resistance training on single muscle fiber contractile function in older men. J Appl Physiol 2000;89:143–52.

[18] Trappe S, Godard M, Gallagher P, et al. Resistance training improves single muscle fiber contractile function in older women. Am J Physiol 2001;281:C398–406.

[19] Larsson L, Li X, Tolback A, et al. Contractile properties in single muscle fibres from chron-ically overused motor units in relation to motoneuron firing properties in prior polio pa-tients. J Neurol Sci 1995;132:182–92.

[20] Krivickas L, Yang J, Kim S, et al. Skeletal muscle fiber function and rate of disease progres-sion in amyotrophic lateral sclerosis. Muscle Nerve 2002;26:636–43.

[21] Atkin J, Scott R, West J, et al. Properties of slow- and fast-twitch muscle fibres in a mouse model of amyotrophic lateral sclerosis. Neuromuscul Dis 2005;15:377–88.

[22] Krivickas LS, Ansved T, Suh D, et al. Contractile properties of single muscle fibers in myo-tonic dystrophy. Muscle Nerve 2000;23:529–37.

[23] O'Cochlain DF, Perez-Terzic C, Reyes S, et al. Transgenic overexpression of human DMPK accumulates into hypertrophic cardiomyopathy, myotonic myopathy and hypotension traits of myotonic dystrophy. Hum Mol Genet 2004;13:2505–18.

[24] Krivickas L, Kim S, Frontera W. Single muscle fiber contractile properties in facioscapulo-humeral dystrophy. Muscle Nerve 2000;23:1632.

[25] Krivickas L, Amato A, Krishnan G, et al. Preservation of in vitro muscle fiber function in dermatomyositis and inclusion body myositis: a single fiber study. Neuromuscul Dis 2005; 15:349–54.

[26] Larsson L, Li X, Edstrom L, Erikson LI, et al. Acute quadriplegia and loss of muscle myosin in patients treated with nondepolarizing neuromuscular blocking agents and corticosteroids: mechanisms at the cellular and molecular levels. Crit Care Med 2000;28:34–45.

[27] Frontera W, Hughes V, Krivickas L, et al. Strength training in older women: early and late changes in whole muscle and single cells. Muscle Nerve 2003;27:601–8.

[28] Trappe S, Costill D, Thomas R. Effect of swim taper on whole muscle and single fiber con-tractile properties. Med Sci Sports Exerc 2000;32:48–56.

[29] Fitts R, Costill D, Gardetto P. Effect of swim exercise training on human muscle fiber func-tion. J Appl Physiol 1989;66:465–75.

[30] Harridge SD, Bottinelli R, Canepari M, et al. Sprint training, in vitro and in vivo muscle function, and myosin heavy chain expression. J Appl Physiol 1998;84:442–9.

[31] Widrick J, Stelzer J, Shoepe T, et al. Functional properties of human muscle fibers after short term resistance exercise training. Am J Physiol 2002;283:R408–16.

ELSEVIER
SAUNDERS

Phys Med Rehabil Clin N Am
16 (2005) 967–979

PHYSICAL MEDICINE
AND REHABILITATION
CLINICS OF
NORTH AMERICA

Electrodiagnostic Studies in a Murine Model of Demyelinating Charcot-Marie-Tooth Disease

Gregg D. Meekins, MD, Michael D. Weiss, MD*

*Department of Neurology, University of Washington School of Medicine, Box 356115,
1959 NE Pacific Street, Seattle, WA 98195, USA*

Charcot-Marie-Tooth disease (CMT) is a form of inherited peripheral neuropathy associated with heterogenous inherited or de novo mutations of genes important for the function of the peripheral nervous system. The phenotype of CMT varies widely in regard to age of onset and physical examination findings, as well as pattern and severity of electrodiagnostic abnormalities [1–5]. In general, CMT involves distal numbness, weakness, and foot deformities such as hammer toes and high arches [6–9]. Standard management for these conditions has focused on improving functional mobility and activities of daily living through assistive devices and medications directed toward symptom relief, although a recent small pilot study of patients with CMT type 1A (CMT1A) has suggested a potential role for neurotrophin-3 in promoting axonal regeneration [10].

The current nomenclature of CMT provides for further subclassification of the hereditary neuropathies into two large groups. Patients with neuropathies inherited in an autosomal dominant pattern and displaying predominantly demyelinating features by nerve conduction studies or nerve biopsies are considered to have CMT type 1 [8]. Neuropathy patients with genetic defects transmitted usually in an autosomal dominant pattern but with evidence of axon loss electrophysiologically or pathologically have a disorder designated as CMT type 2 [9].

Animal models with evolutionarily conserved gene defects shared in common with homologous regions in humans provide a useful observational tool in regard to understanding disease mechanisms and in developing

This study was supported in part by the Neurotrophins Research Fund.
* Corresponding author.
E-mail address: mdweiss@u.washington.edu (M.D. Weiss).

hypothesis-driven treatment studies. Two such murine models, *trembler (tr)* and *trembler-j (tr-j)* mice, have naturally occurring point mutations in the peripheral myelin protein-22 (PMP-22) gene with peripheral nerve demyelination. Due to pathologic and electrodiagnostic similarities shared in common with certain demyelinating forms of CMT neuropathy, the *tr* and *tr-j* have been thought to represent useful models for the study of these forms of human disease [11–14].

This article will discuss current pathophysiologic mechanisms and nerve conduction abnormalities in human CMT1A, as well as review the genetic, pathologic and electrodiagnostic features of the *tr* and *tr-j* strains. *Tr-j* nerve conduction study data from our laboratory is reviewed. Additionally, we report preliminary data regarding the use of stimulated single-fiber electromyography (SSFEMG) to evaluate neuromuscular junction abnormalities and axon loss in *tr-j* mice.

Charcot-Marie-Tooth type 1A

CMT1A denotes the subset of CMT1 patients with duplication or point mutations of the PMP-22 gene located on the short arm of chromosome 17 (17p11.2) [15,16]. Hereditary neuropathy with liability to pressure palsies describes the phenotype associated with an analogous PMP-22 gene deletion, and has traditionally not been classified with CMT1A [17,18]. CMT1A secondary to PMP-22 gene duplication is the most common human form of CMT comprising 52% to 57% of cases [4,19]. Human data suggests that PMP-22 gene duplication comprises approximately 70% to 95% of cases of CMT1A, with the remainder secondary to smaller duplications or point mutations within the PMP-22 gene [4,19–21].

Although found in other organs, PMP-22 gene expression is greatest in Schwann cells and PMP-22 protein expression is highest in Schwann cells and in areas of compact peripheral nerve myelin. PMP-22 is a membrane-bound glycoprotein with four transdomain regions, and plays an important role in the regulation of Schwann cell proliferation [22], growth and maintenance of peripheral nerve myelin, as well as in myelin–axon signaling [23,24]. Pathologic study of peripheral nerves associated with PMP-22 gene defects show evidence of loss of myelinated and unmyelinated axons, increased axon-to-myelin ratio (g-ratio), and aberrant remyelination (onion bulb formation) [25–28].

The phenotypic severity of CMT1A is variable, dependent on whether the PMP-22 gene defect is secondary to a point mutation or gene duplication. Patients with PMP-22 point mutations tend to have more severe weakness, and may present at an earlier age than those with PMP-22 gene duplication [4,25,28,29]. Median and ulnar nerve conduction studies for PMP-22 gene duplication show electrodiagnostic evidence of demyelination with motor conduction velocities in the range of 15 to 30 m/s [19,20,26,30,31], whereas individuals with PMP-22 point mutations have a wide variability of demyelinating features ranging from a greater decrease in nerve conduction velocity slowing [28,32,33] to a degree comparable to PMP-22 gene duplication [19,34,35].

The *trembler* and *trembler-j* mouse

In 1951, Falconer was the first to report a naturally occurring demyelinating mouse line with an autosomal dominant inheritance pattern and a phenotype of tremor, paralysis, and stimulus-induced convulsions, which he designated the *trembler* (*tr*) mouse [11]. Further evaluation suggested the possible use of the *tr* mouse as a model for studying hereditary neuropathy in humans [12]. Subsequent studies demonstrated that the stimulus-sensitive "convulsions" were actually tremors instead of epileptiform activity. Pathologic evaluation of 14-day-old and adult *tr* brain, spinal cord, dorsal root ganglia, sciatic nerve, and muscle with light and electron microscopy revealed evidence of retarded myelin formation, myelin degeneration, and onion bulb formation [36]. No specific central nervous system abnormalities have been found.

Low and McCleod [13] were the first to perform electrophysiologic studies in these mice, recording from the median, sciatic, and tail nerves in *tr* and control mice. Comparison of sciatic motor nerve conduction studies in *tr* and control mice (mean $\pm$ SD) showed significant differences in conduction velocities (2.51 $\pm$ 1.34 versus 45.92 $\pm$ 7.21 m/s), distal latencies (4.16 $\pm$ 2.01 versus 0.6 $\pm$ 1.35 ms), and compound nerve action potential (CMAP) amplitudes (0.21 $\pm$ 0.13 versus 3.18 $\pm$ 1.15 mV), consistent with severe peripheral nerve demyelination in the *tr* group.

A more recent gene mapping study identified a point mutation in the PMP-22 gene on mouse chromosome 11, which causes a glycine to aspartic acid substitution in a putative membrane domain of the PMP-22 protein [37]. Pathologic and nerve conduction studies have suggested that the severity of demyelination in the *tr* mouse is comparable to that seen in human Dejerine-Sottas disease (CMT type 3, CMT3) [13,36]. However, no human cases of demyelinating peripheral neuropathy with a gene defect homologous to that of the *tr* mouse have been reported.

In 1979, Jackson Laboratories demonstrated a mutation coisogenic with the C57BL/6J mouse strain spontaneously occurring in a mouse kindred, independent of the *tr* mutation, called the *trembler-j* (*tr-j*) mouse [38]. As with the *tr* mouse, the *tr-j* has an autosomal dominant inheritance pattern with a phenotype of limb weakness, atrophy, and tremor. Observational studies showed that the severity of gait abnormalities and onion bulb formation in myelinated peripheral nerve fibers are greater in the *tr* mouse than in the *tr-j* mouse (Fig. 1), confirming a more severe demyelinating phenotype in the former [39]. Subsequently, gene sequencing of the *tr-j* mouse revealed a PMP-22 point mutation with a leucine-to-proline substitution in the first transmembrane region of the PMP-22 protein [40]. In 1992, a human

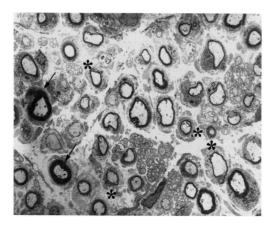

Fig. 1. Ultrastructure of adult *trembler-j* sciatic nerve. Electron microscopy demonstrates mostly hypomyelinated nerve axons with few normally myelinated nerve axons (*arrows*) in a representative section. There is also dramatic reduction in the total number of myelinated nerve fibers, consistent with substantial axonal degeneration. A few "onion bulb" formations (*asterisks*) are seen, signifying repetitive cycles of demyelination and remyelination ($\times 2400$ magnification, then 50% reduction).

kindred with the same point mutation as the *tr-j* mouse was identified [32]. Based on its genetic profile and evidence of peripheral demyelinating disease, the *tr-j* is considered a potential model for the study of CMT1A.

Nerve conduction studies in the *trembler-j* mouse

Peripheral nerve conduction studies provide measurement of physiologic nerve depolarization, termed nerve action potential, along segments of nerve [41,42]. Peripheral nerve may be stimulated via sodium channel activation with exogenous electrical current. Subsequently generated CMAP morphology (ie, amplitude, duration) and the velocity of nerve depolarization (ie, distal latency, conduction velocity) may be measured at recording sites distant to the point of stimulus. This provides information regarding myelin and axon integrity. The CMAP provides a measure of motor unit action potential summation. Reduced CMAP amplitude and area may be suggestive of motor axon loss. Demyelination along motor or sensory nerve fibers may be observed with reduction in conduction velocity, increased distal latency, or abnormal temporal dispersion (ie, abnormally prolonged CMAP duration).

We previously reported on motor nerve conduction in the hindlimb of the *tr-j* mouse [14]. Near nerve stimulation of the sciatic nerve was performed at the knee and sciatic notch in 30- and 72-day-old *tr-j* and C57B1/6 control mice. CMAPs were recorded with steel subdermal needle electrodes at the left foot pad at the base of the second toe (Fig. 2). In comparison to control

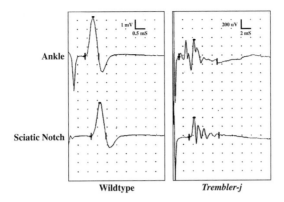

Fig. 2. Representative tracings of sciatic motor nerve conduction from a wild-type and *trembler-j* mouse. Note the difference in display sensitivity and time sweep. The CMAP for the mutant is significantly reduced in amplitude and increased in duration compared with the wild-type CMAP. Motor conduction velocity for the *trembler-j* mouse is reduced about 80% relative to the control mouse shown (approximately 7 m/s versus 35 m/s). The findings are largely consistent with profound demyelination in the mutant.

mice of the same age (mean ± SEM), 30-day-old *tr-j* mice had a statistically significant decrease in CMAP amplitude (0.30 ± 0.03 versus 2.00 ± 0.22 mV), increase in distal motor latency (2.14 ± 0.17 versus 1.01 ± 0.06 milliseconds), decrease in motor conduction velocity (6.3 ± 1.8 versus 33.2 ± 2.4 m/s), and increase in CMAP duration (3.25 ± 0.40 versus 0.92 ± 0.05 milliseconds), consistent with a profound disorder of peripheral nerve myelin. Seventy-two-day-old *tr-j* mice demonstrated nerve conduction findings comparable to the younger animals, suggesting that myelin dysfunction in the mutants remains relatively stable as they age.

Stimulated single-fiber electromyography studies in the *trembler-j* mouse

Single-fiber needle electromyography (EMG) is an electrodiagnostic tool through which the efficiency of neuromuscular transmission (jitter) and ratio of the motor unit innervation (fiber density [FD]) per given area of muscle may be measured [43]. Jitter, as a measurement called mean consecutive difference (MCD), is the summed average interpotential variation in depolarization, per recorded time interval, of two or more voluntarily contracted myofibers innervated by the same motor unit. Jitter can provide a measure of neuromuscular junction failure by recording complete failure of myofiber depolarization (blocking) or reduction in efficiency of neuromuscular transmission as measured by an increase in MCD [44,45]. FD, a measure of the number of the unique single fiber action potentials (SFAPs) observed per given recording area, also provides an estimate of motor unit ratio. Increased FD suggests axon loss, terminal reinnervation, and enlarged motor unit territory [46,47].

SSFEMG allows for direct stimulation of presynaptic motor nerve twigs of close proximity and innervated by the same motor unit [48,49]. As with single-fiber EMG recording from voluntarily contracted muscle, jitter and FD measurements may be obtained. Because SSFEMG is independent of voluntary muscle contraction, it is ideally suited for the study of neuromuscular physiology in patients with decreased level of consciousness, inability to voluntarily contract muscle, or in a laboratory study of animal models where neuromuscular pathology is suspected.

To determine whether SSFEMG can be reliably performed in a murine model of disease and provide information regarding neuromuscular transmission and axonal degeneration, SSFEMG studies were conducted in the *tr-j* mouse. Sixty-day-old wild-type C57B1/6 black and *tr-j* mice were anesthetized using isoflurane and oxygen via nosecone. Body core temperature was maintained between 32°C and 38°C using a heating pad as measured by a rectal thermistor. SSFEMG was performed in a blinded fashion on wild-type (n = 5) and *tr-j* (n = 8) mice using a Viking Quest electromyograph (Nicolet Biomedical, Madison, Wisconsin). Motor nerve axons of the left sciatic nerve were stimulated near the sciatic notch with subdermal steel needle EEG electrodes (Dantec, Copenhagen, Denmark) at a stimulation frequency of 5 Hz, using low amperage and a duration of 0.1 millisecond. A 30-mm single-fiber needle electrode was placed in the left gastrocnemius muscle for recording myofiber potentials. Stimulus intensity was increased to produce a maximal number of individual, myofiber depolarizations. The examiner immobilized the leg manually.

MCD calculations were determined from 100 consecutive discharges. SFAPs accepted for analysis had to be distinct from the stimulus artifact and have a stable waveform morphology, a negative-peak amplitude >200 microvolts, and a baseline to negative-peak rise time of <500 milliseconds. SFAPs with MCD measurements ≤ 5 microseconds were rejected for analysis. FD calculations were determined by counting the number of individual SFAPs per recording that crossed the baseline, had an initial positive depolarization, a rise time <500 microseconds, and a negative-peak amplitude ≥ 200 microvolts. Four to six recordings were obtained in each animal for calculation of average MCD and FD.

All animals were studied in a blinded fashion. Genotyping of animals after electrophysiologic study was performed using previously described methods [14,40]. Statistical analysis for group comparisons of mean MCD and FD measurements were calculated using unpaired Student's *t*-test. A *P*-value <0.05 was considered statistically significant. Representative SSFEMG recordings from *tr-j* and wild-type mice are demonstrated (Fig. 3). In comparison to wild-type mice (mean $\pm$ SEM), 60-day-old *tr-j* mice had an increase in FD (1.65 ± 0.15 versus 1.13 ± 0.05; $P < 0.01$) and average MCD (8.56 ± 0.85 versus 17.29 ± 1.49 microseconds; $P < 0.0005$) (Fig. 4).

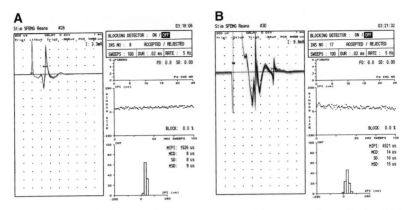

Fig. 3. Representative tracings of stimulated single fiber electromyography studies in wild-type (*A*) and *trembler-j* (*B*) mice. The *trembler-j* mouse studied here shows a substantial increase in jitter compared with the control mouse. The mutant also demonstrates a FD of 2.0 and the wild type of 1.0.

Discussion

Both the *tr* and *tr-j* mouse have naturally occurring point mutations in the PMP-22 gene and have been reported as potential models for the study of CMT neuropathy. The *tr* mouse has a phenotype of severe demyelination, evident by pathologic and electrodiagnostic studies. Several authors have suggested that the *tr* mouse may serve as a model for the study of CMT3 on the basis of phenotypic similarities and the degree of peripheral demyelination. However, CMT3 involves heterogenous genetic defects of the PMP-22 [33,50], myelin protein zero [51,52], early growth response [53], and periaxin [54,55] genes. Based on heterogeneity of genetic mutations, aberrant gene products, and lack of human homolog it is debatable how useful a model the *tr* mouse represents for the study of CMT3 or other forms of CMT neuropathy.

The *tr-j* mouse also has pathologic abnormalities consistent with demyelination of peripheral nerves, although of lesser severity than the *tr* strain. Electrodiagnostic and other functional studies of one human kindred with the same point mutation as the *tr-j* mouse has been reported [56]. When compared with affected members of six CMT1A families with PMP-22 gene duplication, kindred members with the PMP-22 point mutation homologous to the *tr-j* mouse had greater mean neurologic disability scale scores (38 [range 23–56] versus 24 [8–40]), greater mean reduction ($\pm$SD) in nerve conduction velocities (12.3 $\pm$ 6.4 versus 21.7 $\pm$ 6.2 m/s), and nerve biopsies showing a greater degree of small, thinly myelinated fibers consistent with a more severe disease phenotype than commonly seen with PMP-22 gene duplication.

Our laboratory previously reported motor nerve conduction studies in the hindlimb of *tr-j* mice [14]. In comparison to wild type, *tr-j* mice showed

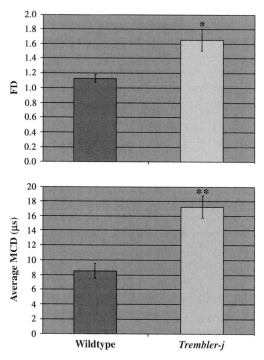

Fig. 4. Grouped average results (mean ± SEM) of SSFEMG for 60-day-old wild-type and *trembler-j* mice including FMD and average MCD. There is a substantial increase in FD and approximately twofold increased in average MCD in the *trembler-j* mice (n = 8) relative to the wild-type animals (n = 5). These findings suggest a degree of impairment of neuromuscular transmission as well as axonal degeneration in the demyelinating mutant. Unpaired Student's *t*-test comparisons for wild-type versus *trembler-j* mice (*P < 0.01, **P < 0.0005).

a statistically significant decrease in CMAP amplitude, increase in distal motor latency, and decrease in motor conduction velocity suggestive of a profound disorder of peripheral myelin. Motor conduction velocities in *tr-j* mice were reduced 87% compared with wild type mice, comparable to the degree of median motor conduction velocity reduction in humans sharing the same point mutations. This suggests that nerve conduction study in the *tr-j* may provide a useful model for studying peripheral nerve demyelination in human CMT1A associated with the homologous point mutation. The *tr-j* mouse, however, may represent a more severe demyelinating phenotype by nerve conduction study than the most common form of CMT1A associated with PMP-22 gene duplication, rendering its utility as a model for this subset of CMT1A less certain.

In 1999, Zielasek and Toyka reported electrodiagnostic evidence of 50- to 150-Hz rhythmic discharges considered neuromytonia by concentric needle EMG in both *tr* and *tr-j* mice [57]. The authors suggested potential etiologies for neuromyotonia including ectopic impulse generation, increased mechanosensitivity, and ephaptic transmission between adjacent axons or impulse reflection. Neuromyotonia detected by EMG, coupled with our findings of a significant decrease in compound muscle action potential amplitudes in 30- and 72-day-old *tr-j* mice, may suggest a component of motor axonal injury beginning at an early age in this strain.

SSFEMG is well suited for evaluating motor axonal denervation and motor unit reinnervation with measurement of FD as well as providing additional information regarding efficiency of neuromuscular transmission through measurement of jitter. Single fiber EMG has been used to study acquired human chronic inflammatory demyelinating polyradiculoneuropathy [58], diabetic neuropathy [59], and familial amyloid peripheral polyneuropathy [60]. To our knowledge, this is the first published report regarding the use of SSFEMG in the study of a murine model of diseases of the peripheral nervous system, in particular, a disease homologous to a form of demyelinating CMT.

In 2001, Gooch and Mosier [61] described normative data in healthy BALB/c, B6/SJL, and C57Bl/6 mouse strains using 2-Hz stimulation of exposed sciatic nerve with SSFEMG recording of the gastrocnemius muscle. Reported MCD measurements, in their study, range from 6 to 8 microseconds for all strains, with a comparable body temperature of 37°C. Mean jitter values for healthy control C57Bl/6 mice obtained in our laboratory are slightly higher than reported by Gooch and Mosier for the identical strain (8.56 ± 0.85 versus 6.1 ± 1.6 microseconds).

The difference in jitter values may reflect methodologic differences between the studies. In our study, general anesthesia was induced with the use of isoflurane and oxygen delivered via nosecone without mechanical ventilatory support, while in the previously described method, anesthesia was induced with intraperitoneal injection of ketamine, xylazine, and acepromazine with respiratory support by tracheal or orotracheal intubation and room air mechanical ventilation. Gooch and Mosier directly stimulated sciatic nerve exposed surgically at a frequency of 2 Hz, whereas in our study, we used subdermal needle electrodes to give near nerve stimulation of the sciatic nerve at a frequency of 5 Hz . Another source of variation could be due to differences in body temperature, as measured jitter values in our study were recorded over a greater range of core body temperature (between 32–38°C) in comparison to the study by Gooch and Mosier (37°C).

SSFEMG in our study produced clearly defined SFAPs for jitter and FD analysis. In comparison to control mice, *tr-j* mice showed a statistically significant increase in average MCD and FD, suggesting impairment of neuromuscular transmission, motor axon loss, and motor unit reinnervation. These single fiber findings in 60-day-old *tr-j* mice suggest that axon loss is a relatively early finding in this mouse model. Defects in neuromuscular transmission have not been reported in animal models or humans with genetic forms of demyelinating peripheral neuropathy. It is postulated that early axon loss and neuromuscular transmission failure, in addition to consequences of motor demyelination, may contribute to muscle weakness in genetic forms of demyelinating peripheral neuropathy.

Summary

Given the increasing number of transgenic murine models of human disease, functional studies are of great importance to demonstrate how closely these animals resemble patients with these diseases. Electrodiagnostic testing is an excellent functional tool for assessing injury to peripheral nerve in these models. Admittedly, there are variables influencing the results of such testing in mice not seen in humans. These include small segmental distances in nerve conduction, which could influence measurements of conduction velocity, and excessive movement in mice in SSFEMG. However, we have found these tests to be generally reproducible in the *tr-j* mouse, providing useful information about the function of peripheral nerve myelin, axon, and neuromuscular transmission in this model for demyelinating CMT.

References

[1] Matsubara S, Tanabe H. A clinico-pathological study of chronic hereditary neuropathy. Acta Neuropathol (Berl) 1983;61(1):43–51.

[2] Yoshioka R, Dyck PJ, Chance PF. Genetic heterogeneity in Charcot-Marie-Tooth neuropathy type 2. Neurology 1996;46(2):569–71.

[3] Gemignani F, Marbini A. Charcot-Marie-Tooth disease (CMT): distinctive phenotypic and genotypic features in CMT type 2. J Neurol Sci 2001;184(1):1–9.

[4] Boerkoel CF, Takashima H, Garcia CA, et al. Charcot-Marie-Tooth disease and related neuropathies: mutation distribution and genotype-phenotype correlation. Ann Neurol 2002;51(2):190–201.

[5] Carvalho AA, Vital A, Ferrer X, et al. Charcot-Marie-Tooth disease type 1A: clinicopathological correlations in 24 patients. J Peripher Nerv Syst 2005;10(1):85–92.

[6] Charcot JM, Marie P. Sur une forme particuliere d'atrophie musculaire progressive souvent familiale debutant par les pieds et les jambs et atteignant plus tard les mains. Rev Med 1886; 6:97–138.

[7] Tooth HH. The peroneal type of progressive muscular atrophy. London: Lewis; 1886. p. 1–43.

[8] Dyck PJ, Lambert EH. Lower motor and primary sensory neuron disease with peroneal muscular atrophy. I. Neurologic, genetic, and electrophysiologic findings in hereditary polyneuropathies. Arch Neurol 1968;18:603–18.

[9] Dyck PJ, Lambert EH. Lower motor and primary sensory neuron disease with peroneal muscular atrophy. II. Neurologic, genetic, and electrophysiologic findings in various neuronal degenerations. Arch Neurol 1968;18:619–25.

[10] Sahenk Z, Nagaraja HN, McCracken BS, et al. NT-3 promotes nerve regeneration and sensory improvement in CMT1A mouse models and in patients. Neurology 2005;65:681–9.

[11] Falconer DS. Two new mutants, "Trembler" and "Reeler," with neurologic actions in the house mouse (*Mus musculus* L.). J Genet 1951;50:192–201.

[12] Braverman IM. Neurological actions caused by the mutant gene Trembler in the house mouse (*Mus musculus*, L.,) an investigation. J Neuropathol Exp Neurol 1953;12(1):64–72.

[13] Low PA, McLeod JG. Hereditary demyelinating neuropathy in the Trembler mouse. J Neurol Sci 1975;26(4):565–74.
[14] Meekins GD, Emery MJ, Weiss MD. Nerve conduction abnormalities in the *trembler-j* mouse: a model for Charcot-Marie-Tooth disease type 1A? J Periph Nerv Syst 2004;9(3): 177–82.
[15] Timmerman V, Raeymaekers P, De Jonghe P, et al. Assignment of the Charcot-Marie-Tooth neuropathy type 1 (CMT 1a) gene to 17p11.2-p12. Am J Hum Genet 1990;47(4):680–5.
[16] Valentijn LJ, Bolhuis PA, Zorn I, et al. The peripheral myelin gene PMP-22/GAS-3 is duplicated in Charcot-Marie-Tooth disease type 1A. Nat Genet 1992;1(3):166–70.
[17] Verhalle D, Lofgren A, Nelis E, et al. Deletion in the CMT1A locus on chromosome 17p11.2 in hereditary neuropathy with liability to pressure palsies. Ann Neurol 1994;3(2):704–8.
[18] Murakami T, Lupski JR. A 1.5-Mb cosmid contig of the CMT1A/HNPP deletion critical region in 17p11.2-p12. Genomics 1996;34(1):128–33.
[19] Wise CA, Garcia CA, Davis SN, et al. Molecular analyses of unrelated Charcot-Marie-Tooth (CMT) disease patients suggest a high frequency of the CMT1A duplication. Am J Hum Genet 1993;53(4):853–63.
[20] Ionasescu VV, Ionasescu R, Searby C. Screening of dominantly inherited Charcot-Marie-Tooth neuropathies. Muscle Nerve 1993;16(11):1232–8.
[21] Nelis E, Van Broeckhoven C, De Joghe P, et al. Estimation of the mutation frequencies in Charcot-Marie-Tooth Type 1 and hereditary neuropathy with liability to pressure palsies: a European collaborative study. Eur J Hum Genet 1996;4(1):25–33.
[22] Giambonini-Brugnoli G, Buchstaller J, Sommer L. Distinct disease mechanisms in peripheral neuropathies due to altered *peripheral myelin protein 22* gene dosage or a *Pmp22* point mutation. Neurobiol Dis 2005;18:656–8.
[23] Robertson AM, King RHM, Muddle JR, et al. Abnormal Schwann cell/axon interactions in the Trembler-j mouse. J Anat 1997;190(pt.3):423–32.
[24] Robertson AM, Huxley C, King RHM, et al. Development of early postnatal peripheral nerve abnormalities in Trembler-J and PMP-22 transgenic mice. J Anat 1999;195(pt.3): 331–9.
[25] Gabreels-Festen AA, Bolhuis PA, Hoogendijk JE, et al. Charcot-Marie-Tooth disease type 1A: morphological phenotype of the 17p duplication versus PMP22 point mutations. Acta Neuropathol (Berl) 1995;90(6):645–9.
[26] Thomas PK, Marques W Jr, Davis MB, et al. The phenotypic manifestations of chromosome 17p11.2 duplication. Brain 1997;120(pt.3):465–78.
[27] Fabrizi GM, Simonati A, Morbin M, et al. Clinical and pathological correlates in Charcot-Marie-Tooth neuropathy type 1A with 17p11.2p12 duplication: a cross-sectional morphometric and immunohistochemical study in twenty cases. Muscle Nerve 1998;21(7): 869–77.
[28] Fabrizi GM, Cavallaro T, Taioli F, et al. Myelin uncompaction in Charcot-Marie-Tooth neuropathy type 1A with a point mutation of peripheral myelin protein-22. Neurology 1999;53(4):846–51.
[29] Roa BB, Garcia CA, Suter U, et al. Charcot-Marie-Tooth disease type 1A. Association with a spontaneous point mutation in the PMP-22 gene. N Engl J Med 1993;329(2):96–101.
[30] Nicholson GA. Penetrance of hereditary motor and sensory neuropathy Ia: assessment by nerve conduction studies. Neurology 1991;41:547–52.
[31] Kaku DA, Parry GJ, Malamutet R, et al. Uniform slowing of conduction studies in Charcot-Marie-Tooth polyneuropathy type 1. Neurology 1993;43(12):2664–7.
[32] Valentijn LJ, Baas F, Wolterman RA, et al. Identical point mutations of *PMP-22* in *Trembler-J* mouse and Charcot-Marie-Tooth disease type 1A. Nat Genet 1992;2(4):288–91.
[33] Roa BB, Dyck PJ, Marks HG, et al. Dejerine-Sottas syndrome associated with point mutation in the peripheral myelin protein 22 (PMP-22) gene. Nat Genet 1993;5(3):269–73.
[34] Roa BB, Garcia CA, Suter U, et al. Charcot-Marie-Tooth disease type 1A. Association with a spontaneous point mutation in the PMP-22 gene. N Engl J Med 1993;324(2):96–101.

[35] Marrosu MG, Vaccargiu S, Marrosu G, et al. A novel point mutation in the peripheral myelin protein 22 (PMP22) gene associated with Charcot-Marie-Tooth disease type 1A. Neurology 1997;48(2):489–93.

[36] Ayers MM, Anderson RM. Onion bulb neuropathy in the Trembler Mouse: a model of hypertrophic interstitial neuropathy in man. Acta Neuropathol (Berl) 1973;25(1):54–70.

[37] Suter U, Welcher AA, Ozcelik T, et al. *Trembler* mouse carries a point mutation in a myelin gene. Nature 1992;356(6366):241–3.

[38] Sidman RL, Cowen JS, Eicher EM. Inherited muscle and nerve diseases in mice: a tabulation with commentary. Ann N Y Acad Sci 1979;317:494–505.

[39] Henry EW, Cowen JS, Sidman RL. Comparison of the Trembler and Trembler-J Mouse phenotypes: varying severity of peripheral hypomyelination. J Neuropathol Exp Neurol 1983;42(6):688–706.

[40] Suter U, Moskow JJ, Welcher AA, et al. A leucine-to-proline mutation in the putative first tansmembrane domain of the 22-kDa peripheral myelin protein in the trembler-J mouse. Proc Natl Acad Sci USA 1992;89(10):4382–6.

[41] Evans BA. Nerve action potentials. In: Daube JR, editor. Clinical neurophysiology. Philadelphia (PA): F.A. Davis Company; 1996. p. 147–56.

[42] Kimura J. Principles and variations of nerve conduction studies. In: Kimura J, editor. Electrodiagnosis in diseases of nerve and muscle: principles and practice. 3rd edition. New York: Oxford University Press; 2001. p. 109–11.

[43] Stalberg E, Ekstedt J, Broman A. The electromyographic jitter in normal human muscles. Electroencephalogr Clin Neurophysiol 1971;31(5):429–38.

[44] Stalberg E, Schiller HH, Schwartz MS. Safety factor in single human motor end-plates studied in vivo with single fiber electromyography. J Neurol Neurosurg Psychiatry 1975;38(8):799–804.

[45] Schiller HH, Stalberg E, Schwarz MS. Regional curare for the reduction of the safety factor in human motor end-plates studied with single fiber electromyography. J Neurol Neurosurg Psychiatry 1975;38(8):805–9.

[46] Stalberg E, Schwartz MS, Trontelj JV. Single fiber electromyography in various processes affecting the anterior horn cell. J Neurol Sci 1975;24(4):403–15.

[47] Thiele B, Stalberg E. Single fiber EMG findings in polyneuropathies of different aetiology. J Neurol Neurosurg Psychiatry 1975;38(9):881–7.

[48] Trontelj JV, Mihelin M, Fernandez JM, et al. Axonal stimulation for end plate jitter studies. J Neurol Neurosurg Psychiatry 1986;49(6):677–85.

[49] Trontelj JV, Stalberg E, Mihelin M, et al. Jitter of the simulated motor axon. Muscle Nerve 1992;15(4):449–54.

[50] Marques W Jr, Neto JM, Barreira AA. Dejerine-Sottas' neuropathy caused by the missense mutation PMP22 Ser72Leu. Acta Neurol Scand 2004;110(3):196–9.

[51] Warner LE, Hilz MJ, Appel SH, et al. Clinical phenotype of different MPZ (0) mutations may include Charcot-Marie-Tooth type 1B, Dejerine-Sottas and congenital hypomyelination. Neuron 1996;17(3):451–60.

[52] Simonati A, Fabrizi GM, Taioli F, et al. Dejerine-Sottas neuropathy with multiple nerve roots enlargement and hypomyelination associated with a missense mutation of the transmembrane domain of MPZ/P0. J Neurol 2002;249(9):1298–302.

[53] Warner LE, Mancias P, Butler IJ, et al. Mutations in the early growth response 2 (EGR2) gene are associated with hereditary myelinopathies. Nat Genet 1998;18(4):382–4.

[54] Timmerman V, De Jonghe P, Ceuterick C, et al. Novel missense mutation in the early growth response gene associated with the Dejerine-Sottas phenotype. Neurology 1999;52(9):1827–32.

[55] Boerkoel CF, Takashima H, Stankiewicz P, et al. Periaxin mutations cause Dejerine-Sottas neuropathy. Am J Hum Genet 2001;68(2):325–33.

[56] Hoogendijk JE, Janssen EAM, Gabreels-Festen AA, et al. Allelic heterogeneity in hereditary motor and sensory neuropathy type Ia (Charcot-Marie-Tooth disease type Ia). Neurology 1993;43(5):1010–5.

[57] Zielasek J, Toyka KV. Nerve conduction abnormalities and neuromyotonia in genetically engineered mouse models of human hereditary neuropathies. Ann N Y Acad Sci 1999; 883:310–20.

[58] Oh SJ. The single-fiber EMG in chronic demyelinating neuropathy. Muscle Nerve 1989; 12(5):371–7.

[59] Shields RW Jr. Single-fiber electromyography is a sensitive indicator of axonal degeneration in diabetes. Neurology 1987;37(8):1394–7.

[60] Blom S, Sten L, Zetterlund B. Familial amyloidosis with polyneuropathy—type 1. A neurophysiological study of peripheral nerve function. Acta Neurol Scand 1981;63(2):99–110.

[61] Gooch CL, Mosier DR. Stimulated single fiber electromyography in the mouse: techniques and normative data. Muscle Nerve 2001;24(7):941–5.

ELSEVIER
SAUNDERS

Phys Med Rehabil Clin N Am
16 (2005) 981–997

PHYSICAL MEDICINE
AND REHABILITATION
CLINICS OF
NORTH AMERICA

Using Electromyography to Assess Function in Humans and Animal Models of Muscular Dystrophy

Jay J. Han, MD[a], Gregory T. Carter, MD[b],*,
Michael D. Weiss, MD[c], Chandra Shekar, MD[b],
Joseph N. Kornegay, DVM, PhD[d]

[a]Department of Physical Medicine and Rehabilitation, University of California, Davis,
4860 Y Street, Suite 3850, Sacramento, CA 95817, USA
[b]Department of Rehabilitation Medicine, University of Washington,
1959 N.E. Pacific Avenue, Seattle, WA 98195, USA
[c]Department of Neurology, University of Washington, 1959 N.E. Pacific Avenue,
Seattle, WA 98195, USA
[d]College of Veterinary Medicine, University of Missouri-Columbia,
Columbia, MO 65211, USA

Electrophysiologic evaluation is a critical component of the diagnosis and management of patients with myopathic disorders. These studies can help guide further diagnostic studies, including muscle biopsy and imaging, as well as help monitor rehabilitation. This article will examine the role of electrophysiologic testing in diagnosing and managing the rehabilitation of patients with myopathic disorders. It is assumed that the reader has a basic understanding of muscle anatomy, physiology, and electrophysiology.

Nerve conduction studies

In the clinical setting, electrodiagnostic testing, which includes electromyography (EMG) and nerve conduction studies (NCS), is a critical extension of the clinician's physical examination and a powerful tool for the evaluation of neuromuscular disorders. However, in the setting of myopathy, the role of NCS is limited. The main use of NCS here is to rule out a neuropathic process. The primary NCS finding in myopathy is decreased

---

* Corresponding author. 1809 Cooks Hill Road, Centralia, WA 98531, USA.
  E-mail address: gtcarter@u.washington.edu (G.T. Carter).

1047-9651/05/$ - see front matter © 2005 Elsevier Inc. All rights reserved.
doi:10.1016/j.pmr.2005.08.001

compound muscle action potential (CMAP) amplitude, along with normal sensory nerve action potential amplitudes and conduction velocities. Abnormal decrement on repetitive stimulation may be seen in some myopathies, particularly notable in some animal models of myotonic myopathy [1]. This is presumably due to sarcolemmal electrical instability and immature end-plates secondary to on-going muscle deterioration. However, this finding is rarely of clinical use.

Surface electromyography

The use of surface EMG (SEMG) as a clinical and research tool in assessing muscle function in myopathy must be approached with some caution. Unlike needle EMG (NEMG), there are several issues of concern that affect the quality of the signal in SEMG, particularly in the setting of myopathy. The primary concern is the signal-to-noise ratio, which is the ratio of the true EMG signal in relation to the noise signal [2–4]. Noise is defined as electrical signals that are not part of the EMG signal. In myopathy there will inherently be less electrical signal coming from the muscle fibers due to atrophy and replacement of muscle fiber with fibrotic, fatty, or necrotic tissue. This may cause distortion of the signal, allowing unwanted frequency components to be mixed in with the true muscle EMG signal [4].

Proper technique and filtering is critical to obtain a signal that contains the maximum amount of information from the EMG signal and the minimum amount of contamination from electrical noise. The amplitude of the CMAP signal can range from 0 to 10 mV (peak to peak), although this trends toward the lower range in myopathy [3]. The desirable components of the signal are usually in the 50- to 500-Hz frequency range, with trending toward the higher frequency in myopathy [4].

Much like in NCS, the bandwidth of the EMG signal is affected by the surface electrode placement and interelectrode spacing, which may effect calculation of the conduction velocity of the action potentials along the muscle fibers [4]. Due to the fact that muscle fibers of motor units are distributed throughout most of the muscle cross-section, the muscle sample size need not be large. Therefore, it is not necessary to cover a large portion of the muscle with the detection surface of the electrode to obtain a representative sample of the EMG signal for a particular set of active motor units. Larger electrodes are more susceptible to detecting crosstalk from other muscles. The risk for this is particularly great in myopathy, where more muscles may be recruited for a given task due to the relative weakness of the individual muscle group [5]. Thus, the electrode should be as small as possible, while still allowing acceptable recording. The electrode should be placed between a motor point and the tendon insertion or between two motor points, and along the longitudinal midline of the muscle.

It is frequently taught in training programs that, for the purpose of detecting an SEMG signal, the electrode should be located on a motor point of the muscle. In reality, due to signal instability at the motor point, this is perhaps the worst location for electrode placement! At the motor point, action potentials travel in several directions along the muscle fibers, creating a potential for phase cancellation of the signal. As the muscle fibers narrow to form the tendon, they become thinner and fewer in number, which also reduces the EMG signal. In the region of the tendon as well as myopathy in general, the physical dimension of the muscle is considerably reduced, making it difficult to properly locate the electrode. These are among the reasons that SEMG is a difficult tool to use in myopathy, where the muscles are usually atrophied.

The SEMG signal is also processed differently than NEMG. Typically, a computer-based EMG will calculate the root-mean-squared (RMS) and the average rectified (AVR) value of the EMG signal. Both of these values reflect a measurement of the area under the signal curve [6,7]. The RMS value is also a relative measure of the power of the signal and is preferred for most applications [8–11].

Currently, the primary application of SEMG is as a research tool. It is the official stance of both the American Academy of Neurology and the American Association of Neuromuscular and Electrodiagnostic Medicine that SEMG is substantially inferior to NEMG for the evaluation of patients with neuromuscular disorders [2,3]. Unfortunately, the SEMG literature consists mainly of class II and III studies that used nonstandardized and dissimilar methods, small sample sizes, and frequently no controls. This does not allow an assessment of the sensitivity and specificity [2]. The American Academy of Neurology gave SEMG a Type E (negative recommendation), based on evidence of ineffectiveness or lack of efficacy, for the diagnosis and evaluation of neuromuscular disorders [2].

Despite the paucity of good literature to support the use of SEMG in the clinical diagnosis and management of myopathy, it is the opinion of this author that SEMG may be of some value to monitor the progression of myopathic disorders and warrants some discussion. SEMG, particularly in a research setting, has several potential applications to monitoring the rehabilitation of a patient with myopathy. SEMG can provide not only an estimate of the force produced by a muscle but also an objective measurement of the rate at which a muscle fatigues through the analysis of the frequency spectrum of the signal. Prior studies have noted a relationship between electromechanical coupling and myopathies. Patients with myopathy have been shown to have impaired muscle fiber electrical conduction and altered ratios of RMS SEMG to force (mechanomyogram) amplitudes, consistent with impaired electromechanical coupling [12–14].

Lindeman et al [15] did a randomized clinical trial the assessing efficacy of strength training in patients with myotonic muscular dystrophy, comparing them to patients with the hereditary neuropathy Charcot-Marie-Tooth (CMT) disease. They recorded SEMG of proximal leg muscles during isometric knee extension at maximal volitional contraction (MVC) and varying degrees thereof. Fatigue was studied by determining the changes in endurance and in the decline of the median frequency of the SEMG during a sustained contraction at 80% MVC. Only the CMT training group showed a gradual significant increase in mean MVC over the training period, as detected by SEMG [15].

Barry et al [16] studied the ratio of SEMG electrical amplitude to acoustic amplitude in children with Duchenne (DMD), Becker, and myotonic muscular dystrophy. The myopathy subjects had significantly higher ratios than the normal control subjects, clearly identifying the disease group. There is also some evidence that muscle fiber conduction velocity (usually around 4.0 m/s) will be slowed or blocked completely in diseased muscle [14,17,18].

Further improvements in SEMG continue to occur, including the ongoing development of high-spatial resolution techniques via computer analysis, which allows for better signal acquisition and resolution [19–22]. In the foreseeable future, it is entirely feasible that the clinical evaluation of a patient with myopathy could include a computer-based SEMG evaluation with measurement of muscle fatigue (force generation and CMAP amplitude) and muscle fiber conduction velocity. This technology would have broad application beyond myopathy. Disability evaluations are becoming increasingly problematic, and this technology could be used as a means to objectively quantify fatigue and effort of maximum voluntary contraction. This could distinguish problems with central activation or central fatigue from true intramuscular fatigue and abnormalities in excitation–contraction coupling [23–27].

Needle electromyography

Significantly more clinical information can be gathered from NEMG studies compared with SEMG. NEMG can initially narrow the differential diagnosis by excluding primarily neurogenic processes such as spinal muscular atrophy, which may sometimes be clinically difficult to distinguish from a myopathy. NEMG will also provide information about the most appropriate muscle site for the biopsy. Typically in myopathies the proximal muscles of the lower extremities exhibit more prominent EMG findings [28]. It is critical to sample a sufficient number of muscles to establish a diffuse myopathic process as opposed to a focal injury. Muscles that are severely weak, that is, less than 2 on manual muscle testing are not good to sample as the muscle tissue may be too deteriorated to provide a good signal [28]. The more revealing findings will be obtained in muscles of intermediate involvement with respect to weakness.

The motor unit action potentials (MUAPs) in patients with myopathic disorders have variable (normal to reduced) amplitudes and are typically polyphasic [29]. This results from the variability in muscle fiber diameters. There may be also a population of short-duration, nonpolyphasic MUAPS as well. Early MUAP recruitment is a hallmark of myopathy, with the inter-ference pattern rapidly filling up. However, if muscle fiber loss is severe, then there may be some motor unit drop out with the appearance of fast firing individual "spikes." This may be distinguished from neurogenic processes by the low amplitudes.

Myopathic disorders will generally display abnormal rest activity on EMG, including fibrillation potentials and positive sharp waves [29]. How-ever, it is important to note that in many metabolic, mitochondrial, and con-genital myopathies, abnormal rest activity may not be present. In the setting of myopathy, fibrillation potentials and positive sharp waves represent spontaneously depolarizing muscle fibers that have been effectively dener-vated due to muscle necrosis destroying the motor endplate or separating it from other portions of the muscle fiber. In long-standing myopathies there may be little residual rest activity due to the loss of muscle fiber. Further, these waveforms may be of smaller amplitude than those seen from a neuro-genic etiology. Thus, the clinician may need to use a higher sensitivity setting on the EMG recording unit.

Other forms of rest activity are critical to note. Increased insertional ac-tivity is common in most myopathies. Myotonic discharges, with waxing and waning of the amplitude and frequency of the motor units, along with a characteristic "dive bomber" sound, are prominent in the myotonic disorders, including myotonic muscular dystrophy. Complex repetitive dis-charges (CRDs), sometimes referred to as "pseudomyotonic" discharges, are a nonspecific finding that may be seen in long standing myopathic or neuropathic conditions.

Using needle electormyography to guide muscle biopsy

The information obtained through NEMG testing can guide the site se-lection for muscle biopsy. Preferably, the EMG should show clear abnor-malities but there should be an abundance of myopathic motor units, assuring an adequate amount of muscle fiber tissue for proper staining and inspection. A muscle that is severely affected will be largely replaced by fat and connective tissue with minimal residual muscle fiber present for evaluation. Muscles that have undergone recent NEMG should be avoided as muscle biopsy sites because of the possibility of cellular changes in the muscle fiber, secondary to the needle study. There may also be some disrup-tion in the architecture of the tissue if needle biopsy technique is used for the biopsy. This can affect histologic evaluation.

The abnormalities noted on NEMG may be correlated to some degree with the pathologic changes noted in diseased muscle on biopsy. The histo-pathologic study will help diagnosis specific disorders, such as a "dystro-phic" versus "inflammatory" myopathy, based on degree of muscle necrosis and presence of inflammatory cells. Inflammatory myopathies typ-ically show more abnormal rest activity on NEMG, presumably due to on-going sarcolemmal instability [29]. Early in a dystrophic myopathy there may be a full interference pattern with small polyphasic MUAPs mixed in with a population of normal appearing MUAP. This "mixed picture" on NEMG is due to the presence of normal fibers, as well as hypertrophied fibers, degenerating fibers, atrophic fibers, and some regenerating fibers. As a dystrophic process progresses, NEMG will show less MUAP activity while the biopsy would show connective tissue and fatty infiltration [30,31].

It is important to note that in some myopathies, the NEMG findings will may be quite subtle. This is true of many of the subtypes of congenital myopathies, a group of structural myopathies whose diagnosis is based on classic histologic characteristics seen on muscle biopsy (eg, centronuclear or myotubular, central core, nemaline rod, and fiber type disproportion myopathies).

Needle electromyography in animal models of muscular dystrophy

In humans with neuromuscular disease, there has been considerable characterization of the NEMG abnormalities. However, there is controversy over what is safe and ethically responsible to do in humans with respect to experimental interventions. Thus, animal models are typically used to investigate responses to therapeutic modalities in diseased muscles. Thus, there is a need for quantitative, physiologic measuring tools, such as EMG, to follow changes after therapeutic interventions. Animal models are usually matched to a human disease by genotype, rather than phenotype. However, the animal muscular dystrophies are a heterogeneous group of disorders that have distinct differences from human disease. Thus, there may be major differences in severity and progression of the disease. The homogous genetic abnormality in humans may have profoundly different phenotypic expression in animals. The same gene deletion may also have a different gene-chromosome location in animals. The most common muscular dystrophy animal models used in research are described in Table 1, which includes type of inheritance, gene location, affected gene product, and the human correlates. EMG findings may be the "deal breaker" in an otherwise reasonable model. The dystrophic chicken is a good example of this. The chicken initially seemed like a reasonable dystrophic model. However, EMG studies revealed that the avian muscles showed electrical myotonia and the dystrophic chicken fell out of favor as a research model for human disease. In rodents and in other animals with dystrophy, such as the cxmd dog, fast-twitch muscles and type 2B fibers are the earliest and most severely affected, and these have EMG characteristics that are similar to human dystrophy. However, there is a marked difference between species in pathology, gene location, and gene product. The autosomal recessive dy/dy mutant mouse (129 ReJ) and the 129B6F$_1$/J hybrid have a deficiency in the laminin alpha 2 chain (merosin). Although phenotypically similar to human DMD, NCS revealed a concomitant peripheral polyneuropathy in

Table 1
Animal models of human muscular dystrophies

Animal models	Inheritance	Human gene location	Affected gene product	Human correlate
mdx mouse and *CXMD* dog	XR	Xp21.2	Dystrophin and associated glycoproteins	DMD/BMD
dy/dy mouse	AR	6q2	Laminin-alpha2 (merosin)	Congenital muscular dystrophy
Hamster	AR	5q33-q34	Delta sarcoglycan	SCARMD
Chicken	AD	Unknown	Unknown	None

Abbreviations: AD, autosomal dominant; AR, autosomal recessive; DMD/BMD, Duchenne and Becker muscular dystrophy; SCARMD, severe childhood autosomal recessive muscular dystrophy; XR, x-linked recessive.

the dy/dy mouse. This mouse model is the most severely impaired, and has the most rapid disease progression of any of the rodent models of muscular dystrophy. However, this may be due in part to the neuropathy, making it a poor model for DMD.

The mdx mouse has provided an animal model well suited to study changes in electrophysiology over time in a dystrophic, myoathic process. The mdx mouse is a well-established, genotypically homologous model of human DMD [32–39]. Both human and murine diseases are caused by deletions at the Xp21 gene loci, leading to an absence of dystrophin, the primary protein product. Dystrophin is a structural protein in the sarcolemmal membrane and its absence produces membrane instability and increased susceptibility to mechanical stress [40–44]. This produces transient breaches of the membrane, allowing leakage of ions and proteins [45–48]. This eventually produces fibrotic replacement of muscle and eventual failure of regeneration with loss of contractility and muscle fiber loss [49–53].

Although mdx muscles show similar histologic changes, phenotypic expression in the mouse is less severe than in human DMD [38,54]. We have studied electrophysiologic changes in the mdx mouse, at various ages and in response to exercise [42,55–58]. Fig. 1A shows a gastrocnemius/soleus H&E muscle section from a 12-week-old, wild-type mouse. In this same mouse, dystrophin immunofluourescent antibody assay showed sarcolemma labeling in all muscle fibers (Fig. 1A). EMG examination of young and middle-aged wild-type mice showed normal insertional activity. There was a trend toward increased insertional activity in muscles from the older (17–24 months) animals. With the exception of one 12-week-old mouse, all control animal muscles showed normal resting activity. Fig. 1C shows a gastrocnemius/soleus H&E muscle section from a 12-week-old mdx mouse. Active muscle fiber degeneration and necrosis, along with central nucleation and inflammatory cells, are readily noticeable. A 24-month-old mdx

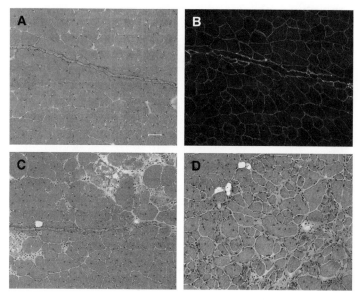

Fig. 1. (*A*) Hematoxylin and esoin (H&E) staining of gastrocnemius/soleus muscle tissue section from a 12-week-old, C57 (wild-type) mouse. (*B*) Corresponding immunofluorescence stain for dystrophin in the same section. (*C*) H&E staining of a gastrocnemius/soleus muscle section from a 12-week-old *mdx* mouse. (*D*) H&E staining of a gastrocnemius/soleus muscle section from a 24-week-old *mdx* mouse. Tracks from the EMG needle electrode are readily visible in the muscle sections.

muscle is shown in Fig. 1D. Compared with 12-week-old mdx muscles (Fig. 1C) there is more fibrosis but less inflammation. EMG showed increased insertional and rest activity (predominantly positive sharp wave [PSW] potentials) in all muscles tested from mdx mice. Although not quantified, there were increased amounts of PSW and fibrillation potentials noted muscles from 10–12-week-old and 24-month-old mdx mice. CRDs were noted in muscles from all mdx animals (Fig. 2). CRDs were also noted in one 10–12-month-old and two 24-month-old control animals. Rare myotonic discharges were also noted (Fig. 3).

Prior in vitro electrophysiologic studies using intracellular micropipette techniques, have demonstrated significant ionic channel abnormalities in mdx muscle [59–62]. Our prior and on-going EMG studies in the mdx mouse have shown significant abnormalities in insertional activity, spontaneous potentials (fibrillations and positive sharp waves), presence of CRDs, and motor unit morphology changes, as noted in Figs. 1 through 4 [55,63]. The prominent spontaneous potentials noted in young mdx mice are likely due to membrane instability secondary to a lack of dystrophin, which mechanically reinforces the sarcolemmal during contraction [64–68]. Insertional and rest activity appear to be most notably increased in the young

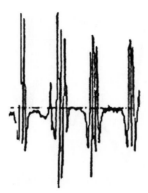

Fig. 2. Complex repetitive discharge recorded from the gastrocneniius muscle of a dystrophic (mdx) mouse. Amplitude is 200 microvolts; firing rate 10 Hz.

mdx mice, likely reflecting the significant amount of muscle degeneration/ regeneration, increase in muscle turnover, and inflammatory changes that are present on muscle biopsy at this stage of the disease.

Although continually present, the amount of the positive sharp waves, and to a lesser extent fibrillation potentials, decrease as the mouse ages. However, these finding increase again in aged mice. The amount of CRDs also increases steadily as the mdx mouse ages, being most notable in the oldest mice. CRDs are thought to be due to ephaptic transmission between adjacent muscle fibers, consistent with muscle membrane instability [55]. Thus, this would be expected to increase as the mdx mouse ages [55,63]. Our studies have shown a consistent increase in CRDs from 20 to 154 days of age [55,63].

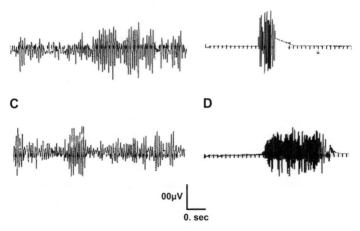

Fig. 3. Insertional activity recorded from gastrocnemius of an mdx mouse. Two types of myotonic insertional activity were occasionally noted. Continuous (C) and discrete (D); continuous discharges were very rate.

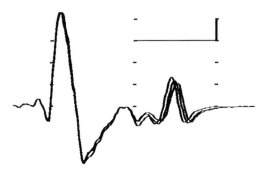

Fig. 4. mdx mouse volitional motor unit action potential with a late component and signficant jitter. Sweep speed is 5 millisconds per division and sensitivity is 200 microvolts per division.

At the University of Washington we have recently developed a method of doing quantitative motor unit analysis in the mdx mouse, which has not been previously done. To do this we used a trigger and delay function to average and quantify MUAPs. In this technique, a single motor unit is captured and then confirmed by showing reproducible waveforms when rastered using the trigger and delay function. To do this, the low- and high-frequency filter settings are set at 20 Hz to 10 kHz, with a sweep speed setting of 5 to 10 ms/division. The sensitivity is adjusted accordingly, to analyze the peak-to-peak amplitude. Only MUAPs that can be reliably reproduced and have a sharp initial rise time (indicating proximity to the recording electrode) are used for analysis. Using this technique we were able to show significant differences in phasicity between mdx and wild-type mice [63]. These polyphasic MUAPs were often accompanied by late components.

In preliminary trials, we found that the combination of a 27-gauge monopolar needle electrode, a nearby 29-gauge reference needle electrode, with an adhesive ground electrode placed at the distal limb, yielded the least background noise and clearly identifiable and reproducible motor units. Concentric (30 gauge) and larger monopolar needle electrodes (28 gauge) did not improve signal-to-noise ratio compared with the 27-gauge monopolar needle electrode, which was ultimately chosen for the study protocol. A needle electrode is much preferable to a surface reference electrode because placement is difficult and impractical due to animals the size of mice. Initial trials with a low-frequency filter of 2 Hz revealed increased baseline noise. The low- and high-frequency filter settings were then set at 20 Hz to 10 kHz, which eliminated some of the noise and improved the baseline.

The depth of anesthesia may also present problems with EMG studies in mice. Increasing the depth of anesthesia decreases the amount of spontaneous, volitional MUAP activity. Proper level of sedation is perhaps the most difficult and critical part of our technique. It is worth noting though, that the pattern of EMG activity did not change with increasing depth of anesthesia. However, it did significantly increase the time it took to complete a study, as the mice were too sedated to produce volitional motor activity.

The findings we noted in the mdx mouse are similar to the NEMG abnormalities observed by Desmedt and Borenstein [30] in the patients with DMD. Much like our mdx mouse studies, they noted the most significant EMG differences between the boys with DMD and the normal boys were increased phasicity of motor units and the presence of late components [30]. The polyphasicity of the MUAPs is likely due to motor unit component dropout secondary to muscle fiber degeneration and focal necrosis, which takes place in both mdx and DMD muscle tissue [30]. Much like the EMG findings in DMD patients, we observed MUAP with late components only in the mdx muscle and but none in the control wild-type mouse muscles. Fig. 4 shows an example of a MUAP recorded from an mdx mouse muscle with late components and significant jitter. These MUAPs with late components are likely due to motor axon sprouting and reinnervation of muscle fibers that are newly formed. This occurs either by segmentation of existing muscle fibers by way of focal necrosis and membrane repair or by muscle regeneration [30,69].

Our findings of increased duration and preserved amplitude of the mdx MUAPs compared with the wild-type mouse is somewhat unexpected from a myopathic process. Typically in a myopathic process, the MUAPs will show increased phasicity due to motor unit component drop out early in the disease [70]. As the disease progresses, EMG will show reduced MUAP amplitude and duration. We did not observe any significant reduction in the mdx MUAP amplitude or reduced duration compared with the control. Furthermore, no significant decrease in MUAP amplitude or reduction in duration was noted, even in the oldest mice. It may be that slight differences in motor unit parameters are beyond the detection level in murine muscle due to the small size of the MUAPs in general. More likely it is due to a different pathophysiology response of murine muscle compared with human muscle in a dystrophin deficient condition.

This hypothesis is be corroborated by the significant phenotypic differences between the mdx mouse and human DMD [35]. Murine muscle, including dystrophin-deficient murine muscle, has considerably more muscle regenerative capacity than human muscle [71–74]. In human DMD, as the disease advances, the muscle fibers are progressively replaced by fibrotic connective and fatty tissue. This is thought to be due to the continued degeneration and regeneration cycle of muscle fiber with attendant inflammatory response that eventually depletes the regenerative capacity. The mdx mouse regenerative capacity is preserved far into the later stages of life, thereby preserving the density and the number of muscle fibers within the motor unit, reflected by normal to slightly increased amplitude and duration of the MUAPs. Histologic evaluation of the old mdx mice shows increased fibrofatty deposition and replacement of muscle mass. However, this is not to the degree witnessed in DMD muscle at a similar stage of the disease

[70,71]. Our emerging mouse data, along with data from other human studies, indicate that an EMG profile can be used to objectively follow the progress of muscular dysfunction as a myopathy progresses [55,63]. Moreover, characterizing longitudinal EMG findings through the course of a muscle disease can establish a baseline data set that may be used as a functional marker for studies involving therapeutic interventions, including gene therapy.

The CXMD dog also is a genetic homolog of human DMD, and shows overt clinical signs of the dystrophy at 6 to 9 weeks of age. The CXMD dog has a clinical progression closer to that of DMD than does the mdx mouse. The dog, being a larger mammal, has a relative biomechanical disadvantage compared with the mouse. Thus, for larger mammals with a dystrophin-deficient condition, locomotion and other less intense forms of activity may place a greater burden on skeletal muscle and induce injury and subsequent necrosis. Valentine et al [75] performed clinical NEMG studies in these dogs (ages 6 weeks to 5.5 years old). Much like our studies in the mdx mouse, they found spontaneous activity, consisting primarily of CRDs, in all dogs tested, but most prominently in dogs greater than or equal to 10 weeks old. They also noted rare myotonic discharges, although the significance of this is not known. They were not present to the degree noted in the chicken model, which clearly has a myotonic disorder. Motor unit potentials were generally abnormally brief and frequently polyphasic.

Single-fiber electromyography studies in myopathy

Single-fiber EMG (SFEMG) has limited practical use in the diagnosis and rehabilitation of patients with myopathy. SFEMG is technically difficult and adds little additional information compared with standard NEMG. Shields et al [76] studied SFEMG in the extensor digitorum communis muscle of 20 patients with limb girdle muscular dystrophy, comparing the finding to patients with spinal muscular atrophy. They concluded that SFEMG added additional diagnostic benefit in patients with an indeterminate diagnoses. However, this study was done over 20 years ago, before the advent of markedly improved biopsy techniques and molecular genetic testing.

Stubgen [77] studied quantitative EMG using different needle techniques in limb girdle muscular dystrophy patients group. He found that standard MUAP analysis correlated with clinical progression. He also found that SFEMG results did not correlate with either clinical measures or standard NEMG findings. His studies supported our finding that show standard NEMG can be used to monitor disease progression in myopathy. However, SFEMG findings do not appear to correleate well with clinical features.

Cruz-Martinez et al [78] did standard NEMG and NCS studies as well as SFEMG in 18 patients with various types of myopathy. Although jitter was abnormal in 10 out of 18 tested patients, the jitter abnormalities did not correlate well with clinical myopathic features. They noted SFEMG abnormalities in muscles without clinical weakness. The results suggest that neuromuscular transmission disturbances likely occur in patients with myopathy. However, SFEMG their study also conluded that SFEMG findings do not correlate well with clinical presentation or progression.

Macro EMG is a technique designed to study total motor unit activity. MacroEMG can give some estimation of the total number and size of component muscle fibers. Several studies have compared NEMG to macro-EMG methods [79–81]. Although macro-EMG seems to be a sensitive and useful electrophysiologic diagnostic method for myopahthy, it does not appear to be more sensitive than standard NEMG.

Magnetic resonance imaging to complement EMG in myopathy

Although still an evolving technology, magnetic resonance imaging MRI is becoming an increasingly useful method of depicting myopathic disorders, and may provide additional, complimentary data to EMG studies. Many advances have occurred in the field of biotechnology over the past decade that has led to tremendous improvement in MRI of muscle [82–89]. From an anatomic and physiologic perspective, the information obtained with MRI is complementary to the data provided by EMG. EMG testing is a time-honored, well-researched, and acknowledged "gold standard" for assessing the physiologic functioning of muscle [83]. The techniques are standardized, with immense amounts of normative data, making it a very reliable procedure. Yet it remains a physiologic test, looking at function primarily and, to a lesser degree, anatomy. Anatomic conclusions based on EMG results must be made indirectly, based on which muscles are involved in the disease. MR imaging is, as of today, a "picture," which looks primarily at anatomy, with assumptions made about the physiologic functioning of structures based on their appearance. Thus, in some regard, it is a mirror of EMG, adding additional information from the opposite orientation. MRI of muscle is covered in more detail in the article by Fritz and colleagues elsewhere in this issue.

Summary

The available studies to date provide evidence of a role for NEMG as an in vivo, objective measurement tool to assess neuromuscular function without endangering the patient or requiring sacrifice of the animal model being studied. Our protocol for capturing and quantifying MUAPs in the mdx mouse support the role of EMG as sutiable objective test for therapeutic intervention trials. SEMG still remains somewhat difficult to quantify due to signal interference from skin and subcutaneous tissues, making it a less desirable tool. However, as computer technology evolves, SEMG may have a growing role in quantifying neuromuscular function, having all the advantages of NEMG plus the added benefit of being completely noninvasive. Coupling EMG findings with MR spectroscopy and imaging techniques in muscle allow a clinicician or investigator to get both physiologic and anatomic information of the neuromuscular system.

References

[1] Carter GT, Longley KJ, Walsh SA, et al. Lack of effect of amitriptyline in murine myotonia. Am J Phys Med Rehabil 1992;71(5):279–82.
[2] Pullman SL, Goodin DS, Marquinez AI, et al. Clinical utility of surface EMG. Report of the Therapeutics and Technology Assessment Subcommittee of the American Academy of Neurology Neurology 2000;55:171–7.
[3] Haig AJ, Gelblum JB, Rechtien JJ, et al. Technology assessment: the use of surface EMG in the diagnosis and treatment of nerve and muscle disorders. Muscle Nerve 1996;19:392–5.
[4] Fuglevand AJ, Winter DA, Patla AE, et al. Detection of motor unit action potentials with surface electrodes: influence of electrode size and spacing. Biol Cybern 1992;67:143–53.
[5] Krivickas LS, Taylor A, Maniar RM, et al. Is spectral analysis of the surface electromyographic signal a clinically useful tool for evaluation of skeletal muscle fatigue? J Clin Neurophysiol 1998;15:138–45.
[6] Bromberg MB, Smith AG, Bauerle J. A comparison of two commercial quantitative electromyographic algorithms with manual analysis. Muscle Nerve 1999;22(9):1244–8.
[7] Huppertz HJ, Disselhorst-Klug C, Silny J, et al. Diagnostic yield of noninvasive high spatial resolution electromyography in neuromuscular diseases. Muscle Nerve 1997;20:1360–70.
[8] Milner-Brown HS, Stein RB. The relation between the surface electromyogram and muscular force. J Physiol 1975;246:549–69.
[9] Inman VT, Ralston HJ, Saunders JB, et al. Relation of human electromyogram to muscular tension. EEG Clin Neurophysiol 1952;4:187–94.
[10] Lippold OCJ. The relation between integrated action potentials in a human muscle and its isometric tension. J Physiol 1952;1:492–9.
[11] Orizio C, Esposito F, Sansone V, et al. Muscle surface mechanical and electrical activities in myotonic dystrophy. Electromyogr Clin Neurophysiol 1997;37:231–9.
[12] Laguency A, Marthan R, Schuermans P, et al. Single fiber EMG and spectral analysis of surface EMG in myotonia congenita with or without transient weakness. Muscle Nerve 1994; 17:248–50.
[13] Priez A, Duchene J, Goubel F. Duchenne muscular dystrophy quantification: a multivariate analysis of surface EMG. Med Biol Eng Comput 1992;30:283–91.
[14] van der Hoeven JH, Links TP, Zwarts MJ, et al. Muscle fiber conduction velocity in the diagnosis of familial hypokalemic periodic paralysis—invasive versus surface determination. Muscle Nerve 1994;17:898–905.
[15] Lindeman E, Spaans F, Reulen J, et al. Progressive resistance training in neuromuscular patients. Effects on force and surface EMG. J Electromyogr Kinesiol 1999;9(6):379–84.
[16] Barry DT, Gordon KE, Hinton GG. Acoustic and surface EMG diagnosis of pediatric muscle disease. Muscle Nerve 1990;13:286–90.
[17] Bigland-Ritchie B, Donovan EF, Roussos CS. Conduction velocity and EMG power spectrum changes in fatigue of sustained maximal efforts. J Appl Physiol 1981;51:1300–5.
[18] Arendt-Nielsen L, Mills KR. The relationship between mean power frequency of the EMG spectrum and muscle fibre conduction velocity. Electroencephalogr Clin Neurophysiol 1985; 60:130–4.
[19] DeAngelis GC, Gilmore LD, DeLuca CJ. Standardized evaluation of techniques for measuring the spectral compression of the myoelectric signal. IEEE Trans Biomed Eng 1990;37(9): 844–9.

[20] Edwards RG, Lippold OCJ. The relationship between force and integrated electrical activity in fatigued muscle. J Physiol 1956;132:677–81.

[21] Hof AL. Errors in frequency parameters of EMG power spectra. IEEE Trans Biomed Eng 1991;38:1077–88.

[22] Hermens HJ, Boon KL, Zilvold G. The clinical use of surface EMG. Acta Belg Med Phys 1986;9:119–30.

[23] Braakhekke JP, Stegeman DF, Joosten EM. Increase in median power frequency of the myo-electric signal in pathological fatigue. Electroencephalogr Clin Neurophysiol 1989;73:151–6.

[24] Klein AB. Comparison of spinal mobility and isometric trunk extensor forces with electro-myographic spectral analysis in identifying low back pain. Phys Ther 1991;1:445–54.

[25] Lind AR, Petrofsky JS. Amplitude of the surface electromyogram during fatiguing isometric contractions. Muscle Nerve 1979;2:257–64.

[26] Bigland-Ritchie B, Cafarelli E, Vollestad NK. Fatigue of submaximal static contractions. Acta Physiol Scand Suppl 1986;556:137–48.

[27] Bazzy AR, Korten JB, Haddad GG. Increase in electromyogram low-frequency power in nonfatigued contracting skeletal muscle. J Appl Physiol 1986;61:1012–7.

[28] Dillingham TR. Electrodiagostic approach to patients with weakness. Phys Med Rehabil Clin N Am 2003;14(2):163–84.

[29] Srinivasan J, Amato AA. Myopathies. Phys Med Rehabil Clin N Am 2003;14(2):403–34.

[30] Desmedt JE, Borenstein S. Regeneration in Duchenne Muscular Dystrophy. Arch Neurol 1976;33(9):642–50.

[31] DiMario JX, Uzman A, Strohman RC. Fiber regeneration is not persistent in dystrophic (MDX) mouse skeletal muscle. Dev Biol 1991;148(1):314–21.

[32] Cohn RD, Campbell KP. Molecular basis of muscular dystrophies. Muscle Nerve 2000;23:1456–71.

[33] Chamberlain JS. Gene therapy of muscular dystrophy. Hum Mol Genet 2002;11(20):2355–62.

[34] Campbell KP, Kahl SD. Association of dystrophin and an integral membrane glycoprotein. Nature 1989;338:259–62.

[35] Abresch RT, Walsh SA, Wineinger MA. Animal models of neuromuscular diseases: patho-physiology and implications for rehabilitation. Phys Med Rehabil N Am 1998;9:285–99.

[36] Allamand V, Campbell KP. Animal models for muscular dystrophy: valuable tools for the development of therapies. Hum Mol Genet 2000;9:2459–67.

[37] Carter GT, Kikuchi N, Abresch RT, et al. Effects of exhaustive concentric and eccentric ex-ercise on murine skeletal muscle. Arch Phys Med Rehabil 1994;75(5):555–9.

[38] Cooper BJ. Animal models of Duchenne and Becker muscular dystrophy. Br Med Bull 1989;45:703–18.

[39] Bulfield G, Siller WG, Wight PA, Moore KJ. X chromosome-linked muscular dystrophy (mdx) in the mouse. Proc Natl Acad Sci USA 1984;81:1189–92.

[40] Wineinger MA, Carter GT, Abresch RT, et al. Effect of aging on the histological, biochem-ical and contractile properties of dystrophin-deficient (mdx) mice. J Cell Biochem 1994;18:525–6.

[41] Carter GT, Kikuchi N, Horasek S, et al. The use of fluorescent dextrans as a marker of sar-colemmal injury. Histo Histopathol 1994;9(3):443–7.

[42] Carter GT, Wineinger MA, Walsh SA, et al. Effect of voluntary wheel-running exercise on muscles of the mdx mouse. Neuromusc Disord 1995;5(4):323–31.

[43] Mallouk N, Jacquemond V, Allard B. Elevated subsarcolemmal Ca2 + in mdx mouse skel-etal muscle fibers detected with Ca2 +-activated K + channels. Proc Natl Acad Sci USA 2000;97(9):4950–5.

[44] Denetclaw WF Jr, Hopf FW, Cox GA, et al. Myotubes from transgenic mdx mice expressing full-length dystrophin show normal calcium regulation. Mol Biol Cell 1994;5(10):1159–67.

[45] Petrof B, Shrager JB, Stedman HH, et al. Dystrophin protects the sarcolemma from stresses developed during muscle contraction. Proc Natl Acad Sci USA 1993;90:3710–4.

[46] McNeil PL, Ito S. Molecular traffic through plasma membrane disruptions of cells in vivo. J Cell Sci 1990;96:549–56.

[47] McNeil PL, Khakee R. Disruptions of muscle fiber plasma membranes. Role in exercise-induced damage. Am J Pathol 1992;140:1097–109.

[48] Fong P, Turner PR, Denetclaw WF, et al. Increased activity of calcium leak channels in my-otubes of Duchenne human and mdx mouse origin. Science 1990;250:673–6.

[49] Lynch GS, Hinkle RT, Chamberlain JS, et al. Force and power output of fast and slow skel-etal muscles from mdx mice 6–28 months old. J Physiol 2001;1(535):591–600.

[50] Lynch GS, Rafael JA, Chamberlain JS, et al. Contraction-induced injury to single permea-bilized muscle fibers from mdx, transgenic mdx, and control mice. Am J Physiol 2000;279(4): 1290–4.

[51] McArdle A, Edwards RH, Jackson MJ. Effects of contractile activity on muscle damage in the dystrophin-deficient mdx mouse. Clin Sci 1991;80:367–71.

[52] Head SI, Williams DA, Stephenson DG. Abnormalities in structure and function of limb skeletal muscle fibres of dystrophic mdx mice. Proc R Soc Lond 1992;248:163–9.

[53] Dellorusso C, Crawford RW, Chamberlain JS, et al. Tibialis anterior muscles in mdx mice are highly susceptible to contraction-induced injury. J Muscle Res Cell Motil 2001;22(5): 467–75.

[54] Straub V, Rafael JA, Chamberlain JS, et al. Animal models for muscular dystrophy show different patterns of sarcolemmal disruption. J Cell Biol 1997;139:375–85.

[55] Carter GT, Longley KJ, Entrikin RK. Electromyographic and nerve conduction studies in the mdx mouse. Am J Phys Med Rehabil 1992;71(1):2–5.

[56] Wineinger MA, Abresch RT, Walsh SA, et al. Effects of aging and voluntary exercise on the function of dystrophic muscle from mdx mice. Am J Phys Med Rehabil 1998;77(1):20–7.

[57] Carter GT, Abresch RT, Fowler WM. Adaptations to exercise training and contraction-induced muscle injury in animal models of neuromuscular disease. Am J Phys Med Rehabil 2002;81:151–9.

[58] Carter GT, Abresch RT, Walsh SA, et al. The mdx mouse diaphragm: exercise-induced injury. Muscle Nerve 1997;20:393–4.

[59] Vilquin JT, Brussee V, Asselin I, et al. Evidence of mdx mouse skeletal muscle fragility in vivo by eccentric running exercise. Muscle Nerve 1998;21:567–76.

[60] McArdle A, Edwards RH, Jackson MJ. Accumulation of calcium by normal and dystro-phin-deficient mouse muscle during contractile activity in vitro. Clin Sci 1992;82:455–9.

[61] Franco A, Lansman JB. Mechanosensitive ion channels in skeletal muscle from normal and dystrophic mice. J Physiol 1994;481:299–309.

[62] Hocherman SD, Bezanilla F. A patch-clamp study of delayed rectifier currents in skeletal muscle of control and mdx mice. J Physiol 1996;493:113–28.

[63] Han JJ, Ra JJ, Abresch RT, Robinson LR, et al. Electromyographic characterization of the mdx mouse, an animal model for Duchenne muscular dystrophy. Am J Phys Med Rehabil 2005;84(3):202 [abstr].

[64] Carnwath JW, Shotton DM. Muscular dystrophy in the mdx mouse: histopathology of the soleus and extensor digitorum longus muscles. J Neurol Sci 1987;80(1):39–54.

[65] Friedrich O, Both M, Gillis JM, et al. Mini-dystrophin restores L-type calcium currents in skeletal muscle of transgenic mdx mice. J Physiol 2004;15:251–65.

[66] Weller B, Karpati G, Carpenter S. Dystrophin-deficient mdx muscle fibers are preferentially vulnerable to necrosis induced by experimental lengthening contractions. J Neurol Sci 1990; 100:9–13.

[67] Dick JR, Vrbova GA. Progressive deterioration of muscles in mdx mice induced by overload. Clin Sci 1993;84:145–50.

[68] Sacco P, Jones DA, Dick JR, et al. Contractile properties and susceptibility to exercise-induced damage of normal and mdx mouse tibialis anterior muscle. Clin Sci 1992;82:227–36.

[69] Reimann J, Irintchev A, Wernig A. Regenerative capacity and the number of satellite cells in soleus muscles of normal and mdx mice. Neuromuscul Disord 2000;10(4–5):276–82.

[70] McDonald CM, Abresch RT, Carter GT, et al. Profiles of neuromuscular disease: Duchenne muscular dystrophy. Am J Phys Med Rehabil 1995;74(5):70–92.

[71] Brooks SV. Rapid recovery following contraction-induced injury to in situ skeletal muscles in mdx mice. J Muscle Res Cell Motil 1998;19:179–87.

[72] Moens P, Baatsen PH, Marechal G. Increased susceptibility of EDL muscles from mdx mice to damage induced by contractions with stretch. J Muscle Res Cell Motil 1993;14:446–51.

[73] Lynch GS, Hayes A, Lam MH, et al. The effects of endurance exercise on dystrophic mdx mice. II. Contractile properties of skinned muscle fibres. Proc R Soc Lond B Biol Sci 1993;253:27–33.

[74] Abresch RT, Fowler WM, Larson DB, et al. Contractile abnormalities in dystrophin-less (mdx) mice. Med Sci Sports Exer 1993;5(5):15–7.

[75] Valentine BA, Kornegay JN, Cooper BJ. Clinical electromyographic studies of canine X-linked muscular dystrophy. Am J Vet Res 1989;50(12):2145–7.

[76] Shields RW Jr. Single fiber electromyography in the differential diagnosis of myopathic limb girdle syndromes and chronic spinal muscular atrophy. Muscle Nerve 1984;7(4):265–72.

[77] Stubgen JP. Limb girdle muscular dystrophy: a quantitative electromyographic study. Electromyogr Clin Neurophysiol 1995;35(6):351–7.

[78] Cruz-Martinez A, Arpa J, Santiago S, et al. Single fiber electromyography (SFEMG) in mitochondrial diseases (MD). Electromyogr Clin Neurophysiol 2004;44(1):35–8.

[79] Szmidt-Salkowska E, Rowinska-Marcinska K, Fidzianska A, et al. Macroemg in manifesting carriers of Duchenne muscular dystrophy. Electromyogr Clin Neurophysiol 1999;39(2): 87–92.

[80] Rowinska-Marcinska K, Szmidt-Salkowska E, Kopec A, et al. Motor unit changes in inflammatory myopathy and progressive muscular dystrophy. Electromyogr Clin Neurophysiol 2000;40(7):431–9.

[81] Cengiz B, Ozdag F, Ulas UH, et al. Discriminant analysis of various concentric needle EMG and macro-EMG parameters in detecting myopathic abnormality. Clin Neurophysiol 2002; 113(9):1423–8.

[82] Constantinides CD, Gillen JS, Boada FE, et al. Human skeletal muscle: sodium MR imaging and quantification-potential applications in exercise and disease. Radiology 2000;216(2): 559–68.

[83] McDonald CM, Carter GT, Fritz RC, et al. Magnetic resonance imaging of denervated muscle: comparison to electromyography. Muscle Nerve 2000;23(9):1431–4.

[84] Argov Z, Arnold DL. MR spectroscopy and imaging in metabolic myopathies. Neurol Clin 2000;18(1):35–52.

[85] Argov Z, Lofberg M, Arnold DL. Insights into muscle diseases gained by phosphorus magnetic resonance spectroscopy. Muscle Nerve 2000;23(9):1316–34.

[86] Meyer RA, Prior BM. Functional magnetic resonance imaging of muscle. Exerc Sport Sci Rev 2000;28(2):89–92.

[87] McCully K, Posner J. Measuring exercise-induced adaptations and injury with magnetic resonance spectroscopy. Int J Sports Med 1992;1:147–9.

[88] McIntosh LM, Baker RE, Anderson JE. Magnetic resonance imaging of regenerating and dystrophic mouse muscle. Biochem Cell Biol 1998;76(2–3):532–41.

[89] Straub V, Donahue KM, Allamand V, et al. Contrast agent-enhanced magnetic resonance imaging of skeletal muscle damage in animal models of muscular dystrophy. Magn Reson Med 2000;44(4):655–9.

ELSEVIER
SAUNDERS

Phys Med Rehabil Clin N Am
16 (2005) 999–1014

PHYSICAL MEDICINE
AND REHABILITATION
CLINICS OF
NORTH AMERICA

Neurotrophic Factors in Neuromuscular Disease

B. Jane Distad, MD, Michael D. Weiss, MD*

*Department of Neurology, University of Washington School of Medicine,
Box 356115, 1959 NE Pacific Street, Seattle, WA 98195, USA*

Neurotrophic factors (NTFs) are small dimeric proteins essential for development, function, maintenance, and plasticity of the vertebrate nervous system [1]. NTFs include glial-derived neurotrophic factor (GDNF), insulin-like growth factor 1 and 2 (IGF-1/2), ciliary neurotrophic factor (CNTF), vascular endothelial growth factor (VEGF) and the neurotrophins nerve growth factor (NGF), brain-derived neurotrophic factor (BDNF), neurotrophin-3 (NT-3), and neurotrophin-4/5 (NT-4/5), and neurotrophin-6 (NT-6). There is considerable evidence demonstrating the importance of NTFs in neuronal maintenance and neural regeneration. NTFs are released following nerve injury by nonneuronal cells in proximity to both neurons and nerve axons. Many of the NTFs then bind with complex membrane receptors. Disruption of NTFs or their receptors resulting from genetic mutations or antibodies to NTFs has been shown to alter neuronal survival [2]. Furthermore, exogenous NTFs at a site of injury have also been found to support survival of various neuronal subpopulations [3].

The neurotrophins BDNF, NT3, and NT4 enhance motor neuron survival through their interactions with tyrosine kinase (Trk) receptors. Other NTFs support motor neurons by exerting their survival-promoting activity through non-Trk, complex membrane receptors. For example, GDNF supports motor neuron survival by acting through receptors involving the c-ret kinase and specific α-receptors. Other growth factors with survival promoting activity for motor neurons include IGF-1/2 and hepatocyte growth factor [4].

In vivo survival of motor neurons often depends on a complex cooperation of more than one factor. NTFs may potentiate each other in supporting motor neuron survival. For example, combining exogenous IGFs with CNTF has an additive effect on enhancing neuronal survival [5]. Also,

---

* Corresponding author.
E-mail address: mdweiss@u.washington.edu (M.D. Weiss).

1047-9651/05/$ - see front matter © 2005 Elsevier Inc. All rights reserved.
doi:10.1016/j.pmr.2005.08.002

although both sympathetic and sensory neurons undergo developmental changes in their responsiveness to NGF, a subpopulation of sensory neurons does not require NGF for survival, but rather BDNF or NT3 [6].

Evidence for the survival effects of NTFs on normal motor neurons has led to a number of experimental studies to determine whether these factors can promote the survival of diseased neurons and nerve regeneration following injury. These studies have involved both in vitro and in vivo models of human diseases involving motor or sensory neurons or peripheral nerves, primarily models for amyotrophic lateral sclerosis (ALS) and peripheral neuropathy. As many of these preclinical studies have demonstrated significant benefit in promoting neuronal survival and function, appropriate NTFs have been tested in a number of clinical trials over the last decade.

Specific neurotrophic factors as therapeutic agents in neuromuscular disease

Nerve growth factor

NGF was identified as a protein influencing nerve growth in the 1950s, and is known to influence sensory neurons of dorsal root ganglia, autonomic sympathetic neurons, and basal forebrain cholinergic neurons [7]. NGF plays a biologic role in the development, maintenance, and survival of sympathetic and small sensory neurons, which express the NGF receptor TrkA [8]. Overexpression of NGF in epidermis in animals has been associated with increased sensory and sympathetic innervation and hypertrophy of sensory and sympathetic ganglia [9]. Also, mutations in the genes for NGF or TrkA have demonstrated a marked reduction in viable sensory and sympathetic neurons [10,11].

Recent evidence suggests a role for NGF in motor neuron disease. NGF is significantly elevated in muscle biopsies [12], lateral columns of spinal cord [13], and spinal motor neurons in ALS. Neurotrophin receptors have shown altered expression in ALS, with an increase in TrkA in motor neurons [14] and decrease in phosphorylated TrkB in spinal cord [15]. Abnormal spinal motor neuron p75 neurotrophic receptor (p75^{NTR}) expression has been identified in studies of transgenic ALS mice [16] and in ALS patients [17]. Recently, elevated reactive astrocyte-derived NGF was linked to accelerated cell death of p75^{NTR}-expressing motor neurons adult transgenic ALS mice [18].

A number of studies in animals and humans have suggested a role for NGF in peripheral neuropathies. Experiments in animals have shown that in the streptozotocin-treated rat model of diabetes mellitus, there is evidence of both decreased NGF production and retrograde transport [19]. Many of the neuronal abnormalities in diabetes can be duplicated by experimental depletion of specific NTFs, especially NGF or other members of the neurotrophin family, their receptors, or their binding proteins. Whether the observed growth factor deficiencies are due to decreased synthesis, or functional, for example, an inability to bind to their receptor, or abnormalities in nerve transport and processing, remains to be established [20]. In patients with vasculitic neuropathy, NGF expression in macrophages has been found to be closely related to the degree of axonal regeneration, suggesting a role in nerve regeneration for this form of neuropathy [21]. NGF has also been demonstrated in animal models to prevent peripheral neuropathies that result from certain chemotherapies, in particular taxol, cisplatin, and vinblastine [22].

Given the findings of preclinical studies of NGF, two randomized, double-blind, placebo-controlled clinical trials of NGF in diabetic neuropathy were recently completed. The first was a phase II trial of 250 patients with painful diabetic neuropathy lasting 6 months [23]. The study used NGF doses of 0.1 and 0.3 µg/kg three times per week. NGF injections caused frequent but mild side effects, mostly injection site hyperalgesia, in more than 90% of patients in both groups. Compared with placebo, NGF-treated patients demonstrated significant improvement in their sensory examination, quantitative sensory tests, and subjective symptom evaluation. However, in a subsequent phase III study of 1019 patients with painful diabetic neuropathy who were followed for 12 months, subcutaneous NGF (0.1 µg/kg 3 days per week) failed to show significant benefit on primary or multiple secondary outcomes that were similar to the phase II trial [24]. In addition to possible effects of lower dose, the results of the phase II study may have been influenced by substantial unblinding of the patients (over 80% in the NGF arm) due to injection site pain. The use of hypertonic saline in the placebo group in the phase III trial is thought to have eliminated this factor.

Conflicting results have also been observed in two randomized, double-blind, placebo-controlled clinical trials with NGF for HIV distal painful sensory neuropathy. In one study, no improvement was seen over 48 weeks in neuropathy severity based on a number of objective and subjective sensory scores [25]. In another recent phase II study of 270 patients followed for 18 weeks, positive treatment effects were observed for global pain assessments and for pin sensitivity [7]. However, as in the phase II diabetic neuropathy NGF trial, a large number of patients (39%) became unblinded due to injection site pain, confounding the results of the study.

Neurotrophin-3

NT-3 plays both a complementary and overlapping role with NGF in the development and maturation of sympathetic neurons. It is also expressed by Schwann cells, and appears to be important for Schwann cell survival and differentiation in adult nerves in the absence of axons [26]. In mice, it is the most abundant neurotrophin during early neuronal development. Sympathetic neuroblasts express both NT-3 and its receptor, tyrosine receptor kinase C (TrkC), and require NT-3 for their proliferation, differentiation, and survival. NT-3 acts in parallel with NGF to promote the survival of postmitotic neurons during late development [2]. NT-3 is synthesized in sympathetic effector tissues and the endogenous factor is retrogradely transported to accumulate within the cell soma. Thus, NT-3, like NGF, is also an effector tissue-derived neurotrophic factor for these neurons in maturity [27].

NT-3 can prevent axotomy-induced sensory neuron loss, and can stimulate sensory neuron differentiation in vitro. Systemic administration of NT-3 has been demonstrated to increase the number of nestin-immunoreactive neurons by two- to threefold in the dorsal root ganglia, following rat sciatic nerve transection. Nestin is a protein produced by neuronal precursor cells, and is involved in differentiation of cells. With systemic administration over 1 month, overall loss of neurons seen at 4 weeks was decreased, but there was no effect on the incidence of apoptotic neurons. NT-3 may prevent neuron loss by stimulating the process of differentiation, rather than by preventing neuron death [28].

NT-3 may play a role in neurodegeneration in ALS. Studies demonstrate it is elevated in ALS muscle [12], but reduced in ALS spinal motor neurons [29]. In studies of gene expression using microarray analysis of laser-captured isolated spinal motor neurons in sporadic ALS autopsied patients, NT-3-TrkC signaling appears to be disrupted. Whereas the expression of TrkC receptor for NT-3 was under expressed and NT-3 was unchanged, the marked downregulation of the transcription factor EGR3 in spinal motor neurons suggests that disruption of sensory-motor connections by decreasing NT-3–TrkC signaling results in motor neuron degeneration [30].

Recent animal studies have suggested that NT-3 might reverse the effects of diabetic neuropathy, neuropathy induced by acrylamide and cisplatin toxicity, and hereditary demyelinating neuropathy. Recombinant adenovirus encoding NT-3 (AdNT-3) was injected intramuscularly into streptozotocin-induced diabetic rats and acrylamide-intoxicated rats partially preventing the slowing of sensory and motor nerve conduction [31]. Administration of recombinant NT-3 by both viral and nonviral vectors showed improvement of cisplatin-induced neuropathy in mice, evident by increased sensory distal latencies electrophysiologically [32]. Another recent study by Sahenk et al [26] looked at the effects of NT-3 injected subcutaneously into nude mice harboring xenografts from patients with Charcot-Marie-Tooth 1A (CMT1A) and into *trembler-j* mice with a peripheral myelin protein-22 mutation following sciatic nerve crush injury. The findings suggested that exogenous NT-3 augmented axonal regeneration in these models for CMT1A, based on morphometric evaluation of myelinated nerve fibers and Schwann cell density. A small, randomized, double-blind, placebo-controlled pilot study by the same investigators of eight patients injected with 150 μg/kg of NT-3 three times a week for 6 months showed significant improvement in Neuropathy Impairment Score and pegboard performance, but not motor function.

Brain-derived neurotrophic factor

BDNF was first purified from porcine brain in 1982, and is widely expressed in the peripheral nervous system and central nervous system (CNS) along with its signaling receptor TrkB [33]. Motor neurons, trigeminal and nodose ganglion sensory neurons, dorsal root ganglia, and populations of CNS neurons are all influenced by BDNF. BDNF clearly affects development of neurons, as mice deficient for the gene for BDNF have substantially reduced numbers of cranial and spinal sensory neurons [34].

BDNF promotes survival of motor neurons after injury, as demonstrated in spinal and cranial neurons [33,35,36]. Previous studies have demonstrated rescue of facial [3,33] and sciatic [36,37] motor neurons from axotomy-induced death following injections of BDNF. In one recent study, over expression of BDNF and GDNF, induced in avulsed and reimplanted animal ventral roots using gene transfer techniques, resulted in an increased survival of motoneurons, most prominent at 1 month, and persistent expression of these NTFs in spinal cord for 16 weeks [38].

Preclinical studies using BDNF in animal models for human disease have been performed in the *wobbler* mouse, a model for motor neuron disease [39,40]. *Wobbler* mice treated with subcutaneous injections of BDNF at doses of 5.0 mg/kg three times per week demonstrated slowing of the rate of decline of grip strength compared with placebo-treated mice. Following 4 weeks of treatment, grip strength was increased twofold, and in vivo muscle twitch tension 30%, compared with controls. As the number of viable motor neurons did not appear changed relative to controls, it was concluded that BDNF does not just promote motor neuron survival but also enhances the function of preserved motor neurons [39].

Based on the findings in animal studies, three randomized double blind, placebo-controlled trials of BDNF in ALS have been performed [41–43]. In the phase I/II study [41], 283 patients were given subcutaneous injections of placebo or BDNF at doses between 10 and 300 µg/kg/day and followed for 6 months. The BDNF-treated patients showed a significant decrease in the decline in walking speed compared with the placebo-treated group. Additionally, patients injected with BDNF at doses ranging from 25 to 150 µg/kg/day demonstrated a smaller decline in forced vital capacity (FVC) of 11.5% to 15.5% compared with a 20% decline in the placebo-treated patients. Overall the medication was well tolerated, although mild injection site irritation was seen in a number of patients. No change in survival or muscle strength was noted in the BDNF-treated group.

Given the promising results of the phase I/II trial, a phase III study of BDNF in ALS was performed in which 1135 patients were treated with placebo or BDNF at doses ranging from 25 to 100 µg/kg/day [42]. No significant differences between the placebo and BDNF-treated patients were noted for the primary endpoints of survival, FVC, walking speed, and other ALS measures. The statistical power of the phase III trial may have been diminished due to a higher survival rate of 85% for the placebo group in that study compared with a survival rate of 73% in the phase I/II trial. However, post hoc analysis did show that BDNF injections increased 9-month survival in patients with more advanced ALS receiving 100 µg/kg/day with FVC $\geq 91\%$ of predicted and those with serum chloride ≤ 100 mEq. Additionally, for the 20% of patients receiving 100 µg/kg/day of BDNF who suffered altered bowel function as a consequence of therapy, suggesting an effective medication dose, 9-month survival was significantly increased compared with that of placebo-treated patients (97.5% versus 85%).

In an attempt to improve delivery of BDNF to the CNS, a recent 12-week phase I/II randomized double-blind placebo-controlled trial of intrathecal BDNF in 25 patients with ALS was completed [43]. Patients were given escalating doses of BDNF ranging from 25 to 1000 µg/day. Mild side effects were common, especially at higher doses (>150 µg/day), and included paresthesias or a sense of increased warmth that often necessitated dose reductions. Although treatment of ALS patients with intrathecal BDNF was concluded to be feasible, given the study design, no conclusions could be made in regard to efficacy.

Ciliary neurotrophic factor

CNTF is a neuroactive cytokine found in Schwann cells, likely released in the setting of nerve injury. CNTF binds to complexes that exert their survival-promoting activity through complex membrane receptors involving gp130 and LIFR-α [4]. CNTF reduces motor neuron cell death in various rodent models. At adequate concentrations, CNTF supports the survival of embryonic rat and human motor neurons in tissue culture [44]. CNTF also appears to have a role in sensory neuron function. For example, thermal hypoalgesia, produced in rats with streptozotocin-induced diabetes, is prevented by treatment with CNTF [45].

Given evidence for neuroprotection by CNTF in rodents, two randomized double-blind placebo-controlled trials of CNTF in ALS were recently conducted. In one trial of 730 patients with ALS, no benefit was noted for subcutaneous injections of CNTF at doses of either 15 µg/kg or 30 µg/kg, and dose-limiting toxicity, including anorexia, weight loss, and cough, was seen at the higher dose [46]. No beneficial effect was seen in a second study of 570 patients randomized to receive placebo or 0.5, 2, or 5 µg/kg/day of CNTF in primary or secondary endpoints, including limb megascores and pulmonary function [47].

Glial cell line-derived neurotrophic factor

GDNF is a member of the GDNF family ligands, which are important for the development, survival, and maintenance of distinct populations of central and peripheral neurons. These factors signal through a multicomponent receptor complex comprising a glycosylphosphatidylinositol-anchored cell surface molecule (GDNF family receptor α) and Ret Trk, triggering the activation of multiple signaling pathways in responsive cells. GDNF is expressed in skeletal muscle, Schwann cells, neurons, astrocytes, and oligodendrocytes, and promotes embryonic motor neuron survival in vitro and in vivo [48].

Many studies have supported the role of GDNF as a survival factor for motor neurons and midbrain dopaminergic neurons. For example, in mice deficient for GDNF receptors, a 20% to 30% loss of motor neuron subpopulations has been reported [35,49]. Markedly increased survival of brachial, lumbar, and thoracic motor neurons following neonatal facial nerve axotomy has been observed in transgenic mice overexpressing GDNF [48]. Overexpression of GDNF using gene transfer is associated with a reduction of motor neuron loss following axotomy in neonatal rodents, although the effect may be transient or incomplete [36,49]. GDNF has also been shown to induce axonal outgrowth in vitro using organotypic spinal cord cultures and is neuroprotective against excitotoxic motor neuron degeneration [50].

A number of recent preclinical studies have explored a possible role for gene delivered GDNF as a treatment for motor neuron disease. Intramuscular injection of adeno-associated viral vector containing the gene for GDNF (AAV-GDNF) has been shown to result in substantial expression of transgenic GDNF persisting for months, and its delivery to spinal motoneurons by retrograde transport [51]. Additionally, injection of AAV-GDNF was found to prevent motor neuron loss, postpone disease onset, delay the progression of motor dysfunction, and prolong life span when injected into transgenic ALS mice [52–54]. A single clinical trial of intrathecal administration of GDNF in ALS failed to show any benefit [55].

Insulin-like growth factor-1

IGF-1, a member of the insulin and proinsulin family of structurally related proteins, has endocrine, paracrine, and autocrine effects on cells. It acts through a receptor that is structurally and functionally similar to the insulin receptor. The IGF signaling system is complex, involving several cell surface receptors, circulating and bound binding proteins, and specific proteases that recognize and cleave individual binding proteins. Recent evidence suggests that IGF-1 acts not only on nonneuronal cells but is also a neurotrophic factor. IGF-1 has been shown to affect developing sympathetic and sensory neurons to increase neurite outgrowth and promote survival [56]. The IGF-1 receptor is widely expressed in the nervous system. IGF-1 mRNA has been identified in mammalian nerve, motor, and sensory neurons, autonomic ganglion neurons, and skeletal muscle [57]. IGF-I likely affects all components of the motor unit: spinal cord motor neuron, axon, neuromuscular synapse, and muscle fiber, and IGF-I probably acts as a potent life signal on such cells [58].

IGF appears to have survival-promoting activity for motor neurons as demonstrated in a number of animal studies. In mice, IGF-1 and IGF-1 mRNA has been shown to be upregulated in the facial nucleus follow facial nerve axotomy [59], and in the segment of sciatic nerve at and distal to a site of injury [60,61]. Subcutaneous injections of IGF-1 following lesioning of sciatic nerve may enhance axonal regeneration in adult rodents [62] and prevent motoneuron death in neonatal mice [37]. Additionally, antibodies to IGF-1 and IGF-2 were found to inhibit axonal regeneration after crush injury of ventral root in rodents [63]. The ability of IGF-1 to reduce atrophy resulting from denervation was recently examined after transection of the sciatic nerve in transgenic mLC/mIGF-1 mice that overexpress mIGF-1 specifically in differentiated myofibers. Overexpression of mIGF-1 reduced the rate of denervation-induced myofiber atrophy by approximately 30% and preserved myofibers with larger cross-sectional area, compared with wild-type muscles [64].

A number of animal studies have focused on survival effects of IGF-1 in motor neuron disease. *Wobbler* mice treated with subcutaneous IGF-1 at doses of 1.0 mg/kg/day for 6 weeks demonstrated a 40% increase in grip strength and a significant increase in muscle fiber diameter compared with controls, although no difference in the number of spinal motor neurons was noted [65]. Coadministration of subcutaneous IGF-1 and glycosaminoglycans was found to delay the onset of disease and motor neuron death in *wobbler* mice by 9 to 12 weeks [66]. Mice expressing the gene for a mutated form of superoxide dismutase-1 (SOD1) given intramuscular injections of AAV-IGF-1 had prolongation of life and delayed disease progression [67]. In another recent study, transgenic ALS mice were treated by continuous IGF-1 delivery into the intrathecal space of the lumbar spinal cord. The treated mice demonstrated improved motor performance, delayed onset of clinical disease, and extended survival, as well as a reduction of motor neuron loss [68].

Two randomized double-blind placebo-controlled phase III studies of IGF-1 in ALS have been completed. In a North American study [69], 266 ALS patients were administered twice daily subcutaneous injections for 9 months of IGF-1 at doses of 0.05 mg/kg/day or 0.1 mg/kg/day or placebo. Although IGF-1 was well-tolerated, some patients did experience a mild injection site reaction. The primary endpoint was a difference in the rate of change of the Appel ALS Rating Scale (AALS), which is a measure of clinical function. The group treated with the higher dose exhibited a significantly slower rate of decline (26% decrease compared with placebo) and about half the relative risk for a 20-point deterioration on the AALS or for progressing to the early terminal stage. Additionally, the high dose-treated patients had a significantly higher score on the Sickness Impact Profile scale.

In a phase III trial conducted in Europe [70], 183 patients were injected twice a day with subcutaneous IGF-1 at doses of 0.1 mg/kg/day of IGF-1 or placebo for 9 months in a study design similar to the North American trial. No significant differences were noted in IGF-1–treated patients compared with placebo-treated in progression of disease, measured by the AALS score or Sickness Impact Profile scale. In fact, there was a greater number of deaths in the IGF-1 treatment group than in the control group (15% versus 8%), although not statistically significant. The discrepancy between the two phase III studies has been suggested to relate to the smaller sample size of the European Study, likely decreasing statistical power. Another phase III, randomized, double-blind placebo-controlled North American study of IGF-1 in ALS is currently enrolling patients.

Vascular endothelial-derived growth factor

Although VEGF has long been considered to be an endothelial cell-specific factor important for angiogenesis, there is emerging evidence that it has a direct protective effect on neural cells [71]. VEGF exerts its neuroprotective actions through the inhibition of programmed cell death and the stimulation of neurogenesis [72]. Recent studies suggest that VEGF may be an important neurotrophic/survival factor in motor neuron disease. In a model of X-linked spinobulbar muscular atrophy, a reduction of VEGF was noted. Additionally, mutant androgen receptor-induced death of motor neuron-like cells was rescued by VEGF [73]. Intracerebroventricular delivery of VEGF in a rat model of ALS was associated with delayed onset of paralysis, improved motor performance, and substantially increased [74]. In another recent study, intramuscular injection of a VEGF-expressing lentiviral vector was shown to delay the onset and slow the progression of ALS in SOD1 mice. VEGF treatment increased the life expectancy of the ALS mice by 30% without causing toxic side effects [75].

In studies of ALS patients, VEGF was recently found to have a role as a modifier of motor neuron degeneration. In a meta-analysis of 1900 Northern European ALS patients, subjects homozygous for certain mutations in the VEGF promoter/leader sequence had a 1.8 times greater risk of ALS ($P = 0.00004$) [71]. In the same study, SOD1(G93A) mice crossbred with transgenic mice deficient for VEGF were shown to die substantially earlier due to more severe motor neuron degeneration. These mice were unusually susceptible to persistent paralysis after spinal cord ischemia. Treatment with exogenous VEGF was able to protect the VEGF-deficient mutants against ischemia-induced motor neuron cell death [71].

Future directions

To date, human studies involving the treatment of neurologic diseases by NTFs have been limited in their success. There are many potential reasons for the failure of these agents, including inadequate drug delivery, difficulty crossing the blood–brain barrier, bioavailability, and toxicity. Additionally, it is difficult to extrapolate the results of treatment trials in animal models to neuromuscular diseases in humans. For instance, the most commonly used animal model for sporadic ALS is the SOD1 transgenic mouse, yet this mutant is really a model for familial ALS.

Uncovering the functions as well as interactions of an ever increasing number of growth factors, especially those that support neuronal survival, could lead to more opportunities for therapeutic intervention in the future. For instance, hepatocyte growth factor is a heterodimeric protein with similarities to plasminogen, and influences survival only of subpopulations of motor neurons. Pigment epithelium-derived factor (PEDF) is a retinal trophic and antiangiogenic factor for the eye that is present in the CNS and is also a motor neuron protectant. In ALS, PEDF levels were found to be significantly elevated in the CSF compared with neurologic controls [76]. Fibroblast growth factor-1 is one of a family of fibroblast growth factors that regulates cell growth, differentiation, inflammation, and angiogenesis, and is selectively expressed in certain neuronal populations. It has potent neurotrophic and neurite-stimulating activity in vitro, and exerts beneficial effects in models of spinal cord injury and axon regeneration. FGF-1 released as a result of oxidative stress may have a role in activating astrocytes, which could initiate motor neuron apoptosis in ALS through a $p75^{NTR}$-dependent mechanism mutation [77]. Blockage of its release might decrease neuronal injury.

Other approaches to implementing NTFs as therapy need to be considered. Combining different NTFs could be of value. There is some experimental evidence that motor neuron survival may require the synergistic effect of NTFs. For instance, the combination of BDNF and GDNF reduced motor neuron death after axotomy more than either factor alone [78]. In another study, a combination of exogenous CNTF and BDNF in *wobbler* mice was found to arrest paw deformity [39].

NTFs have a short half-life when injected peripherally, sometimes lasting only for a few hours. They are also often significantly metabolized before they cross the blood–brain barrier or have great difficulty in getting into the CNS. Finding the optimal approach to delivering exogenous NTFs into the CNS is of great importance. In addition to gene transfer techniques already mentioned earlier, xenogenic cells, which release bioactive substances when implanted into animals, may be a useful therapeutic technique as they can be directly implanted into the CNS. For example, a recent study demonstrated that baby hamster kidney cells releasing human CNTF can survive up to 20 weeks when implanted intrathecally [79].

Other novel approaches to employing NTFs as therapy include the use of neural stem cells (NSCs). In addition to giving rise to neurons and or glia, neural stem cells in vitro have been shown to release GDNF and NGF into culture media, which could benefit injured neurons [50]. NSCs are capable of being implanted into lesioned areas of brain and replacing damaged neurons

Table 1
Clinical trials of neurotrophic factors

Neurotrophic factor	Phase[a]	Neurologic disease	Number of subjects	Benefit	Reference
NGF	II	Neuropathy (DM)	250	Positive	[23]
NGF	II	Neuropathy (HIV)	270	Positive	[7]
NGF	II	Neuropathy (HIV)	200	Negative	[25]
NGF	III	Neuropathy (DM)	1019	Negative	[24]
NT-3	II	Neuropathy (CMT1A)	8	Possible	[26]
BDNF	I/II	ALS	283	Positive	[41]
BDNF	III	ALS	1135	Possible	[42]
CNTF	III	ALS	730	Negative	[46]
CNTF	III	ALS	570	Negative	[47]
GDNF	I/II-intraventricular	ALS	?	Negative	[55]
IGF-1	III	ALS	266	Positive	[69]
IGF-1	III	ALS	183	Negative	[70]

Abbreviations: BDNF, brain-derived neurotrophic factor; CMT1A, Charcot-Marie-Tooth disease type 1A; CNTF, ciliary neurotrophic factor; DM, diabetes mellitus; GDNF, glial-derived neurotrophic factor; HIV, human immunodeficiency virus; IGF-1; insulin-like growth factor 1; NGF, nerve growth factor; NT-3, neurotrophin-3.

[a] Neurotrophic factors were administered subcutaneously unless indicated. Only trials that assessed efficacy are shown.

or delivering therapeutic gene products [80–84]. Targeting neurotrophic receptors could also be important for therapy. Neurotrophic receptors may be key regulators in promoting neuronal survival and neurite outgrowth via complex signaling pathways. For example, the Shc adapter proteins can couple trk-signaling to the Ras/MAP-kinase pathway, which has been shown to be involved in promoting neuronal survival and neurite outgrowth [4]. Agents that can mimic specific NTFs and activate neurotrophic receptors directly could have therapeutic potential.

Summary

Over the last decade, much has been learned about the effects of NTFs in both animals and humans. Preclinical studies have led to a more sophisticated understanding of the role of these agents in supporting neurons and peripheral nerve. A number of small clinical trials have demonstrated modest benefit of certain NTFs (Table 1), in particular IGF-1 and NGF, for peripheral neuropathies and motor neuron disease. However, the results of the few large trials that have been conducted have been disappointing, either due to lack of efficacy or drug toxicity. Although NTFs remain promising therapeutic agents, additional research is required to bring them to the bedside.

References

[1] Chao MV. Trophic factors: an evolutionary cul-de-sac or door into higher neuronal function? J Neurosci Res 2000;59(3):353–5.

[2] Farinas I, Jones KR, Backus C, et al. Severe sensory and sympathetic deficits in mice lacking neurotrophin-3. Nature 1994;369(6482):658–61.

[3] Serpe CJ, Byram SC, Sanders VM, et al. Brain-derived neurotrophic factor supports facial motoneuron survival after facial nerve transection in immunodeficient mice. Brain Behav Immun 2005;19(2):173–80.

[4] Sendtner M, Pei G, Beck M, et al. Developmental motoneuron cell death and neurotrophic factors. Cell Tissue Res 2000;301(1):71–84.

[5] Arakawa Y, Sendtner M, Thoenen H. Survival effect of ciliary neurotrophic factor (CNTF) on chick embryonic motoneurons in culture: comparison with other neurotrophic factors and cytokines. J Neurosci 1990;10(11):3507–15.

[6] Vogel KS. Development of trophic interactions in the vertebrate peripheral nervous system. Mol Neurobiol 1993;7(3–4):363–82.

[7] McArthur JC, Yiannoutsos C, Simpson DM, et al. A phase II trial of nerve growth factor for sensory neuropathy associated with HIV infection. AIDS Clinical Trials Group Team 291. Neurology 2000;54(5):1080–8.

[8] Dyck PJ, Peroutka S, Rask C, et al. Intradermal recombinant human nerve growth factor induces pressure allodynia and lowered heat-pain threshold in humans. Neurology 1997; 48(2):501–5.

[9] Albers KM, Wright DE, Davis BM. Overexpression of nerve growth factor in epidermis of transgenic mice causes hypertrophy of the peripheral nervous system. J Neurosci 1994; 14(3 Pt 2):1422–32.

[10] Crowley C, Spencer SD, Nishimura MC, et al. Mice lacking nerve growth factor display perinatal loss of sensory and sympathetic neurons yet develop basal forebrain cholinergic neurons. Cell 1994;76(6):1001–11.

[11] Smeyne RJ, Klein R, Schnapp A, et al. Severe sensory and sympathetic neuropathies in mice carrying a disrupted Trk/NGF receptor gene. Nature 1994;368(6468):246–9.

[12] Kust BM, Copray JC, Brouwer N, et al. Elevated levels of neurotrophins in human biceps brachii tissue of amyotrophic lateral sclerosis. Exp Neurol 2002;177(2):419–27.

[13] Anand P, Parrett A, Martin J, et al. Regional changes of ciliary neurotrophic factor and nerve growth factor levels in post mortem spinal cord and cerebral cortex from patients with motor disease. Nat Med 1995;1(2):168–72.

[14] Nishio T, Sunohara N, Furukawa S. Neutrophin switching in spinal motoneurons of amyotrophic lateral sclerosis. Neuroreport 1998;9(7):1661–5.

[15] Mutoh T, Sobue G, Hamano T, et al. Decreased phosphorylation levels of TrkB neurotrophin receptor in the spinal cords from patients with amyotrophic lateral sclerosis. Neurochem Res 2000;25(2):239–45.

[16] Lowry KS, Murray SS, McLean CA, et al. A potential role for the p75 low-affinity neurotrophin receptor in spinal motor neuron degeneration in murine and human amyotrophic lateral sclerosis. Amyotroph Lateral Scler Other Motor Neuron Disord 2001;2(3):127–34.

[17] Kerkhoff H, Jennekens FG, Troost D, et al. Nerve growth factor receptor immunostaining in the spinal cord and peripheral nerves in amyotrophic lateral sclerosis. Acta Neuropathol (Berl) 1991;81(6):649–56.

[18] Turner BJ, Murray SS, Piccenna LG, et al. Effect of p75 neurotrophin receptor antagonist on disease progression in transgenic amyotrophic lateral sclerosis mice. J Neurosci Res 2004; 78(2):193–9.

[19] Brewster WJ, Fernyhough P, Diemel LT, et al. Diabetic neuropathy, nerve growth factor and other neurotrophic factors. Trends Neurosci 1994;17(8):321–5.

[20] Pittenger G, Vinik A. Nerve growth factor and diabetic neuropathy. Exp Diabesity Res 2003; 4(4):271–85.

[21] Mitsuma N, Yamamoto M, Iijima M, et al. Wide range of lineages of cells expressing nerve growth factor mRNA in the nerve lesions of patients with vasculitic neuropathy: an implication of endoneurial macrophage for nerve regeneration. Neuroscience 2004;129(1): 109–17.

[22] Yuen EC, Howe CL, Li Y, et al. Nerve growth factor and the neurotrophic factor hypothesis. Brain Dev 1996;18(5):362–8.

[23] Apfel SC, Kessler JA, Adornato BT, et al. Recombinant human nerve growth factor in the treatment of diabetic polyneuropathy. NGF Study Group. Neurology 1998;51(3):695–702.

[24] Apfel SC, Schwartz S, Adornato BT, et al. Efficacy and safety of recombinant human nerve growth factor in patients with diabetic polyneuropathy: a randomized controlled trial. rhNGF Clinical Investigator Group. JAMA 2000;284(17):2215–21.

[25] Schifitto G, Yiannoutsos C, Simpson DM, et al. Long-term treatment with recombinant nerve growth factor for HIV-associated sensory neuropathy. Neurology 2001;57(7):1313–6.

[26] Sahenk Z, Nagaraja HN, McCracken BS, et al. NT-3 promotes nerve regeneration and sensory improvement in CMT1A mouse models and in patients. Neurology 2005;65:681–9.

[27] Zhou XF, Chie ET, Deng YS, et al. Rat mature sympathetic neurones derive neurotrophin 3 from peripheral effector tissues. Eur J Neurosci 1997;9(12):2753–64.

[28] Kuo LT, Simpson A, Schanzer A, et al. Effects of systemically administered NT-3 on sensory neuron loss and nestin expression following axotomy. J Comp Neurol 2005;482(4): 320–32.

[29] Duberley RM, Johnson IP, Anand P, et al. Neurotrophin-3-like immunoreactivity and Trk C expression in human spinal motoneurones in amyotrophic lateral sclerosis. J Neurol Sci 1997;148(1):33–40.

[30] Jiang YM, Yamamoto M, Kobayashi Y, et al. Gene expression profile of spinal motor neurons in sporadic amyotrophic lateral sclerosis. Ann Neurol 2005;57(2):236–51.

[31] Pradat PF, Kennel P, Naimi-Sadaoui S, et al. Continuous delivery of neurotrophin 3 by gene therapy has a neuroprotective effect in experimental models of diabetic and acrylamide neuropathies. Hum Gene Ther 2001;12(18):2237–49.

[32] Pradat PF, Finiels F, Kennel P, et al. Partial prevention of cisplatin-induced neuropathy by electroporation-mediated nonviral gene transfer. Hum Gene Ther 2001;12(4):367–75.

[33] Koliatsos VE, Clatterbuck RE, Winslow JW, et al. Evidence that brain-derived neurotrophic factor is a trophic factor for motor neurons in vivo. Neuron 1993;10(3):359–67.

[34] Jones KR, Farinas I, Backus C, et al. Targeted disruption of the BDNF gene perturbs brain and sensory neuron development but not motor neuron development. Cell 1994;76(6): 989–99.

[35] Henderson CE, Camu W, Mettling C, et al. Neurotrophins promote motor neuron survival and are present in embryonic limb bud. Nature 1993;363(6426):266–70.

[36] Yan Q, Elliott J, Snider WD. Brain-derived neurotrophic factor rescues spinal motor neurons from axotomy-induced cell death. Nature 1992;360(6406):753–5.

[37] Li L, Oppenheim RW, Lei M, et al. Neurotrophic agents prevent motoneuron death following sciatic nerve section in the neonatal mouse. J Neurobiol 1994;25(7):759–66.

[38] Blits B, Carlstedt TP, Ruitenberg MJ, et al. Rescue and sprouting of motoneurons following ventral root avulsion and reimplantation combined with intraspinal adeno-associated viral vector-mediated expression of glial cell line-derived neurotrophic factor or brain-derived neurotrophic factor. Exp Neurol 2004;189(2):303–16.

[39] Mitsumoto H, Ikeda K, Klinkosz B, et al. Arrest of motor neuron disease in wobbler mice cotreated with CNTF and BDNF. Science 1994;265(5175):1107–10.

[40] Mitsumoto H, Bradley WG. Murine motor neuron disease (the wobbler mouse): degeneration and regeneration of the lower motor neuron. Brain 1982;105(Pt 4):811–34.

[41] Bradley WG. A phase I/II study of recombinant brain-derived neurotrophic in patients with ALS. Ann Neurol 1995;38:971.

[42] The BDNF Study Group (Phase III). A controlled trial of recombinant methionyl human BDNF in ALS. Neurology 1999;52(7):1427–33.

[43] Ochs G, Penn RD, York M, et al. A phase I/II trial of recombinant methionyl human brain derived neurotrophic factor administered by intrathecal infusion to patients with amyotrophic lateral sclerosis. Amyotroph Lateral Scler Other Motor Neuron Disord 2000;1(3): 201–6.

[44] The ALS CNTF Treatment Study (ACTS) Phase I–II Study Group. The pharmacokinetics of subcutaneously administered recombinant human ciliary neurotrophic factor (rHCNTF) in patients with amyotrophic lateral sclerosis: relation to parameters of the acute-phase response. Clin Neuropharmacol 1995;18(6):500–14.

[45] Calcutt NA, Freshwater JD, Mizisin AP. Prevention of sensory disorders in diabetic Sprague-Dawley rats by aldose reductase inhibition or treatment with ciliary neurotrophic factor. Diabetologia 2004;47(4):718–24.

[46] The ALS CNTF Treatment Study Group. A double-blind placebo-controlled clinical trial of subcutaneous recombinant human ciliary neurotrophic factor (rHCNTF) in amyotrophic lateral sclerosis. Neurology 1996;46(5):1244–9.

[47] Miller RG, Petajan JH, Bryan WW, et al. A placebo-controlled trial of recombinant human ciliary neurotrophic (rhCNTF) factor in amyotrophic lateral sclerosis. rhCNTF ALS Study Group. Ann Neurol 1996;39(2):256–60.

[48] Zhao Z, Alam S, Oppenheim RW, et al. Overexpression of glial cell line-derived neurotrophic factor in the CNS rescues motoneurons from programmed cell death and promotes their long-term survival following axotomy. Exp Neurol 2004;190(2):356–72.

[49] Oppenheim RW, Houenou LJ, Johnson JE, et al. Developing motor neurons rescued from programmed and axotomy-induced cell death by GDNF. Nature 1995;373(6512):344–6.

[50] Llado J, Haenggeli C, Maragakis NJ, et al. Neural stem cells protect against glutamate-induced excitotoxicity and promote survival of injured motor neurons through the secretion of neurotrophic factors. Mol Cell Neurosci 2004;27(3):322–31.

[51] Lu YY, Wang LJ, Muramatsu S, et al. Intramuscular injection of AAV-GDNF results in sustained expression of transgenic GDNF, and its delivery to spinal motoneurons by retrograde transport. Neurosci Res 2003;45(1):33–40.

[52] Wang LJ, Lu YY, Muramatsu S, et al. Neuroprotective effects of glial cell line-derived neurotrophic factor mediated by an adeno-associated virus vector in a transgenic animal model of amyotrophic lateral sclerosis. J Neurosci 2002;22(16):6920–8.

[53] Manabe Y, Nagano I, Gazi MS, et al. Adenovirus-mediated gene transfer of glial cell line-derived neurotrophic factor prevents motor neuron loss of transgenic model mice for amyotrophic lateral sclerosis. Apoptosis 2002;7(4):329–34.

[54] Acsadi G, Anguelov RA, Yang H, et al. Increased survival and function of SOD1 mice after glial cell-derived neurotrophic factor gene therapy. Hum Gene Ther 2002;13(9):1047–59.

[55] Muscular Dystrophy Association. Available at: http://mdausa.org/publications/Quest/q71research.html. Accessed July 15, 2005.

[56] Ishii DN, Glazner GW, Pu SF. Role of insulin-like growth factors in peripheral nerve regeneration. Pharmacol Ther 1994;62(1–2):125–44.

[57] Lewis ME, Neff NT, Contreras PC, et al. Insulin-like growth factor-I: potential for treatment of motor neuronal disorders. Exp Neurol 1993;124(1):73–88.

[58] Festoff BW. The preclinical rationale for the use of insulin-like growth factor-I in amyotrophic lateral sclerosis. Drugs Today (Barc) 1998;34(1):65–77.

[59] Gehrmann J, Yao DL, Bonetti B, et al. Expression of insulin-like growth factor-I and related peptides during motoneuron regeneration. Exp Neurol 1994;128(2):202–10.

[60] Hansson HA, Dahlin LB, Danielsen N, et al. Evidence indicating trophic importance of IGF-I in regenerating peripheral nerves. Acta Physiol Scand 1986;126(4):609–14.

[61] Glazner GW, Morrison AE, Ishii DN. Elevated insulin-like growth factor (IGF) gene expression in sciatic nerves during IGF-supported nerve regeneration. Brain Res Mol Brain Res 1994;25(3–4):265–72.

[62] Contreras PC, Steffler C, Vaught JL. rhIGF-I enhances functional recovery from sciatic crush. Time-course and dose–response study. Ann N Y Acad Sci 1993;692:314–6.

[63] Nachemson AK, Lundborg G, Hansson HA. Insulin-like growth factor I promotes nerve regeneration: an experimental study on rat sciatic nerve. Growth Factors 1990;3(4):309–14.

[64] Shavlakadze T, White JD, Davies M, et al. Insulin-like growth factor I slows the rate of denervation induced skeletal muscle atrophy. Neuromuscul Disord 2005;15(2): 139–46.

[65] Hantai D, Akaaboune M, Lagord C, et al. Beneficial effects of insulin-like growth factor-I on wobbler mouse motoneuron disease. J Neurol Sci 1995;129(Suppl):122–6.

[66] Gorio A, Lesma E, Madaschi L, et al. Co-administration of IGF-I and glycosaminoglycans greatly delays motor neurone disease and affects IGF-I expression in the wobbler mouse: a long-term study. J Neurochem 2002;81(1):194–202.

[67] Kaspar BK, Llado J, Sherkat N, et al. Retrograde viral delivery of IGF-1 prolongs survival in a mouse ALS model. Science 2003;301(5634):839–42.

[68] Nagano I, Ilieva H, Shiote M, et al. Therapeutic benefit of intrathecal injection of insulin-like growth factor-1 in a mouse model of amyotrophic lateral sclerosis. J Neurol Sci 2005; 235(1–2):61–8.

[69] Lai EC, Felice KJ, Festoff BW, et al. Effect of recombinant human insulin-like growth factor-I on progression of ALS. A placebo-controlled study. The North America ALS/IGF-I Study Group. Neurology 1997;49(6):1621–30.

[70] Borasio GD, Robberecht W, Leigh PN, et al. A placebo-controlled trial of insulin-like growth factor-I in amyotrophic lateral sclerosis. European ALS/IGF-I Study Group. Neurology 1998;51(2):583–6.

[71] Lambrechts D, Storkebaum E, Morimoto M, et al. VEGF is a modifier of amyotrophic lateral sclerosis in mice and humans and protects motoneurons against ischemic death. Nat Genet 2003;34(4):383–94.

[72] Gora-Kupilas K, Josko J. The neuroprotective function of vascular endothelial growth factor (VEGF). Folia Neuropathol 2005;43(1):31–9.

[73] Sopher BL, Thomas PS Jr, LaFevre-Bernt MA, et al. Androgen receptor YAC transgenic mice recapitulate SBMA motor neuronopathy and implicate VEGF164 in the motor neuron degeneration. Neuron 2004;41(5):687–99.

[74] Storkebaum E, Lambrechts D, Dewerchin M, et al. Treatment of motoneuron degeneration by intracerebroventricular delivery of VEGF in a rat model of ALS. Nat Neurosci 2005;8(1): 85–92.

[75] Azzouz M, Ralph GS, Storkebaum E, et al. VEGF delivery with retrogradely transported lentivector prolongs survival in a mouse ALS model. Nature 2004;429(6990):413–7.

[76] Kuncl RW, Bilak MM, Bilak SR, et al. Pigment epithelium-derived factor is elevated in CSF of patients with amyotrophic lateral sclerosis. J Neurochem 2002;81(1):178–84.

[77] Cassina P, Pehar M, Vargas MR, et al. Astrocyte activation by fibroblast growth factor-1 and motor neuron apoptosis: implications for amyotrophic lateral sclerosis. J Neurochem 2005;93(1):38–46.

[78] Iwasaki Y, Ikeda K. Cotreatment of amyotrophic lateral sclerosis patients. Rinsho Shinkei-gaku 1999;39(12):1253–5.

[79] Zurn AD, Henry H, Schluep M, et al. Evaluation of an intrathecal immune response in amyotrophic lateral sclerosis patients implanted with encapsulated genetically engineered xenogeneic cells. Cell Transplant 2000;9(4):471–84.

[80] Martinez-Serrano A, Bjorklund A. Protection of the neostriatum against excitotoxic damage by neurotrophin-producing, genetically modified neural stem cells. J Neurosci 1996;16(15): 4604–16.

[81] Park KI, Teng YD, Snyder EY. The injured brain interacts reciprocally with neural stem cells supported by scaffolds to reconstitute lost tissue. Nat Biotechnol 2002;20(11): 1111–7.

[82] Rosario CM, Yandava BD, Kosaras B, et al. Differentiation of engrafted multipotent neural progenitors towards replacement of missing granule neurons in meander tail cerebellum may help determine the locus of mutant gene action. Development 1997;124(21):4213–24.

[83] Snyder EY, Taylor RM, Wolfe JH. Neural progenitor cell engraftment corrects lysosomal storage throughout the MPS VII mouse brain. Nature 1995;374(6520):367–70.

[84] Snyder EY, Yoon C, Flax JD, et al. Multipotent neural precursors can differentiate toward replacement of neurons undergoing targeted apoptotic degeneration in adult mouse neocortex. Proc Natl Acad Sci USA 1997;94(21):11663–8.

ELSEVIER
SAUNDERS

Phys Med Rehabil Clin N Am
16 (2005) 1015–1032

PHYSICAL MEDICINE
AND REHABILITATION
CLINICS OF
NORTH AMERICA

Electrodiagnostic Automation: Principles and Practice

Shai N. Gozani, MD, PhD[a],*, Morris A. Fisher, MD[b,c],
Xuan Kong, PhD[a], J. Thomas Megerian, MD, PhD[a,d],
Seward B. Rutkove, MD[e]

[a]NeuroMetrix, Inc., 62 Fourth Ave. Waltham, MA 02451, USA
[b]Department of Neurology (127), Hines Veterans Administration Hospital,
P.O. Box 5000, Hines, IL 60141-5199, USA
[c]Loyola University Stritch School of Medicine, Maywood, IL, USA
[d]Department of Neurology, Children's Hospital, 300 Longwood Avenue,
Boston, MA 02115, USA
[e]Department of Neurology, Beth Israel Deaconess Medical Center, 330 Brookline Avenue,
TCC-810, Boston, MA 02215, USA

With the dramatic advances in microprocessor technology over the past 2 decades, many diagnostic tests have incorporated varying degrees of automation, ranging from simple data collection protocols to more complex analysis and interpretation methods. Examples include computerized tomography and magnetic resonance imaging systems, which use automated scanning procedures, and electrocardiography systems, which provide an automatic assessment of rhythm and ischemic changes. Nerve conduction studies (NCS) have also incorporated a number of automated features, such as preliminary cursor assignment for motor responses, sensory responses, and F-waves. These features have become so commonplace as to be considered necessary components of any NCS/electromyography (NCS/EMG) system purchased today. Other aspects of automation are also embedded in modern NCS systems, including preset protocols that allow the operator to simply click a button to initiate a testing paradigm and advanced single fiber EMG data analysis. This automation has proven

This work was supported by NeuroMetrix, Inc.

Disclosures: Drs. Rutkove and Fisher serve on the NeuroMetrix, Inc. Neurology Advisory Board and receive compensation from the company; Drs. Kong, Megerian and Gozani are employed by NeuroMetrix, Inc.

* Corresponding author.

E-mail address: gozani@neurometrix.com (S.N. Gozani).

useful by accelerating the completion of NCS/EMG procedures and reporting while also improving the consistency of measurements. Nearly all NCS and EMG procedures performed by neurologists, physiatrists, and other physicians today use instrumentation with embedded automation.

Given the substantial benefits of automation to date, further progress in the automation of many aspects of peripheral electrodiagnosis is likely to occur in the coming years. The utility of such automation has already been proposed [1–6]. As applied to NCS, the role of electrodiagnostic automation is to facilitate, simplify, and increase the reliability of NCS data, as well as to provide decision support [7]. The potential advantages of such automation extend beyond the simple mechanics of performing individual studies and include: (1) standardization of data acquisition and analysis so that large reference and disease databases can be widely deployed to clinicians and researchers increasing both sensitivity and specificity of the tests; (2) establishment of equivalence so that studies performed on the same patient by two different physicians at different times can be directly compared, as well as facilitating national NCS registries for epidemiologic and phase IV clinical trials; and (3) expansion of NCS by increasing the number of nonspecialist physicians who may use NCS in appropriate clinical situations, such as in the evaluation of peripheral neuropathy in patients with diabetes.

NCS automation may be defined as the process of automating one or more steps in the performance, analysis, or reporting of an NCS. This definition does not include actual interpretation and diagnosis, which is beyond the scope of this review, and is best performed by a physician in the broad context of the patient's clinical history and examination. Electrodiagnostic automation can be characterized by the degree of human operator involvement required, the nature of the automation (eg, physiologic, algorithmic, programmatic), the level of scientific and clinical validation, and the demonstrated clinical utility. We propose a classification scheme for NCS automation primarily according to the degree of human (ie, physician or technician) involvement required (see Table 1).

In this review, we present a brief history of NCS automation followed by an overview of current examples of automation. A detailed description of automation features implemented in a commercial system (NC-stat, NeuroMetrix, Inc., Waltham, Massachusetts) with which the authors have extensive experience follows. Next, a review of the challenges and limitations of electrodiagnostic automation are discussed. The article concludes with a discussion of statistical approaches to automated system validation and the authors' thoughts on future directions of NCS automation and its implications for neuromuscular subspecialists.

History of automation in nerve conduction studies

From the 1950s, when the first commercial NCS/EMG systems became available, until the 1980s, performing and interpreting electrodiagnostic

Table 1
Electrodiagnostic automation classification system, with specific application to nerve conduction studies

Automation level	Type of automation	Human involvement required
0	None	Manual performance, no automation
1	• Limited automatic data acquisition • Preliminary cursor assignment • Basic report generation in the form of measured parameters, reference ranges and abnormalities	Comprehensive physician oversight on all components of study
2	• Complete automation in data acquisition including stimulation control • Validated real-time waveform analysis of latency, amplitude, and other parameters • Real-time automatic report generation including all Level 1 features plus decision support analysis	Human oversight limited to random sampling (10% or less) for technical quality control and ongoing confirmation of effectiveness of decision support
3	• Same as Level 2 • Real-time feedback to assist physician in optimizing the study	Human oversight limited to random sampling (5% or less) for technical quality control and ongoing confirmation of effectiveness of decision support

studies was a slow and laborious process. Physicians were required to set everything from filter settings to the sweep speeds for each individual study. Data analysis was performed manually using film or paper images of the waveforms recorded on the oscilloscope [8,9]. In the late 1970s, the first digital NCS/EMG instruments were introduced, but these supported a low level of automation, with most analyses still performed manually on paper. In the 1980s, microprocessor control was introduced and by the early 1990s NCS/EMG instruments became add-ons to personal computers. With these later advances, increasing automation in the form of preset testing protocols, automatic cursor assignment, and report generation became commonplace, and thus most systems achieved Level 1 automation. However, the introduction of digital and PC based instruments did not usher in a host of additional automated features, likely because the equipment was used primarily by specialized physicians for diverse applications and using varying techniques. As a result, there was little demand and economic incentive to invest in more advanced automation. In 1999, the first generation NC-stat System was introduced [2,3] which, unlike its predecessors, was designed for use by nonspecialist physicians but for common clinical applications such as carpal tunnel syndrome. This was the first instrument to provide Level 2 automation in that the entire process of performing a median nerve study including electrode placement, determination of the appropriate stimulus intensity, real-time latency and amplitude determination, and report generation was automated. Since that time, further enhancements have been made to the NC-stat System, as discussed further below, but to our knowledge no additional Level 2 or Level 3 systems have been developed.

Examples of electrodiagnostic automation

As previously noted, all commercially available NCS/EMG instruments offer automation. To simplify the analysis of automation, electrodiagnostic testing can be divided into four phases: data collection, data analysis, data reporting, and clinical diagnosis, with the first three as potential targets for automation.

Most NCS/EMG equipment employs some degree of automation in data collection in that virtually all modern machines are computer-based and use software specifically developed to control electrical stimulation and waveform recording. All motor, sensory, F-wave, repetitive stimulation and basic EMG procedures are to some extent automated, in that only a single button needs to be pressed to acquire data. However, outside of having preset programs that can acquire and display data, most other aspects of data collection remain manual, such as increasing stimulation intensity or adjusting the sweep or sensitivity to visualize and analyze the waveform fully.

Because of waveform digitization, some degree of data analysis automation is also available on most NCS/EMG systems. These components are usually relatively straightforward, but nonetheless offer time-saving benefits to the physician and include automatic amplitude and latency marker placements on waveforms, with automated calculation of secondary parameters such as duration and area. When acquiring a series of F-waves, the latency markers may all be set and a minimum, maximum, and mean value provided with relatively little effort on the part of the physician. Unfortunately, although these waveform analysis routines generally perform well on clean waveforms, their performance degrades rapidly with stimulus artifact, non-flat baselines, low amplitude and absent signals, unusual response morphology, and noise. Furthermore, although widely used, the accuracy and reproducibility of these algorithms have not been evaluated in peer-reviewed published clinical studies. Rather, they are intended as initial assignments that must be reassessed and often modified by the electromyographer physician (or supervised technician) performing the study.

Other commonplace automated features include: repetitive stimulation programs allowing for the decrement or increment in amplitude and area to be measured immediately. Motor unit number estimation (MUNE) programs are also available on some systems [10], although this technique remains mainly confined to research uses. Most systems also have some automation in needle EMG data analysis, including automated quantitative analysis via signal decomposition (eg, multimotor unit potential analysis) [11–13], interference pattern analysis [14,15], and single-fiber EMG [16]. With the exception of single-fiber EMG, most physicians in day-to-day electrodiagnostic practice continue to perform mainly qualitative analysis of the EMG data [17]. Nonetheless, these automated protocols can be helpful in some clinical situations, such as assessing mild myopathic disease.

Reporting of the NCS/EMG data remains a relatively undeveloped area of automation, although in most currently available systems, the collected data can be transformed into a tabular form with normal reference values included. The waveforms themselves can also be included, printed in a smaller summary report form. These reporting features have provided substantial time savings as well as increased the legibility and clarity of the reports. These improvements in reporting have been followed by several efforts to develop NCS and EMG decision support systems to increase diagnostic standardization [6]. These software systems generally use probability models, rule-based expert systems, or other pattern-matching techniques to assign probabilities to possible neuromuscular disorders based on the patterns of the electrodiagnostic findings. These innovative efforts are presently limited to research studies and have not found widespread use.

In summary, all modern NCS/EMG instruments contain some degree of automation in data collection, analysis, and in reporting. However, much of the work remains the responsibility of the physician or technician performing the study including adjustments of stimulus intensity, determining when a waveform is supramaximal, cursor placement in low amplitude or abnormal waveforms, and creating a written summary of the findings.

Case study in Level 2 electrodiagnostic automation: the NC-stat

The NC-stat, in conjunction with the onCall system, is an instrument that performs NCS with Level 2 automation and has undergone substantial development and expansion of its clinical application since its introduction in 1999. Unlike other NCS/EMG equipment, the NC-stat is intended to completely automate an NCS up to the point of physician interpretation and diagnosis. The device has FDA 510(k) clearance for the performance of motor studies of the median, ulnar, peroneal, and tibial nerves, and sensory studies of the median, ulnar, and sural nerves (FDA 510[k] #K041320). The comparability of NCS data generated by the NC-stat and NCS/EMG equipment under neurologist or physiatrist supervision has been evaluated for motor studies of the median, ulnar, and peroneal nerves [2–5,18]. The clinical utility of the NC-stat has been demonstrated in the diagnosis of carpal tunnel syndrome [2–4], tracking of electrophysiologic response to carpal tunnel release surgery [4,19], and, by using novel F-wave analysis methods, confirmation of suspected lumbosacral radiculopathy [20].

The system is comprised of "biosensors," a monitor, and the onCall reporting system. The biosensor is a spatially fixed configuration of electrodes (stimulating, recording, and common reference), microelectronic components, and printed embedded electrical circuits (traces). Biosensors are tailor made for each nerve and are often left/right specific as well. The biosensors are designed for placement by health care personnel with modest training using readily identifiable anatomic landmarks (eg, wrist crease or malleoli) and have some adaptive capabilities that account for residual neuroanatomic variability following landmark-based placement. The biosensors also include a temperature sensor that records the skin surface temperature allowing normalization of the data obtained to standard temperatures. The electrical traces are attached through a single keyed connector that ensures secure and correct equipment connection. The monitor is a digital device with three microprocessors (two controlling the amplifiers and performing waveform analysis, one controlling the stimulator). The software-guided device has technical specifications consistent with standard NCS/EMG equipment [21].

Upon initiation of a test, the monitor software determines the supramaximal stimulus intensity using a sequence of electrical stimuli of increasing magnitude (range 5-100 milliamps and duration 100-500 microseconds). To efficiently identify the supramaximal intensity, the algorithm uses a priori knowledge of the nerve tested and patient characteristics. For example, nerves stimulated at the wrist typically require lower intensity than those stimulated at the ankle. Similarly, patients with high BMI generally require higher intensity stimuli than those with low BMI. This information is used by the stimulus control algorithm to determine an optimal starting point as well as to chart out a stimulation sequence, and the control algorithm determines when the supramaximal intensity is attained. This is accomplished by identifying a plateau in the amplitude of the motor or sensory evoked response. "False" early plateaus that are narrow or unstable are ignored. If the stimulus intensity reaches the maximal current output (100 mA) before attaining the supramaximal level, the control algorithm continues with longer duration stimuli that satisfy the strength–duration behavior of peripheral nerves [22]. The quantitative stimulus–response data is stored and can be used in real-time for submaximal stimulation paradigms, such as for acquisition of F-waves at low stimulation intensity [23,24].

Following determination of the supramaximal stimulus intensity, the monitor software controls acquisition of the motor (compound muscle action potential, CMAP), F-wave, and sensory (sensory nerve action potential, SNAP) responses. Filter, gain, and other data acquisition parameters are automatically adjusted and digital averaging is automatically triggered for sensory studies because of their low signal-to-noise ratio. The software limits the number of stimuli to the minimum number consistent with a predetermined level of data reliability, which is defined by the parameter characteristics (eg, lower extremity F-wave latencies may require as many as 20 to 40 stimuli), response variability (eg, consistency of stimulus to stimulus latencies), and signal-to-noise ratio. Throughout acquisition, the monitor continually runs quality controls checks to verify that the acquired waveforms are physiologically realistic. These quality control checks include detection of saturation, excessive stimulus artifact, noise levels, and unexpected changes in waveform morphology. Once acquired, the waveforms are analyzed in real-time by signal processing algorithms that convert the evoked waveforms into nerve conduction response parameter values, such as latencies/velocities (ie, distal motor latency, F-wave latency, distal sensory latency, motor and sensory conduction velocity), amplitudes (ie, CMAP amplitude, SNAP amplitude), and waveform configurations (eg, CMAP duration and area, SNAP duration). The response parameters are adjusted to standardized skin surface temperatures (32°C in the upper extremity and 30°C in the lower extremity) using linear regression equations as long as the temperatures are within predetermined ranges (25°C–36.5°C in the upper extremity and 23°C–36°C in the lower extremity). If the skin surface temperature is outside this range, then the operator is instructed to warm or cool the patient's limb, as appropriate, before proceeding.

The NC-stat waveform analysis algorithms perform a higher level cursor assignment than those found in other NCS/EMG instruments because they are specifically designed to incorporate the complexities of stimulus artifact, baseline variation, noise, and complex waveform morphology. F-wave latency assignment provides a good example of this feature. On other NCS/EMG systems available today, algorithms used for cursor assignment are typically designed to detect the first deflection from baseline exceeding a preset threshold as the latency. This method works well when the trace is flat, free of contamination from noise and other sources of artifact, and the F-wave morphology is simple and clearly differentiated from the trace baseline (eg, the F-wave has large amplitude and sharp leading edge). However, F-wave parameters recorded under many clinical conditions can be challenging to evaluate. The onset latency is often embedded in the terminal slow negative decay portion of the M-wave, there is external noise (both high frequency and 60 Hz), there are various artifacts such as surface-recorded voluntary motor unit potentials from unstimulated muscles, and F-wave latencies may overlap with A-waves. Indeed, F-wave latency markings on commercial NCS/EMG equipment require frequent manual correction. In the NC-stat F-wave algorithm (see Fig. 1 as an example), the residual component of the M-wave is first removed from all traces by fitting the trace baseline to a function that models the non–F-wave portion of the trace. Digital filters are dynamically selected and applied to further reduce environmental and background muscle noise, while preserving the original F-wave morphology. A-waves are detected using a clustering approach that operates simultaneously across the entire ensemble of F-wave traces. One or more windows are then defined for the F-wave latency search. These windows are based on the expected range of F-wave latencies from reference

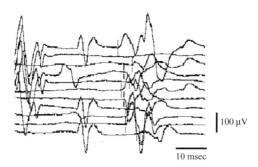

Fig. 1. F-wave traces obtained by stimulation of deep peroneal nerve at the ankle and recording from the extensor digitorum brevis muscle, using the NC-stat. Each trace represents a sequential supramaximal stimulation. Traces start at 27 milliseconds poststimulation. Short vertical lines on each trace designate latency assigned by F-wave algorithm. As shown, activity preceding F-waves is ignored.

data as well as the location of identified A-waves, which otherwise would interfere with latency detection. F-wave latency is then assigned within a temporal window preceding the most prominent peak within each trace. The F-wave latency assignment method operates in an iterative fashion to address complex waveform morphology effectively. The reliability of this F-wave latency assignment method has been demonstrated [5]. This computerized ability to accurately analyze F-waves should meaningfully enhance their clinical usefulness.

The monitor has an LCD screen that displays the nerve conduction response parameters in real time. The user may also view comparisons of the measured values to normative ranges that were obtained with the NC-stat using identical methodology. The normative database is embedded in the device and is adjusted according to the patient's age and height. The operator may also choose to send the data to the onCall system, located at the company headquarters in Waltham, Massachusetts, which is accomplished through a docking station containing a high-speed modem. The docking station-onCall communications protocol is secure and has extensive error checking. The nerve conduction data is archived in the onCall database, and a detailed report is automatically generated and returned within several minutes. An onCall report includes display of all the response waveforms with identification of the waveform features (eg, latency, amplitude, duration, area) determined by the NC-stat in real time, summary of patient characteristics (eg, age, height, body mass index) and the study purpose, a customized description of the methodology (eg, nerves tested, distances, equipment specifics), a reference table listing all the parameters with identification of reference ranges, abnormalities and percentiles of those parameters that are normally distributed, and a decision support section that summarizes key findings. The onCall decision support algorithm is a multilayer rule-based expert system [25], which is constantly undergoing further development and refinement to provide the most complete and helpful decision support analysis. The report is automatically faxed or emailed to the physician performing the study for his/her use in the patient's clinical diagnostic assessment and can be directly placed in the patient's medical record for future reference. The real-time turnaround allows physicians to obtain reports during the NCS study, if needed, and a complete report within minutes of completing the study.

Challenges and limitations to electrodiagnostic automation

Even if electrodiagnostic automation is improved to the point of Level 3 sophistication, certain issues present continuing challenges. Moreover, there are limitations that for both practical and theoretic reasons automated electrodiagnostic techniques may not be able to overcome. These challenges and limitations highlight the continued central role of physicians in overseeing electrodiagnostic testing.

The biggest challenges for automated electrodiagnostic testing fall within the realm of reporting and decision support, and one of the most apparent challenges for any Level 2 or 3 system is that of appropriately ordering identified abnormalities by clinical relevance, relegating relatively trivial issues to their appropriate status. For example, a median neuropathy at the wrist should be relegated to the status of "incidental finding" in a patient who also has motor neuron disease. In automated systems, such categorization is challenging because of the large number of possible findings and the difficulty in codifying physician clinical reasoning [26,27]. The system, unable to assess which abnormality is most relevant to the patient, provides a list of electrodiagnostic abnormalities from which the physician must choose for their clinical relevance.

A similar issue arises if the initial testing paradigm chosen by physician using the automated technology is misdirected or incomplete. For example, a patient with bilateral hand numbness might be considered clinically to have carpal tunnel syndrome. A study is performed in that light, but in addition to prolonged median distal latencies, focal conduction velocity slowing in the ulnar nerves across both elbows is also found. The report and decision support system list bilateral median neuropathies at the wrists, bilateral ulnar neuropathies at the elbows, and the possibility of an underlying polyneuropathy. However, because the clinical question asked was whether there was focal upper extremity nerve compression, the possibility that this constellation of findings could represent a demyelinating polyneuropathy with disproportionate slowing at sites of compression might not be included. Thus, an important challenge for a decision support system is to integrate findings so as not to focus on multiple individual abnormalities when a single, more comprehensive explanation might be more germane. This further confirms the importance of viewing the NCS as an extension of the clinical examination of the patient, regardless of the level of automation employed.

In all cases, the physician must correlate the patient's presentation with the individual findings and use the information only as one component of their diagnostic analysis.

Another challenge is the elderly patient. All electrodiagnostic testing in the elderly is difficult because robust normative data is not readily available and is demanding to develop. In fact, differentiating normal age-associated changes from disease states is often quite arbitrary. What is meant by "normal" in an 80- or 90-year-old is not straightforward, and is often left to the judgment of the clinician performing and interpreting the study. Nonetheless, this issue may be overcome to some extent with sufficient normative data in the older age group. In this respect, automated techniques have the potential to use large databases that cannot be applied without standardized approaches to testing.

Relying on NCS alone, without needle EMG, makes it virtually impossible to assess cervical radiculopathy at the most common levels of C5, C6, and C7, even with sophisticated automation. This is because motor nerve conduction parameters that assess the cervical spine are the median and ulnar F-responses, which can only evaluate the C8 and T1 roots. Although H-reflexes from the flexor carpi radialis [28–30] could theoretically be used to test these roots, it is likely that these techniques will be insufficient. By contrast, assessment of common lumbosacral radiculopathies (ie, L5 and S1 roots) is enabled by automation technology. These methods facilitate rapid acquisition, standardization (ie, temperature, age, and height normalization) and processing of large ensembles of peroneal and posterior tibial nerve F-waves using multiple statistical parameters (eg, mean, chronodispersion), which leads to high detection sensitivity [20,31–33]. Needle EMG is also useful in the assessment of disease severity, information that may be helpful in deciding upon surgical intervention or for establishing prognosis [34]. Sensory and motor response amplitudes [35–37] and specialized nerve conduction techniques, such as MUNE [38,39], however, may also be useful in this role.

There are also physician and technician challenges. Some inappropriate clinical use may occur, particularly as nonspecialist physicians start using the technology. This situation is not unique to electrodiagnosis [40], and can generally be addressed with high-quality continuing education. Regardless, occasional poor or inconsistent electrode application is inevitable, and could degrade the quality of the studies. Still, some amount of placement variability can be addressed using prefabricated electrode configurations such as those with adaptive capabilities (in fact, the NC-Stat system currently incorporates such a feature). The possibility of electrodiagnostic automation leading to diagnostic errors needs to be considered, and any system using Level 2 or 3 automation should have sophisticated quality-control measures that detect most errors. Furthermore, the automation algorithms must have quality control checks built into them to detect physiologic responses with questionable morphology and to assess whether an absent response is technical or pathologic in origin. Finally, it is important that the physicians assessing the patient use appropriate clinical judgment when interpreting the relevance of abnormalities. At the same time, errors also occur in traditional studies performed by subspecialists [41–43], and automation and standardization of NCS has the potential for actually improving overall study quality.

In addition to these challenges and limitations, there are some hurdles that probably cannot be overcome due to technologic complexity and economic considerations. One such issue is that the need for predesigned electrode configurations precludes assessment of every nerve that can possibly be evaluated in an NCS. For example, the medial and lateral antebrachial cutaneous nerves of the arms, the lateral femoral cutaneous nerve of the thigh, and the saphenous nerve of the lower leg are not readily studied by automated techniques. Although technically feasible, product development for electrodiagnostic automation of these nerves is not economically practical because they are studied infrequently. In addition, some nerves, such as the saphenous and lateral femoral cutaneous, are technically challenging even for experienced specialized physicians.

A final limitation is that the evaluation of children would be difficult because a wide array of electrodes would need to be developed. Because electrodiagnostic techniques are used in children infrequently, practical economic factors would not support their development. Similarly, the need for uniform sizes and shapes in electrode design would make certain automated technology impractical for use in individuals with nonstandard anatomy such as patients with amputated digits, severe obesity, surgical transpositions, or traumatic wounds.

This review has focused on NCS automation because complete automation of needle EMG, while possible, remains unlikely. From a theoretic perspective, it is conceivable that an automated needle EMG device could be developed. However, such a device would have to be responsive to many factors including being exquisitely sensitive to endplate noise and spikes (so as to avoid causing inadvertent pain to the patient), the rise time of motor unit action potentials, so as to have accurate duration/amplitude measurements, and to fibrillation potentials and positive sharp waves. Moreover, such an apparatus would require some form of force transducer to allow for accurate motor unit action potentials recruitment analysis. But even if these obstacles could be overcome, it is difficult to envision a patient feeling comfortable with the absence of a human hand guiding the needle. Rather, noninvasive approaches for obtaining limited EMG information are more likely targets for automation, such as MUNE [38,39], quantitative surface EMG [44], electrical impedance myography [45,46], and power spectral analysis of passive electrical muscle recordings [47].

In summary, many of the potential challenges and even some of the limitations may be theoretically surmountable, but ultimately, the economics and physician education necessary will dictate the limits of electrodiagnostic automation. Automated techniques employed by physicians without subspecialized training will be most effective when applied to the evaluation of relatively common clinical conditions in anatomically normal adults. Ultimately, the flexibility of having a variety of electrodes for stimulating and recording and the associated experience and knowledge of a trained neuromuscular physician specialist will be essential for the evaluation of individuals with complex problems.

Statistical issues in validating electrodiagnostic automation

Demonstrating the statistical validity and reliability of automated electrodiagnostic instruments is critical to their acceptance and ultimate success. Statistical validity is the extent to which an instrument or method measures what it is intended or purported to measure. As applied to neurophysiologic measurements, this definition may be extended to confirm that the method is capable of measuring nerve function over a wide spectrum from normal to highly abnormal. Statistical reliability is the degree of agreement between two methods. When applied to neurophysiologic measurements, high reliability implies that two methods will yield nearly the same value (eg, latency) when applied to the same subject.

Examination of validity and reliability requires a reference measurement that is itself regarded as valid and reliable (ie, a "gold-standard"). A well-defined and accepted electrodiagnostic reference does not exist as substantial interexaminer and intraexaminer variability has been observed among highly qualified and experienced physicians specializing in EMG for both specific nerve conduction parameters [48–53] and overall diagnostic assessments [54,55]. Even the use of apparently identical methodology does not eliminate interexaminer variability [53]. In light of these results, the reference measurements should meet several criteria: (1) they should be performed by a qualified high-volume neuromuscular laboratory such as in academic centers; (2) the laboratory should use standardized, documented, and well-accepted procedures meeting applicable published practice parameters [56]; (3) measurement procedures and definitions of abnormalities must be applied in a consistent manner and independent of a priori data such as the referral diagnosis; and (4) the reference and instrument measurements should be performed in close temporal proximity to avoid the introduction of physiologic variability.

It is important to note that both the instrument under study and the references have inherent measurement variability, so intermethod differences cannot be assigned entirely to either method alone [57]. Ideally, an instrument will have high validity and reliability. However, measurement of reliability requires that the instrument and the reference use nearly identical methods. Because NCS measurements are strongly dependent on the exact technique used and forcing the instrument and reference to be identical may cause one or both to deviate from their normal mode of operation, reliability assessment can be challenging.

Statistical validity is usually quantified by the Pearson product moment correlation between the instrument and reference measurements. A strong correlation establishes that the instrument is statistically valid. Because there are no specific correlation levels that establish validity, the results should be compared against correlation values obtained comparing individual physicians regarded as experts in the performance of electrodiagnosis. Statistical reliability may be quantified in a number of ways. The intraclass correlation coefficient (ICC) [58] ranges from 0 to 1, and assesses the agreement between two methods by comparing the variability between measurements (eg, latency) on the same subject to the total variance across all measurements and all subjects. If the variance between the instrument and reference measurements in each subject is small relative to the total variance, then the two methods have high agreement (ICC close to 1) and the instrument is regarded as reliable. On the other hand, if the variance between the instrument and reference measurements is high, the technique is considered to have poor reliability. Criterion levels for acceptable reliability should be obtained from ICCs observed between expert physicians performing NCS on the same subjects, in a fashion similar to that used to assess validity. Another standard method for assessing reliability is to use Bland-Altman analysis [59]. This procedure consists of calculating and plotting differences between measurements against the mean of the measurements. The mean difference is called the bias, and the standard deviation of the differences may be termed the intermethod precision. The precision quantifies the reliability of a measurement as judged against a reference.

The accuracy of electrodiagnostic automation techniques can also be measured by the reproducibility or consistency of the results obtained on the same subjects over a period of time (intraexaminer variability). Outcome studies demonstrating that instruments using electrodiagnostic automation yield useful clinical outcomes are difficult to perform but valuable. In all studies designed to evaluate electrodiagnostic automation, evidence-based medicine should be used to guide study design. The goal would be to have Class I and II clinical studies to confirm the accuracy and utility of automation techniques [60].

Future trends in electrodiagnostic automation

Currently, most commercial NCS/EMG instruments have achieved Level 1 automation, incorporating limited automated functions in data acquisition, data analysis, and report generation. The NC-Stat System, in conjunction with the onCall system, includes substantial data acquisition automation and waveform analysis capabilities, as well as advanced report generation including waveform visualization, demographic-matched reference range comparison, and decision support analysis, and thus reaches Level 2. Achieving Level 3 automation, in which there is real-time data analysis helping to provide interactive decision support, will eventually become available.

Further progress and dissemination of automated electrodiagnosis should have a positive impact in a number of areas. For example, automated electrodiagnosis could serve a valuable role in underserved areas both within the United States and throughout the world. Potential uses include evaluating at-risk individuals for diabetic peripheral neuropathy [61], assessing employees for carpal tunnel syndrome [62,63], and evaluating field workers for insecticide exposure secondary to organophosphates [64]. Moreover, such systems could be used to advantage in multicenter clinical trials where electrodiagnostic measurement variation could be significantly reduced through standardization [65]. Finally, allowing a wider group of physicians to perform NCS will increase the visibility of electrodiagnosis, which should contribute to a greater recognition for its value in peripheral nerve assessment and benefit all who work in the field.

The impact of increasing use of automated technology, however, may raise concern for physicians specializing in electrodiagnostic medicine. These concerns are likely based on several issues including the potential for the technology being used by nonphysicians, the fact that such technology could have a direct negative economic impact (ie, fewer patients referred to subspecialists for evaluation), and perhaps most importantly, the sense that the subspecialist's authority and expertise are being undermined. The wide use of NCS by nonphysicians has already been documented [66,67]. We believe it is imperative that electrodiagnostic procedures, regardless of the level of automation, are only performed by physicians or under direct physician supervision. Moreover, whereas it may be inevitable that some referrals will decrease, overall, we anticipate that more widespread access to NCS technology will create new referral patterns rather than simply encroaching on already established ones. For example, patients who previously would have been taken to surgery for suspected lumbosacral radiculopathy based on history, examination, and magnetic resonance imaging data but without an electrodiagnostic assessment may now also be given an NCS using automated multiparameter F-wave analysis [5,20] to further confirm the diagnosis before operating.

The single most important issue likely to impede the acceptance of advanced automated peripheral electrodiagnostic techniques by subspecialists in neuromuscular disease is the impression that advanced automation may render their expertise unnecessary. But advanced automated techniques by their very nature are best used in the assessment of common disorders for which the pretest probability of a positive result is reasonably high, such as in diabetic patients, patients with clinical evidence of carpal tunnel syndrome, and patients with signs and symptoms of lumbosacral radiculopathy. But for those patients with more difficult problems or unusual presentations, the expertise of physicians with specialized neuromuscular training will continue to be invaluable. Ultimately, given the possibility of an increased number of patient studies, reduced technician training, and simplified record keeping and standardization of results, increasing numbers of electrodiagnostic specialists may choose to incorporate some degree of Level 2 or 3 automated technology into their own practices. Just as we have found that automatic cursor placement and latency determination help us perform more rapid and consistent studies, it remains possible that advanced automation in NCS may enhance our ability to provide more efficient and better care to our patients.

Summary

Development and use of electrodiagnostic automation methods are an inevitable consequence of advances in microelectronic and computer technology over the past several decades. In fact, although not widely recognized, automation is an important component of nearly all NCS performed using modern instrumentation. This review provides an overview of electrodiagnostic automation, primarily as it relates to NCS, and includes a simple classification scheme, basic history, and a number of examples. Recent efforts to extend automation are described, along with limitations and appropriate use of such technology. Fundamentally, electrodiagnostic automation is a tool to be used by physicians when clinically appropriate. The expansion of NCS use to a wider group of physicians, through increasingly sophisticated automation technology, has many potential benefits for both physicians and patients alike.

References

[1] Gitter A, Lin V. Automated sensory nerve conduction testing using fuzzy logic. Am J Phys Med Rehabil 1999;78(5):425–34.

[2] Leffler CT, Gozani SG, Nguyen ZQ, et al. An automated electrodiagnostic technique for detection of carpal tunnel syndrome. Neurol Clin Neurophysiol 2000;3A.

[3] Leffler CT, Gozani SN, Cros D. Median neuropathy at the wrist: diagnostic utility of clinical findings and an automated electrodiagnostic device. J Occup Environ Med 2000;42:398–409.

[4] Vinik AI, Emley MS, Megerian JT, et al. Median and ulnar nerve conduction measurements in patients with symptoms of diabetic peripheral neuropathy using the NC-stat system. Diabetes Technol Ther 2004;6:816–24.

[5] Fisher MA. Comparison of automated and manual F-wave latency measurements. Clin Neurophys 2005;116(2):264–9.

[6] Pattichis CS, Schofield I, Merletti R, et al. Introduction to this special issue. Intelligent data analysis in electromyography and electroneurography. Med Eng Phys 1999;21(6–7):379–88.

[7] Vingtoft S, Fuglsang-Frederiksen A, Ronager J, et al. KANDID—an EMG decision support system—evaluated in a European multicenter trial. Muscle Nerve 1993;16(5):520–9.

[8] Bonner FJ Jr, Devleschoward AB. AAEM minimonograph #45: the early development of electromyography. Muscle Nerve 1995;18(8):825–33.

[9] Ladegaard J. Story of electromyography equipment. Muscle Nerve 2002;Suppl 11:S128–33.

[10] Henderson RD, McClelland R, Daube JR. Effect of changing data collection parameters on statistical motor unit number estimates. Muscle Nerve 2003;27(3):320–31.

[11] Nandedkar SD, Barkhaus PE, Charles A. Multi-motor unit action potential analysis (MMA). Muscle Nerve 1995;18(10):1155–66.

[12] Stewart CR, Nandedkar SD, Massey JM, et al. Evaluation of an automatic method of measuring features of motor unit action potentials. Muscle Nerve 1989;12(2):141–8.

[13] Stalberg E, Nandedkar SD, Sanders DB, et al. Quantitative motor unit potential analysis. Clin Neurophysiol 1996;13(5):401–22.

[14] Sanders DB, Stalberg EV, Nandedkar SD. Analysis of the electromyographic interference pattern. J Clin Neurophysiol 1996;13(5):385–400.

[15] Nandedkar SD, Sanders DB, Stalberg EV. Automatic analysis of the electromyographic interference pattern. Part II: findings in control subjects and in some neuromuscular diseases. Muscle Nerve 1986;9(6):491–500.

[16] Stalberg E, Trontelj JV. Single fiber electromyogaphy. New York: Raven Press; 1994.

[17] Bromberg MB, Smith AG, Bauerle J. A comparison of two commercial quantitative electromyographic algorithms with manual analysis. Muscle Nerve 1999;22(9):1244–8.

[18] Rotman MB, Enkvetchakul BV, Megerian JT, et al. Time course and predictors of median nerve conduction after carpal tunnel release. J Hand Surg [Am] 2004;29:367–72.

[19] Guyette TM, Wilgis EF. Timing of improvement after carpal tunnel release. J Surg Orthop Adv 2004;13:206–9.

[20] Wells MD, Myers AP, Emley M, et al. Detection of lumbosacral nerve root compression with a novel composite nerve conduction measurement. Spine 2002;27:2811–9.

[21] Bischoff C, Fuglsang-Fredriksen A, Vendelbo L, et al. Standards of instrumentation of EMG. In: Deuschl G, Eisen A, editors. Recommendations for the practice of clinical neurophsyiology: guidelines of the International Federation of Clinical Physiology (EEG Suppl. 52). New York: Elsevier Science B.V.; 1990. p. 199–211.

[22] Burke D, Kiernan MC, Bostock H. Excitability of human axons. Clin Neurophysiol 2001; 112(9):1575–85.

[23] Clinchot DM, Colachis SC, Kaplansky BD, et al. Effects of stimulus parameters on characteristics of the F-response in normal subjects. Am J Phys Med Rehabil 1994;73:313–8.

[24] DiBenedetto M, Gale SD, Adarmes D. F-Wave acquisition using low-current stimulation. Muscle Nerve 2003;28:82–6.

[25] Perry CA. Knowledge bases in medicine: a review. Bull Med Libr Assoc 1990;78(3):271–82.

[26] Forde R. Competing conceptions of diagnostic reasoning—is there a way out? Theor Med Bioeth 1998;19(1):59–72.

[27] Kassirer JP. Diagnostic reasoning. Ann Intern Med 1989;110(11):893–900.

[28] Christie AD, Inglis JG, Boucher JP, et al. Reliability of the FCR H-reflex. J Clin Neurophysiol 2005;22(3):204–9.

[29] Schimsheimer RJ, Ongerboer de Visser BW, Kemp B. The flexor carpi radialis H-reflex in lesions of the sixth and seventh cervical roots. J Neurol Neurosurg Psychiatry 1985;48: 445–9.

[30] Schimsheimer RJ, Ongerboer de Visser BW, Kemp B. Digital nerve somatosensory evoked potentials and flexor carpi radialis H reflexes in cervical disc protrusion and involvement of the sixth or seventh cervical root: relations to clinical and myelographic findings. Electroencephalalogr Clin Neurophysiol 1988;70:313–24.

[31] Fisher MA. Electrophysiology of radiculopathies. Clin Neurophysiol 2002;113(3):317–35.

[32] Berger AR, Sharma K, Lipton RB. Comparison of motor conduction abnormalities in lumbosacral radiculopathy and axonal polyneuropathy. Muscle Nerve 1999;22(8):1053–7.

[33] Toyokura M, Murakami K. F-wave study in patients with lumbosacral radiculopathies. Electromyogr Clin Neurophysiol 1997;37(1):19–26.

[34] Daube JR. AAEM minimonograph #11: needle examination in clinical electromyography. Muscle Nerve 1991;14(8):685–700.

[35] Wilbourn AJ. Sensory nerve conduction studies. J Clin Neurophysiol 1994;11(6):584–601.

[36] Verhamme C, van Schaik IN, Koelman JH, et al. Clinical disease severity and axonal dysfunction in hereditary motor and sensory neuropathy Ia. J Neurol 2004;251(12):1491–7.

[37] Scelsa SN, Berger AR, Herskovitz S. Electrophysiologic correlates of weakness in L5/S1 radiculopathy. Electromyogr Clin Neurophysiol 2001;41(3):145–51.

[38] Shefner JM, Gooch CL. Motor unit number estimation. Phys Med Rehabil Clin N Am 2003; 14(2):243–60.

[39] Daube JR, Gooch C, Shefner J, et al. Motor unit number estimation (MUNE) with nerve conduction studies. Clin Neurophysiol Suppl 2000;53:112–5.

[40] Bodenheimer T, Fernandez A. High and rising health care costs. Part 4: can costs be controlled while preserving quality? Ann Intern Med 2005;143(1):26–31.

[41] Dumitru D, Walsh NE. Practical instrumentation and common sources of error. Am J Phys Med Rehabil 1988;67(2):55–65.

[42] Landau ME, Diaz MI, Barner KC, et al. Changes in nerve conduction velocity across the elbow due to experimental error. Muscle Nerve 2002;26(6):838–40.

[43] Padua L, Padua R, Nazzaro M, et al. Errors in diagnosis of polyneuropathy: three cases of chronic lumbosacral root impairment. J Peripher Nerv Syst 1998;3(3):224–6.

[44] Zwarts MJ, Stegeman DF. Multichannel surface EMG: basic aspects and clinical utility. Muscle Nerve 2003;28(1):1–17.

[45] Rutkove SB, Esper GJ, Lee KS, et al. Electrical impedance myography in the detection of radiculopathy. Muscle Nerve 2005;32(3):335–41.

[46] Rutkove SB, Aaron R, Shiffman CA. Localized bioimpedance analysis in the evaluation of neuromuscular disease. Muscle Nerve 2002;25(3):390–7.

[47] Keller SP, Sandrock AW, Gozani SN. Noninvasive detection of fibrillation potentials in skeletal muscle. IEEE Trans Biomed Eng 2002;49(8):788–95.

[48] Chaudhry V, Corse AM, Freimer ML, et al. Inter- and intraexaminer reliability of nerve conduction measurements in patients with diabetic neuropathy. Neurology 1994;44: 1459–62.

[49] Chaudhry V, Cornblath DR, Mellits ED, et al. Inter- and intra-examiner reliability of nerve conduction measurements in normal subjects. Ann Neurol 1991;30:841–3.

[50] Dyck PJ, Kratz KM, Lehman KA, et al. The Rochester Diabetic Neuropathy Study: design, criteria for types of neuropathy, selection bias, and reproducibility of neuropathic tests. Neurology 1991;41:799–807.

[51] Husstedt IW, Evers ST, Grotemyer KH. Reproducibility of different nerve conduction velocity measurements in healthy test subjects and patients suffering from diabetic neuropathy. Electromyogr Clin Neurophysiol 1997;37:359–63.

[52] Valensi P, Attali JR, Gagant S, et al. Reproducibility of parameters for assessment of diabetic neuropathy. Diabetes Med 1993;10:933–9.

[53] Salerno DF, Werner RA, Albers JW, et al. Reliability of nerve conduction studies among active workers. Muscle Nerve 1999;22:1372–9.

[54] Fuglsang-Frederiksen A, Johnsen B, de Carvalho M, et al. Variation in diagnostic strategy of the EMG examination—a multicentre study. Clin Neurophysiol 1999;110(10): 1814–24.

[55] Tankisi H, Johnsen B, Fuglsang-Frederiksen A, et al. Variation in the classification of polyneuropathies among European physicians. Clin Neurophysiol 2003;114(3):496–503.

[56] Jablecki CK, Andary MT, Floeter MK, et al. Second AAEM Literature review of the usefulness of nerve conduction studies and needle electromyography for the evaluation of patients with carpal tunnel syndrome. Muscle Nerve 2002;26:S1–53.

[57] Bland JM, Altman DG. Comparing methods of measurement: why plotting difference against standard method is misleading. Lancet 1995;346:1085–7.

[58] Rosner B. Fundamentals of biostatistics. 4th edition. New York: Wadsworth Publishing; 1995. p. 518–20.

[59] Bland JM, Altman DG. Statistical methods for assessing agreement between two methods of clinical measurement. Lancet 1986;i:307–10.

[60] England JD, Gronseth GS, Franklin G, et al. Distal symmetrical polyneuropathy: definition for clinical research. Neurology 2005;64(2):199–207.

[61] Perkins BA, Bril V. Diabetic neuropathy: a review emphasizing diagnostic methods. Clin Neurophysiol 2003;114(7):1167–75.

[62] Werner RA, Gell N, Franzblau A, et al. Prolonged median sensory latency as a predictor of future carpal tunnel syndrome. Muscle Nerve 2001;24(11):1462–7.

[63] Gell N, Werner RA, Franzblau A, et al. A longitudinal study of industrial and clerical workers: incidence of carpal tunnel syndrome and assessment of risk factors. J Occup Rehabil 2005;15(1):47–55.

[64] Pilkington A, Buchanan D, Jamal GA, et al. An epidemiological study of the relations between exposure to organophosphate pesticides and indices of chronic peripheral neuropathy and neuropsychological abnormalities in sheep farmers and dippers. Occup Environ Med 2001;58(11):702–10.

[65] Bril V, Ellison R, Ngo M, et al. Electrophysiological monitoring in clinical trials. Roche Neuropathy Study Group. Muscle Nerve 1998;21(11):1368–73.

[66] Dillingham TR, Pezzin LE. Under-recognition of polyneuropathy in persons with diabetes by nonphysician electrodiagnostic services providers. Am J Phys Med Rehabil 2005;84(6): 399–406.

[67] Dillingham TR, Pezzin LE, Rice JB. Electrodiagnostic services in the United States. Muscle Nerve 2004;29(2):198–204.

ELSEVIER
SAUNDERS

Phys Med Rehabil Clin N Am
16 (2005) 1033–1051

PHYSICAL MEDICINE
AND REHABILITATION
CLINICS OF
NORTH AMERICA

Physiological and Anatomical Basis of Muscle Magnetic Resonance Imaging

Russell C. Fritz, MD[a], Mark E. Domroese, MD, PhD[b],
Gregory T. Carter, MD[b],*

[a]*National Orthopaedic Imaging Associates, 1260 South Eliseo Drive,
Greenbrae, CA 94904, USA*
[b]*Department of Rehabilitation Medicine, University of Washington,
1959 N.E. Pacific Avenue, Seattle, WA 98195, USA*

Over the past decade, MRI has become a widely used technique for imaging the brain and spinal cord. MRI has also become an important tool for evaluating the spine and musculoskeletal system. Ongoing research and clinical experience with MRI is further defining the role of this technique in evaluating disorders of the neuromuscular system. There have been numerous case series and reports documenting the usefulness of MRI in this area [1–10]. Although still evolving, MRI is becoming an increasingly useful method of depicting disorders of muscle and nerve.

Clinical evaluation of neuromuscular disorders typically consists of obtaining a detailed clinical history, physical examination, and electrophysiologic examinations. Electrodiagnostic examinations significantly aid in distinguishing between myopathy, neuropathy, and neuromuscular disorders. Electrodiagnostic examinations also assist in determining the severity and extent of disease. Progress can also be monitored on follow-up testing. The benefit of MRI in neuromuscular disease evaluation lies primarily in identifying a specific underlying gross pathologic cause and its anatomic location [10]. MRI is also helpful in identifying associated secondary findings. In some cases, MRI may be particularly helpful when a solitary, small, deep muscle is affected. Imaging can be useful in assessing clinical progress in some cases. Causes of muscle denervation include mass lesions and trauma as well as infectious, autoimmune, and idiopathic causes. In cases in which

---

* Corresponding author. 1809 Cooks Hill Road, Centralia, WA 98531, USA.
E-mail address: gtcarter@u.washington.edu (G.T. Carter).

1047-9651/05/$ - see front matter © 2005 Elsevier Inc. All rights reserved.
doi:10.1016/j.pmr.2005.08.004   *pmr.theclinics.com*

a mass is responsible for denervation, MRI can directly illustrate the lesion and aid in treatment planning. This manuscript will focus on the anatomic and physiologic aspects of MRI in evaluating muscle function., including both clinical and experimental denervation and primary myopathic conditions.

Techniques for MRI of muscle

Many advances have occurred in the field of biotechnology over the past decade that have led to tremendous improvement in MRI of muscle. Technical developments in magnetic surface coil design and newer pulse sequences have resulted in higher quality MR images that can be obtained rapidly. With respect to accurate interpretation of images, ultimately quality is the most important factor. Although dynamic, kinematic MRI studies are currently being developed, most scanners still require the patient to be motionless to obtain high-quality images. Thus, the patient must be placed in a comfortable position to avoid motion artifact. MR scans are usually done with the patient in a supine position, although sometimes when imaging the upper limb it is necessary to put the patient in a prone position with the arm extended overhead. Now there are newer, wrap-around, surface coils that allow for imaging the arm in the supine position [11,12]. These new surface coils appear similar to a blood pressure cuff, and are excellent for obtaining clear images of smaller limb muscles regardless of the MR field strength and pulse sequences chosen. Different types of surface coils are continually being developed to improve the signal-to-noise ratio from a specific parts of the body. Phased-array coils and higher field strength magnets with modern gradient systems typically provide the greatest amount of signal to work with for a given amount of imaging time [11]. The more signal that is available, the better the resolution that is obtained before unacceptable noise appears in the image. Patients scanned on older machines with lower field systems will require a longer amount of imaging time to obtain the same quality images compared with higher field systems and newer machines. Longer imaging times entail a greater risk of motion artifact that may result in degraded images.

Physiology of MRI

The signal that generates the image is derived from protons in the hydrogen atoms within body tissues [11,13]. Pulse sequences are chosen that create contrast between the signal intensities of these various tissues. The hydrogen atoms within fat generate the most signal on T1-weighted images; thus, fat appears brightest on these images. The hydrogen atoms within water generate the most signal on T2-weighted images. Accordingly, tissue with lots of free water appears brightest on these images. Fat will also appear bright on T2-weighted images, particularly on newer fast spin-echo or turbo spin-echo, T2-weighted images when compared with older conventional T2-weighted images. Fat-suppression pulses may be applied to T2-weighted images to remove the signal from the hydrogen atoms within fat that would otherwise contribute to the signal intensity (SI) of the image [11,14–16]. Hence, the contrast between tissues of differing water content is improved with fat suppression. The fat-suppressed, T2-weighted images are essentially a map of water content within the body.

Anatomy is best depicted on pulse sequences in which fat is the brightest tissue in the image. Fat is abundant throughout the body and surrounds muscle. The high-signal intensity of fat on T1-weighted images allows tissue planes in muscles to be identified. Thus, morphologic changes such as fatty infiltration and loss of bulk of a chronically denervated, atrophic muscle are best seen on T1-weighted images.

Pathology is most accurately depicted on pulse sequences in which the hydrogen atoms within free water are the brightest tissue in the image. The high signal intensity of fluid on fat-suppressed, T2-weighted images allows edema within muscle to be identified. For example, subacute denervation of muscle is characterized by an increase in signal intensity within affected muscles on fat-suppressed, T2-weighted images [17–19]. The signal intensity is increased relative to the signal intensity of unaffected normal muscles seen on the same images.

Conventional spin-echo, pulse sequences are the oldest and most familiar. These pulse sequences include T1-weighted images, proton density images (also referred to as balanced or intermediate weighted images), and T2-weighted images [11]. T1-weighted images are characterized by a short repetition time (TR) and a short echo time (TE). Proton density images are characterized by a long TR and a short TE. T2-weighted images are characterized by long TR and a long TE [11,14,20]. Newer pulse sequences, such as the fast spin-echo or turbo spin-echo sequence, can produce images with similar tissue contrast in a much shorter amount of time.

A high-resolution fast spin-echo, proton density sequence with a long TR (2000–3000 milliseconds) and a short TE (25 milliseconds) is often used for anatomic definition. The other sequence used extensively on high-field MR systems is a fat-suppressed, fast spin-echo T2-weighted image. Locally we use a long TR (3000–4000 milliseconds) and an intermediate TE (40–60 milliseconds) with chemical shift fat suppression on a 1.5 Tesla high-field system. These fat-suppressed images are adequately T2-weighted to detect edema within muscles and have an adequate amount of signal present to obtain high resolution quickly. Using longer echo times on these sequences to obtain greater T2-weighting will decrease the signal-to-noise ratio, thus degrading the quality of the image.

The short-time-inversion-recovery (STIR) pulse sequence is a very useful technique. Newer MR systems have a fast version of the STIR pulse sequence that is better than the conventional STIR pulse sequence, and should be used when it is available. An inversion time, depending on the field strength of the magnet, is chosen to null the signal from fat. Due to more complete suppression of signal from fat, the STIR sequence has a relatively poor signal-to-noise ratio when compared with the chemical shift method of fat suppression discussed above. Despite this, pathology may be more evident with STIR because of the more complete fat suppression and the effects of additive T1 and T2 contrast that characterize the STIR technique. The primary disadvantage of the STIR sequence is that there is less available signal to work with to generate ample resolution without undesirable noise. STIR images with lower resolution are adequate when imaging larger muscles and soft tissue masses. For example, one may use STIR to image the legs in cases of lumbar radiculopathy [2,13,21]. However, fat-suppressed, fast spin-echo, T2-weighted images are better when evaluating small muscles in the distal limbs due to the higher resolution obtained.

It should be noted that the same pulse sequences may appear different, depending on the particular machine. Many older MR units have poor magnetic field homogeneity in the periphery of the magnet, requiring that the patient be positioned off to the side of the magnet's bore when imaging a limb. This places the area of interest within the magnet's most homogeneous field. The STIR pulse sequence is less dependent on a homogeneous magnetic field to obtain uniform fat suppression throughout the image. Therefore, the STIR sequence may be used in place of the fat-suppressed, fast spin-echo, T2-weighted images whenever there is heterogeneous fat suppression [11,22]. T1-weighted or proton density, fast spin-echo images are also good for anatomic definition. However, as noted previously, STIR should be used for detecting pathology characterized by relative increases in tissue water content.

MR image analysis

Several sets of images are obtained from the pulse sequences described above. Both anatomic and pathologic images in three perpendicular planes of section should be obtained for a total of six separate pulse sequences. Both types of images are obtained in the axial, sagittal, and coronal planes. The images should be angled so they are perpendicular to each other. Intravenous gadolinium may provide additional details when imaging neoplastic, ischemic, or inflammatory processes of muscles [23,24]. T1-weighted images with fat suppression are typically obtained whenever gadolinium is administered This results in more than 100 individual cross-sectional images in a typical examination. Muscle, normally surrounded by fat, is best visualized on cross-sectional images. In the limbs, these images are in the axial or transverse plane of section. Grossly edematous or atrophic muscles are easiest to identify when there is a large amount of surrounding fat. It is most difficult to identify small, normal muscles that are the same signal intensity as other muscles in a muscular individual with little surrounding fat.

After anatomic identification, muscles should be evaluated for morphologic changes like atrophy or enlargement. The T1-weighted or proton density images excel at anatomic definition due to relative brightness of fat. The muscle is then assessed for edema, illustrated by a increased signal intensity on the T2-weighted, fat-suppressed T2-weighted, or STIR images obtained at the same slice locations.

Just as computer-based electromyography (EMG) units are now common, interpretation of MR images on a computer workstation is currently the state of the art, and will increasingly become the norm. Doing this makes it much easier to derive the information contained within the images. At a computer workstation the anatomy and pathology images are still viewed side by side on monitors similar to what is done with films on viewboxes. Images are grouped together so that scrolling through one set of images moves the matching images along synchronously. This allows a structure to be identified on anatomic images and then evaluated for relative edema on the matching pathology images. Computer software also provides a colored line that moves its location on the other two sets of images each time a viewer scrolls from one image to the next. This makes it possible to remain oriented as to the location of each slice as sequential images are viewed on the monitor. Moreover, this makes it much easier to confirm abnormalities in multiple planes of a given section.

A computer workstation also allows for control of the grayscale, which is a tremendous advantage when interpreting subtleties on the images. Although some imaging abnormalities are striking, frequently the edema within muscles is more subtle and is characterized by the variations between shades of gray. Although there may be changes in morphology that can be recognized on MRIs, the nature of the technique involves pathology manifesting itself as a change in relative signal intensity [25]. Much like changing the gain or filter settings on an EMG machine, modifying and adjusting the grayscale on an MR unit is extremely valuable when trying to decide if a given muscle is abnormal.

Comparing MRI with electrodiagnostic testing

From an anatomic and physiologic perspective, the information obtained with MRI is complementary to the data provided by electrodiagnostic testing (EDx). EDx testing is a time-honored, well-researched, and acknowledged "gold standard" for assessing the physiologic functioning of muscle and nerve [13]. The techniques are standardized, with immense amounts of normative data, making it a very reliable procedure. Yet it remains a physiologic test, looking at function primarily and, to a lesser degree, anatomy. Anatomic conclusions based on EDx results must be made indirectly, based on which muscles and nerve are involved in the lesion. MRIs are, as of today, a "picture," which looks primarily at anatomy, with assumptions made about the physiologic functioning of structures based on their appearance.

Thus, in some regards, it is a mirror of EDx, adding additional information from the opposite orientation.

Pathology of muscle can be detected and characterized with MRIs through characteristic changes in the morphology and signal intensity. As noted previously, denervated skeletal muscle shows increased signal intensity on T2-weighted and STIR MRI sequences. This is due to longer T1 and T2 relaxation times from the increased size of extracellular fluid relative to intracellular fluid spaces [26–29]. Normal muscle has intermediate to long T1 and short T2 relaxation times relative to surrounding soft tissues and appears gray on most pulse sequences [30–32]. The increased extracellular water content of subacutely denervated or inflamed muscle results in increased signal intensity that is easily visualized on the STIR images. Fig. 1 shows the leaks that appear in the muscle membrane of dystrophinless mdx mice following running exercise. These leaks allowing for significant increases in intracellular water. The same process occurs in human muscular dystrophy. Fig. 2 shows calf muscles from an ambulatory patient with limb girdle muscular dystrophy who overexercised on his treadmill, severely straining his right calf musculature, with resultant increased intracellular edema. This is easily detected with STIR MR images. The patient still had persistent pain and increased calf weakness 2 weeks later. However, his MR images now showed only the expected muscle atrophy. He agreed to a small biopsy, which is shown in Fig. 3. Clearly, the edema had resolved, consistent with his MR findings. This time pattern of recovery from exercise-induced muscle injury is similar to what we have previously observed in dystrophic mice [33].

Denervation presents a somewhat different temporal sequence. Although this increase in relative signal intensity has been reported as early as 4 days

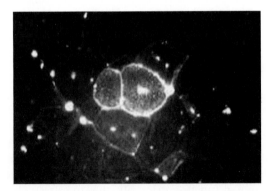

Fig. 1. This illustration is a photomicrograph of quadriceps muscle from an adult mdx mouse 3 days following running exercise and subsequent tail vein injection of 10,000 molecular weight fluorescent dextran. Significant intracellular staining exists in several fibers (center), indicating membrane damage. Central nuclei, present in regenerating fibers, are shown in focal-intense areas of fluorescence.

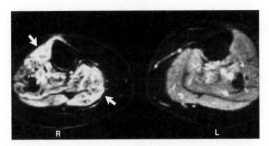

Fig. 2. Axial MRI of the calf musculature. There is significant atrophy and increased signal intensity (*arrows*) throughout the anterior and posterior compartment muscles of the right calf, and atrophy in the left calf. This image was taken from an adult ambulatory patient with limb girdle muscular dystrophy who strained his right leg after strenuous treadmill exercise. The image was taken 2 days after the injury, when the patient presented to the clinic with severe pain and increased leg weakness, primarily in the right leg.

after a severe nerve injury, it is typically seen after 2 to 3 weeks of denervation on STIR or fat-suppressed T2-weighted images [13]. In subacute denervation the affected muscles are relatively bright on T2-weighted images secondary to muscle fiber shrinkage and associated increases in extracellular water [33]. These signal abnormalities seen with MR images may then be followed to resolution or progressive atrophy and fatty infiltration [34,35]. However, it should be noted that increased signal is not specific to denervation, and may also be seen in any condition that causes muscle edema,

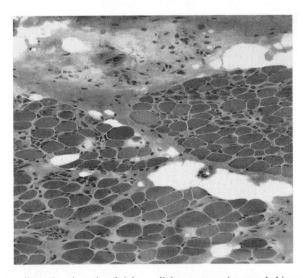

Fig. 3. Hematoxylin and eosin stain of right medial gastrocnemius muscle biopsy from leg imaged in Fig. 2. Now, 2 weeks after the injury, the initial edema noted on the MRI has resolved. Biopsy reveals significant fatty infiltration of the muscle and replacement of muscle with fibrosis. The remaining muscle fibers are irregular in shape, with scattered distribution of fiber size.

including severe muscle strains, blunt trauma, and acute myositis [36–38]. Nonetheless, there is typically perifascial edema present in muscle strain injury that is absent in subacute denervation that allows differentiation of these two entities on MRIs [39]. As with EDx, the clinical history and examination are critical to the interpretation of the findings. We have previously assessed the usefulness of STIR MR images in detecting denervation of skeletal muscle compared with needle EMG [13]. Ninety subjects with clinical evidence of peripheral nerve injury or radiculopathy underwent STIR MRI and EMG of the affected limb. In 74 (82%) of these subjects, a positive correlation was found between STIR MR images and EMG ($P < 0.009$). In our study, STIR MRI had a relative sensitivity of 84% and specificity of 100% for detecting denervation. STIR MRI findings were also analyzed in a semiquantitative fashion by creating a signal intensity ratio (SIR) that compared the signal intensity of the abnormal muscle with that of normal-appearing adjacent muscle and background using the formula: SIR = (SI of abnormal muscle minus SI of background) divided by (SI of normal muscle minus SI background). To assess whether degree of abnormal signal intensity could be correlated with extent of abnormal spontaneous rest activity we randomly chose a subset of 28 subjects and compared SIR and EMG findings in 76 muscles. Spearman Rho rank order correlation coefficients were used to evaluate the relationship between SIR and EMG findings. In the random set of 76 muscles evaluated with the SIR, the Spearman Rho rank order correlation coefficient between SIR and abnormal EMG rest activity was 0.70 ($P < 0.001$). ANOVA-protected pairwise comparisons showed significantly higher mean SIR values in those muscles whose abnormal spontaneous EMG activity was 2+ or greater [13].

The time course of T2-relaxation time changes in denervation and subsequent reinnervation was studied in a rat model by Wessig et al [6] They showed a prolongation of the T2 relaxation time in muscles was present 48 hours after experimental denervation, which was paralleled by spontaneous activity on EMG [6]. Histologically, there was a marked enlargement of the capillaries at that time point, indicating increased blood volume. The relaxation time changes peaked 3 weeks after beginning of nerve regeneration identified by EMG. Subsequently, the T2 prolongation normalized until 10 weeks after beginning of regeneration, which was associated with a histologic regression of the capillary enlargement. This study confirms our clinical findings indicating that MRI closely mirrors the electrophysiologic changes following denervation and reinnervation, and may thus be used as adjunct to electrophysiology. This study adds to our data in that it provides evidence that the pathophysiologic basis for the MR relaxation time changes is predominantly the enlargement of the capillary bed.

Recently Jonas et al [40] looked at quantitative EMG data and the amount of abnormal spontaneous rest activity and compared that with MR image signal intensities in the tibialis anterior muscles of 20 patients with axonal polyneuropathy and 14 normal subjects. Using hierarchical regression analysis, the mean motor unit action potential (MUAP) size index and the amount of abnormal spontaneous rest activity were accurate predictors of T1-weighted signal intensity in MR images. The MUAP SI was superior to MUAP amplitude in explaining the variance of T1 signal intensity. A high correlation was found between the amount of abnormal spontaneous rest activity and the T2-weighted signal intensity in the STIR sequence.

We have previously determined that STIR MRI is a useful tool in assessing lower limb (LL) denervation in subacute lumbar radiculopathy [2]. We had 25 subjects undergo lumbar spine MRIs, LL STIR MRIs, and EMG. In 23 (92%) subjects there was a positive correlation between LL STIR MRI and EMG ($P < 0.009$). However, the time window for MR image changes is smaller than EMG. By 3 months postsymptom onset, MR images showed primarily atrophy as opposed to increased signal intensity (Fig. 4). MRI is also useful at detecting denervation in other peripheral nerve entrapments (Fig. 5), but the clinical history is important as a muscle contusion may look similar to denervation edema (Fig. 6).

Price et al [41] compared MRI and surface EMG (SEMG) to evaluate the effect of knee angle upon plantar flexion activity in the medial and lateral gastrocnemius and soleus muscle. Their group was able to consistently show that soleus activity is measurable by MRI, and that MRI and EMG

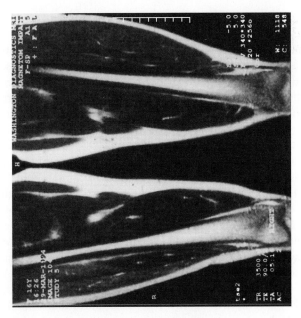

Fig. 4. Coronal T2-weighted MR image of the thighs showing decreased muscle mass in the right quadriceps, compared to the left, in a patient with a chronic L4 radiculopathy.

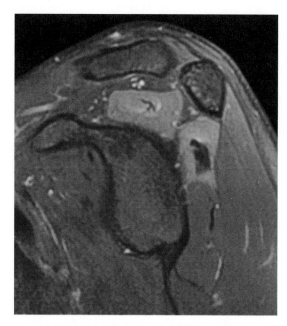

Fig. 5. Suprascapular nerve entrapment in a 24-year-old volleyball player. A fat-suppressed T2-weighted sagittal image reveals increased signal (*whittened areas*) within the spuraspinatus and infraspinatus muscles secondary to repetitive entrapment of the suprascapular nerve. Note that there is an absence of surrounding fluid that is typically seen in muscle strain or contusion injury.

produce similar results from different physiologic sources. This study further confirms that these are complementary tools for evaluating muscle activity.

Despite this promising data, there are still many unanswered questions regarding the use of MRIs to detect muscle denervation. The reasons why MRI exhibits decreased sensitivity in detecting muscle denervation are not clear. It may be that there is a smaller time window of abnormality for MRI relative to EMG in detecting denervation, or perhaps there is a threshold of muscle edema induced by denervation that is required to increase signal intensity sufficiently to be visualized as an abnormality on MR images. Moreover, the time course of changes in signal intensity seen on STIR images of denervated muscles is not well studied. Longitudinal studies on larger populations of subjects are needed to better define the specificity and sensitivity of STIR MRI at different intervals following onset of denervation. Although our studies confirm that STIR MRI is less sensitive than EMG in detecting muscle denervation, some caution should be taken in interpretation of the data. With respect to sensitivity, if a novel technique, that is, STIR MRI, is compared against a gold standard, that is, EMG, the gold standard will always come out superior. Further, better, less subjective, methods of quantifying STIR signal intensity need to be developed. The

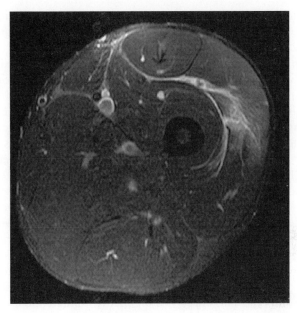

Fig. 6. Thirty-two-year-old prefessional football player with pain and weakness after an injury. This offensive lineman was injured from a direct blow to the thigh with a football helmet the day before. A STIR axial image reveals increased signal within the vestus lateralis muscle (*top of image*) as well as a small amount of fluid deep to the muscle. There is no evidence of a large defect in the muscle or large hematoma.

degree of STIR abnormality in complete versus incomplete axonal lesions, and the imaging changes occurring with reinnervation, have not been systematically studied. Presently, electrodiagnostic studies are still necessary to differentiate a complete from an incomplete axonal lesion.

Functional MRI of muscle

There have been many recent advances in the use of MRI to functionally assess both skeletal and cardiac muscle [42–44]. Functional MRI in real time is an emerging tool for the assessment of dynamic changes in brain and muscle activation. A recent study demonstrated a method to evaluate motion and realign functional images in real time implemented on standard imaging hardware [34,35,45]. Muscle functional MRI (mfMRI) is used to compare the relative involvement of different muscles recruited during exercise. The method relies on the activity-induced increase in T2 relaxation times of muscle water, which is caused by osmotically driven shifts of fluid into the myofibrillar space. During vigorous exercise the water content of muscle increases transiently, which can be observed using MRI via prolonged T2 relaxation times and visualized on the STIR sequences. In addition to imaging of whole-muscle recruitment, muscle MRI may reveal changes in motor unit organization during disease.

Although mfMRI has been widely used to study muscle recruitment during exercise in young healthy subjects, it has not been validated or used with older subjects. Ploutz-Snyder et al [34] recently demonstrated the use of mfMRI in the geriatric setting by comparing older women with healthy sedentary younger women. T2-weighted MR image scans were obtained of the quadriceps femoris at rest and immediately following three bouts of knee extension exercise (50%, 75%, and 100% of untrained 5 × 10 repetition maximum [RM]). Older subjects performed knee extension training for 12 weeks and repeated the MR image scan protocol using the same absolute loads. Training induced a 13% increase in one RM and a 25% increase in 5 × 10 RM. Older subjects had higher resting T2 values compared with younger subjects; however, the T2 response to exercise (slope) was similar among groups. In all cases, T2 increased linearly with load. Trained older subjects showed a lower T2 response when lifting the same absolute load compared with before training, which is consistent with results previously obtained from young subjects. This study was the first to validate the use of mfMRI in an older population. The noninvasiveness of mfMRI offers significant benefits over other techniques of studying muscle function in the elderly.

Recently, MRI has been applied to exercise physiology to investigate mass specific blood flow in human dynamic knee-extensor exercise [43]. Prior studies have suggested that the perfusion-to-muscle mass ratio can reach enormously high levels in the human quadriceps. However, in these studies mass specific blood flows were calculated based on the assumption that the quadriceps are the only muscles involved in the knee-extensor exercise, which is difficult to verify using an in vivo human model. Previous validations of this assumption have been performed using EMG and assessments of strain gauge tracings, but neither has been able to completely assess the involvement of all thigh muscles in this exercise. MRI was used to answer this question by having four subjects exercise at 90% of their work rate maximum for 2 minutes and then a transverse section of the thigh was studied using T2-weighted MRI to distinguish active from nonactive muscles by the increased signal intensity. On a separate occasion, measurements followed 2 minutes of conventional two-legged cycle ergometry at 90% of maximum work rate in the same subjects [43]. Following knee-extensor exercise there was a clearly visible change in T2-weighted signal intensity only in the four muscles of the quadriceps. After bicycle exercise, signal intensity changes revealed a varied muscle use across all muscles. From the MRI data it was concluded that, unlike cycle exercise in which all muscles are recruited to varying extents, single leg knee-extensor exercise is limited to the four muscles of the quadriceps. Thus, the common practice of normalizing blood flow and metabolic data to the quadriceps muscle mass in human knee-extensor exercise studies appears appropriate.

Saab et al [44] determined the effects of intense exercise on the T2 relaxation of human skeletal muscle. The flexor digitorum profundus muscles of 12 male subjects were studied by using MRI (six echoes, 18-millisecond echo time) and in vivo MR relaxometry (1000 echoes, 1.2-millisecond echo time), before and after an intense handgrip exercise. MRI of resting muscle produced a single T2 value of 32 milliseconds that increased by 19% with exercise. In vivo relaxometry showed at least three T2 components for all subjects with mean values of 21, 40, and 137 milliseconds and respective magnitudes of 34, 49, and 14% of the total MR signal. These component magnitudes changed with exercise by −44%, +52%, and +23%, respectively. These results demonstrate that intense exercise has a profound effect on the multicomponent T2 relaxation of muscle. They concluded that changes in the magnitudes of all the T2 components synergistically increase MRI T2 signal, but changes in the two shortest T2 components predominate.

Automated MRI texture analysis was compared with visual MRI analysis for the diagnosis of muscular dystrophy in 14 healthy and 17 diseased subjects [14]. MRI texture analysis was performed on eight muscle regions of interest using four statistical methods (histogram, co-occurrence matrix, gradient matrix, run-length matrix) and one structural (mathematic morphology) method. Nonparametric tests were used to compare diagnoses based on automated texture analysis and visual analysis. Texture analysis methods discriminated between healthy volunteers and patients with a sensitivity of 70%, and a specificity of 86%. Compared with visual analysis, texture analysis of MR images may provide additional useful information contributing to the diagnosis of skeletal muscle disease.

MRI of cardiac muscle

Newer MRI techniques, including spin-echo, cine MR angiography, and contrast enhanced spin-echo MRI have shown promise in detecting heart muscle disorders. Clearly, there is a need for a noninvasive tool that can aid prognosis and follow-up in this setting. In a recent study, focal myocardial enhancement with associated regional wall motion abnormality correlated with myocarditis in 10 out of 12 patients, and two patients with abnormal focal enhancement alone also clinically had myocarditis [46]. None of the nonmyocarditis patients showed abnormal focal enhancement. In the correct clinical context, focal myocardial enhancement on spin-echo MR image strongly supports a diagnosis of myocarditis, especially when associated with regional wall motion abnormality.

A new real-time MRI technique (acquisition duration, 62 ms/image) for the determination of left ventricular end-diastolic volume, end-systolic volume, ejection fraction, and muscle mass was compared with turbo gradient echo imaging as the reference standard [47]. Thirty-four patients were examined with digital echocardiography, standard, and real-time MRI. A close correlation was found between the results of real-time imaging and the reference standards for end-diastolic volume, end-systolic volume, and ejection fraction. Real-time MRI enables the acquisition of high-quality cine loops of the entire heart in minimal time. Compared with echocardiography, patient setup and scan time can be reduced considerably.

MRI for primary muscle disease

We have previously demonstrated large sarcolemmal leaks in exercise-damaged and diseased muscle using fluorescent labeled dextrans in mouse models [42]. This required tail vein injections that are very difficult technically. In normal control muscles, strong fluorescence is seen between fibers (intercellular), confirming sarcolemmal integrity. In muscles from mice run exhaustively downhill and dystrophinless (mdx) mice there were increased numbers of fibers with intracellular fluorescence compared with the controls. Using new albumin-targeted contrast agent-enhanced MRI one may study essentially the same thing in a much easier fashion. Straub et al [29] studied mdx and sarcoglycan-deficient mice, demonstrating a significant accumulation of contrast material in skeletal muscle. The results suggest that contrast agent-enhanced MRI could serve as a common, noninvasive imaging procedure for evaluating the localization, extent, and mechanisms of skeletal muscle damage in muscular dystrophy.

Allamand et al [36] used the same technique to investigate sarcolemmal integrity in animals who had a single intramuscular injection of a first generation gene carrying adenovirus that led to sustained expression of alpha-sarcoglycan at the sarcolemma. The morphology of transduced muscles was consequently preserved. They provided strong evidence that early virus-mediated gene transfer of a sarcoglycan protein constitutes a promising therapeutic strategy for treating these forms of limb-girdle muscular dystrophy, and that the benefits of this approach can easily and effectively be monitored by noninvasive methodologies such as contrast agent-enhanced MRI. This method is expected to facilitate assessment of therapeutic approaches in muscle diseases.

McIntosh et al [24] used MRI to follow dystrophy and regeneration in the mdx mouse. It was hypothesized that MR images would distinguish normal control from mdx muscle, and that regenerating areas (spontaneous and after an imposed injury) would be evident and evolve over time. T2-weighted images of hind-limb mdx muscle appeared heterogeneous in comparison to homogeneous images of control muscle. Foci of high intensity in mdx images corresponded to dystrophic lesions observed in the histologic sections of the same muscles. In addition, it was possible to follow chronologically the extent of injury and repair after an imposed crush injury to mdx muscle. These results further confirm that it is possible to obtain meaningful MR images from particular regions of interest in muscle (i.e, regenerating, degenerating, normal muscle) acquired during neuromuscular diseases and treatment regimens).

Messineo et al [15] showed a good correlation between clinical EMG studies and and spin-echo T1, T2-weighted, multiple-echo, and STIR sequences MRI data. Specifically, in a group of 23 patients with slowly progressive myopathy, Sperman's index was found to be 0.63 in its correlation between the clinical examination and MRI. The T2-weighted and STIR sequences had great sensitivity in showing initial changes in the muscles. The spin-echo T1-weighted sequence was especially useful in detecting degeneration in the muscle tissue. As in our studies, the STIR sequence, because of its high sensitivity and greater speed of response, could be used instead of the SE T2-weighted, particularly in patients who were unable to tolerate a prolonged period of scanning. However, because these sequences have a low signal-to-noise ratio, they must always be associated with a spin-echo sequence.

EMG is traditionally used to measure the electrical activity of a muscle and can be used to estimate muscle contraction intensity. This approach, however, is limited not only in terms of the volume of tissue that can be monitored, but must be invasive if deep lying muscles are studied. Heers et al [48] used MR elastography in an attempt to noninvasively determine muscle activity. This novel approach uses a conventional MRI system. However, in addition to the imaging gradients, an oscillating, motion sensitizing field gradient is applied to detect mechanical waves that have been generated within the tissue. The wavelength correlates with the stiffness of the muscle, and hence with the activity of the muscle. The wavelengths of mechanically generated shear waves in this study were then measured measured as subjects resisted ankle plantar- and dorsi-flexing. The findings were then compared with EMG data collected under the same loading conditions. MR elastography wavelengths were linearly correlated to the muscular activity as defined by EMG, and a high correlation was found [48]. This study showed that MR elastography may be a promising tool for the noninvasive determination of muscle activity, and has potential as the basis for a new noninvasive approach to study in vivo muscle function.

MRI and spectroscopy as a basic science research tool

MRI and MR spectroscopy (MRS) are both useful basic science research tools. Metabolic capacity of muscle may be measured as the rate of phosphocreatine (PCr) recovery following exercise. PCr levels can be assessed using MRS [49–52]. Phosphorus MRS (P-MRS) has now been used in the investigation of muscle energy metabolism in health and disease for over 15 years. We have done prior assessments of metabolic capacity in exhaustive exercise using muscle biopsies [33,42,43]. Short-term endurance training results in significant increases in metabolic capacity. However, this adaptation to exhaustive exercise training is also associated with muscle injury. Muscle injury may be seen as a transient elevation of Pi/PCr at rest in response to an acute bout of exercise. This elevation of resting Pi/PCr will usually persist during continued training [21]. Metabolic capacity as measured by the rate of phosphocreatine recovery will increase with endurance training and decrease with normal aging and metabolic disease. Small levels of persistent muscle injury is a natural by product of strenuous endurance training and muscle disease [42,43]. This may all be assessed with MRS.

Constantinides et al [50] used sodium 23 (Na-23) MRI to quantify non-invasively total sodium in human muscle. Total sodium was determined from the ratio of the relaxation-corrected Na-23 signal intensities measured from short echo-time (0.4 milliseconds) Na-23 images to those from an external saline solution reference. Na-23 MRI also was performed in two healthy subjects after exercise, two patients with myotonic dystrophy, and two patients with osteoarthritis. The Na-23 MRI yielded a total sodium value of 28.4 mmol/kg of wet weight ± 3.6 (SD) in normal muscle, consistent with prior biopsy data. Mean signal intensity elevations were 16% and 22% after exercise and 47% and 70% in dystrophic muscles compared with those at normal resting levels. In osteoarthritis, mean signal intensity reductions were 36% and 15% compared with those in unaffected knee joints. The authors concluded that Na-23 MRI can be used to quantify total sodium in human muscle. The technique may facilitate understanding of the role of the sodium–potassium pump and perfusion in normal and diseased muscle. MRS and MRI of muscle also offers new possibilities for non-invasive diagnosis of metabolic myopathies. These functional techniques may allow assessment of the pathophysiology of mitochondrial encephalo-myopathies, glycolytic disorders, and hypothyroidism [37,38]. Estimation of body composition is possible with MRI. Gong et al [39] did a detailed systematic series of axial MR images (T1-weighted) throughout the whole body of normal and muscular dystrophy subjects. The mean normalized volumes of muscle in the muscular dystrophy patients was significantly decreased and total fat was increased relative to controls. MR images may have an application in assessing body composition, particularly with respect to treatment efficacy in patients with various types of neuromuscular disorders.

Summary

MRI of muscle is becoming an increasingly useful diagnostic tool. Multiple studies have now indicated that increased signal intensity noted on MR images of specific denervated muscles corresponds closely with abnormalities on EMG. Further, there are many newer forms of MRI and applied MR technology, including functional MRI, contrast enhanced spin-echo

MRI, and more modern MRS. These techniques are allowing MR to play a growing role in the functional and dynamic evaluation of skeletal muscle pathology and injury, body composition, and cardiac disease.

Despite these advances in the use of MRI, there are definite limitations. Clinically available MRI still requires the subject to be relatively motionless. This limits its usefulness as a functional assessment tool. Further, available data confirm that MRI is less sensitive in detecting muscle denervation than needle EMG. The degree of abnormality in complete versus incomplete axonal lesions, and the imaging changes occurring with reinnervation, have not been systematically studied. Presently, electrodiagnostic studies are still necessary to differentiate a complete from an incomplete axonal lesion. Better, less subjective, methods of quantifying MR signal intensity need to be developed. With respect to denervation, longitudinal, serial studies in the same patient over an extended time are needed to better define the usefulness of MRI in terms of sensitivity and specificity in relation to time after nerve injury.

References

[1] Bredella MA, Tirman PF, Fritz RC, et al. Denervation syndromes of the shoulder girdle: MR imaging with electrophysiologic correlation. Skeletal Radiol 1999;28(10):567–72.

[2] Carter GT, Fritz RC. Electromyographic and lower extremity STIR MRI findings in lumbar radiculopathy. Muscle Nerve 1997;20:1191–3.

[3] Carter GT, McDonald CM, Chan TT, et al. Isolated femoral mononeuropathy to the vastus lateralis: EMG and MRI findings. Muscle Nerve 1995;18:341–4.

[4] Sofka CM, Lin J, Feinberg J, et al. Teres minor denervation on routine magnetic resonance imaging of the shoulder. Skeletal Radiol 2004;33(9):514–8.

[5] Elsayes KM, Shariff A, Staveteig PT, et al. Value of magnetic resonance imaging for muscle denervation syndromes of the shoulder girdle. J Comput Assist Tomogr 2005;29(3):326–9.

[6] Wessig C, Koltzenburg M, Reiners K, et al. Muscle magnetic resonance imaging of denervation and reinnervation: correlation with electrophysiology and histology. Exp Neurol 2004; 185(2):254–61.

[7] Bendszus M, Wessig C, Solymosi L, et al. MRI of peripheral nerve degeneration and regeneration: correlation with electrophysiology and histology. Exp Neurol 2004;188(1):171–7.

[8] Fritz RC, Breidahl WH. Radiographic and special studies: recent advances in imaging of the elbow. Clin Sports Med 2004;23(4):567–80.

[9] Fritz RC. Magnetic resonance imaging of sports-related injuries to the shoulder: impingement and rotator cuff. Radiol Clin N Am 2002;40(2):217–34.

[10] Carter GT, Kilmer DD, Szabo RM, et al. Focal posterior interosseus neuropathy in the presence of hereditary motor and sensory neuropathy, type I. Muscle Nerve 1996;19:644–8.

[11] Fritz RC, Boutin RA. Magnetic resonance imaging of the peripheral nervous system. Phys Med Rehabil Clin N Am 2001;12(2):190–224.

[12] Qayyum A, MacVicar AD, Padhani AR, et al. Symptomatic brachial plexopathy following treatment for breast cancer: utility of MR imaging with surface-coil techniques. Radiology 2000;214(3):837–42.

[13] McDonald CM, Carter GT, Fritz RC, et al. Magnetic resonance imaging of denervated muscle: comparison to electromyography. Muscle Nerve 2000;23(9):1431–4.

[14] Herlidou S, Rolland Y, Bansard JY, et al. Comparison of automated and visual texture analysis in MRI: characterization of normal and diseased skeletal muscle. Magn Reson Imaging 1999;17(9):1393–7.

[15] Messineo D, Cremona A, Trinci M, et al. MRI in the study of distal primary myopathopies and of muscular alterations due to peripheral neuropathies: possible diagnostic capacities of MR equipment with low intensity field (0.2 T) dedicated to peripheral limbs. Magn Reson Imaging 1998;16(7):731–41.

[16] Fritz RC, Breidahl WH. Radiograph and special studies: recent advances in imaging of the elbow. Clin Sports Med 2004;23(4):567–80.

[17] Fleckenstein JL, Watumull D, Conner KE, et al. Denervated human skeletal muscle: MR imaging evaluation. Radiology 1993;187(1):213–8.

[18] Kullmer K, Sievers KW, Reimers CD, et al. Magnetic resonance tomography and histopathologic findings after muscle denervation. A comparative animal experiment study during a two month follow-up. Nervenarzt 1996;67(2):133–9.

[19] Kullmer K, Sievers KW, Reimers CD, et al. Changes of sonographic, magnetic resonance tomographic, electromyographic, and histopathologic findings within a 2-month period of examinations after experimental muscle denervation. Arch Orthop Trauma Surg 1998; 117(4–5):228–34.

[20] Hamano T, Mutoh T, Hirayama M, et al. MRI findings of benign monomelic amyotrophy of lower limb. J Neurol Sci 1999;165(2):184–7.

[21] McCully K, Posner J. Measuring exercise-induced adaptations and injury with magnetic resonance spectroscopy. Int J Sports Med 1992;13(Suppl 1):S147–9.

[22] Mathiak K, Posse S. Evaluation of motion and realignment for functional magnetic resonance imaging in real time. Magn Reson Med 2001;45(1):167–71.

[23] Marras WS, Jorgensen MJ, Granata KP, et al. Female and male trunk geometry: size and prediction of the spine loading trunk muscles derived from MRI. Clin Biomech Bristol, Avon 2001;16(1):38–46.

[24] McIntosh LM, Baker RE, Anderson JE. Magnetic resonance imaging of regenerating and dystrophic mouse muscle. Biochem Cell Biol 1998;76(2–3):532–41.

[25] Meyer RA, Prior BM. Functional magnetic resonance imaging of muscle. Exerc Sport Sci Rev 2000;28(2):89–92.

[26] Fritz RC, Helms CA, Steinbach LS, et al. Suprascapular nerve entrapment: evaluation with MR imaging. Radiology 1992;182(2):437–44.

[27] Sallomi D, Janzen DL, Munk PL, et al. Muscle denervation patterns in upper limb nerve injuries: MR imaging findings and anatomic basis. AJR Am J Roentgenol 1998;171(3):779–84.

[28] Shabas D, Gerard G, Rossi D. Magnetic resonance imaging examination of denervated muscle. Comput Radiol 1987;11:9–13.

[29] Straub V, Donahue KM, Allamand V, et al. Contrast agent-enhanced magnetic resonance imaging of skeletal muscle damage in animal models of muscular dystrophy. Magn Reson Med 2000;44(4):655–9.

[30] Uetani M, Hayash K, Matosunaga N, et al. Denervated skeletal muscle: MR imaging. Radiology 1993;189:511–5.

[31] West GA, Haynor DR, Goodkin R, et al. Magnetic resonance imaging signal changes in denervated muscles after peripheral nerve injury. Neurosurgery 1994;35(6):1077–85 [discussion 1085–6].

[32] Zamani AA, Moriarty T, Hsu L, et al. Functional MRI of the lumbar spine in erect position in a superconducting open-configuration MR system: preliminary results. J Magn Reson Imaging 1998;8(6):1329–33.

[33] Carter GT, Kikuchi N, Abresch RT, et al. Effects of exhaustive concentric and eccentric exercise on murine skeletal muscle. Arch Phys Med Rehabil 1994;75(5):555–9.

[34] Ploutz-Snyder LL, Yackel-Giamis EL, Rosenbaum AE, et al. Use of muscle functional magnetic resonance imaging with older individuals. J Gerontol A Biol Sci Med Sci 2000;55(10): B504–11.

[35] Polak JF, Jolesz FA, Adams DF. Magnetic resonance imaging examination of skeletal muscle prolongation of T1 and T2 subsequent to denervation. Invest Radiol 1988;23:365–9.

[36] Allamand V, Donahue KM, Straub V, et al. Early adenovirus-mediated gene transfer effectively prevents muscular dystrophy in alpha-sarcoglycan-deficient mice. Gene Ther 2000; 7(16):1385–91.

[37] Argov Z, Arnold DL. MR spectroscopy and imaging in metabolic myopathies. Neurol Clin 2000;18(1):35–52.

[38] Argov Z, Lofberg M, Arnold DL. Insights into muscle diseases gained by phosphorus magnetic resonance spectroscopy. Muscle Nerve 2000;23(9):1316–34.

[39] Gong QY, Phoenix J, Kemp GJ, et al. Estimation of body composition in muscular dystrophy by MRI and stereology. J Magn Reson Imaging 2000;12(3):467–75.

[40] Jonas D, Conrad B, Von Einsiedel HG, et al. Correlation between quantitative EMG and muscle MRI in patients with axonal neuropathy. Muscle Nerve 2000;23(8):1265–9.

[41] Price TB, Kamen G, Damon BM, et al. Comparison of MRI with EMG to study muscle activity associated with dynamic plantar flexion. Magn Reson Imaging 2003;21(8):853–61.

[42] Carter GT, Kikuchi N, Horasek S, et al. The use of fluorescent dextrans as a marker of sarcolemmal injury. Histo Histopathol 1994;9(3):443–7.

[43] Richardson RS, Frank LR, Haseler LJ. Dynamic knee-extensor and cycle exercise: functional MRI of muscular activity. Int J Sports Med 1998;19(3):182–7.

[44] Saab G, Thompson RT, Marsh GD. Effects of exercise on muscle transverse relaxation determined by MR imaging and in vivo relaxometry. J Appl Physiol 2000;88(1):226–33.

[45] Petersilge CA, Yoo JU, Boswell MV, et al. MR imaging in pyriformis syndrome. Radiology 1998;209:193–4.

[46] Roditi GH, Hartnell GG, Cohen MC. MRI changes in myocarditis—evaluation with spin echo, cine MR angiography and contrast enhanced spin echo imaging. Clin Radiol 2000; 55(10):752–8.

[47] Schalla S, Nagel E, Lehmkuhl H, et al. Comparison of magnetic resonance real-time imaging of left ventricular function with conventional magnetic resonance imaging and echocardiography. Am J Cardiol 2001;87(1):95–9.

[48] Heers G, Jenkyn T, Dresner MA, et al. Measurement of muscle activity with magnetic resonance elastography. Clin Biomech (Bristol, Avon) 2003;18(6):537–42.

[49] Green RA, Wilson DJ. A pilot study using magnetic resonance imaging to determine the pattern of muscle group recruitment by rowers with different levels of experience. Skeletal Radiol 2000;29(4):196–203.

[50] Constantinides CD, Gillen JS, Boada FE, et al. Human skeletal muscle: sodium MR imaging and quantification-potential applications in exercise and disease. Radiology 2000;216(2): 559–68.

[51] Fleckenstein JL, Shellock FG. Exertional muscle injuries: magnetic resonance imaging evaluation. Top Magn Reson Imaging 1991;3:50–70.

[52] Bendszus M, Wessig C, Solymosi L, et al. MRI of peripheral nerve degeneration and regeneration: correlation with electrophysiology and histology. Exp Neurol 2004;188(1): 171–7.

ELSEVIER
SAUNDERS

Phys Med Rehabil Clin N Am
16 (2005) 1053–1062

PHYSICAL MEDICINE
AND REHABILITATION
CLINICS OF
NORTH AMERICA

Obesity, Physical Activity, and the Metabolic Syndrome in Adult Neuromuscular Disease

David D. Kilmer, MD[a,b,*], Holly H. Zhao, MD[a,b]

[a]Department of Physical Medicine and Rehabilitation, University of California,
Davis Medical Center, 4860 Y Street, Suite 3850, Sacramento, CA 95817, USA
[b]VA Northern California Health Care System, Sacramento, CA 95817, USA

In the United States, there is an epidemic of obesity and the development of type 2 diabetes mellitus and cardiovascular disease. Investigators have identified a constellation of factors that increases the risk for these diseases, termed the *metabolic syndrome*. Obesity and reduced physical activity are associated strongly with metabolic syndrome, and primary therapy consists of increasing physical activity and dietary modification. In able-bodied populations, interventions targeting these factors lead to improvement in measures associated with metabolic syndrome.

In individuals with slowly progressive hereditary neuromuscular diseases (NMDs), common disabilities include muscular weakness, decreased physical working capacity, and fatigability. Because of these issues, a sedentary lifestyle is common. Ability to exercise varies among specific disorders, but is generally reduced in all NMDs. Presumably, individuals with NMDs should be at even greater risk for metabolic syndrome than the general population. Obesity does seem to be more prevalent in adults with physical disabilities, particularly lower extremity mobility difficulties [1]. About 70% of older (> 50 years old) physically disabled adults do not obtain the recommended amount of physical activity to maintain health [2].

Life span in many individuals with NMDs and other disabilities now may be similar to life span in able-bodied individuals. Secondary conditions, such as diabetes mellitus and cardiovascular disease, play an important role in

This article was supported by grants H133B031118 and H133B980008 from the National Institute on Disability and Rehabilitation Research, US Department of Education.

* Corresponding author. Department of Physical Medicine and Rehabilitation, University of California, Davis Medical Center, 4860 Y Street, Suite 3850, Sacramento, CA 95817, USA.
    E-mail address: ddkilmer@ucdavis.edu (D.D. Kilmer).

reducing quality of life. Until definitive treatment for the primary disease of nerve or muscle becomes available, improving quality of life should be a major focus of treating patients with NMDs and other physical disabilities. This article discusses risk factors and assessment methods for these diseases in individuals with NMDs and highlights more recent research investigating methods to identify and prevent complications of obesity and reduced physical activity.

Body composition in neuromuscular diseases

Obesity is a major issue in individuals with disability. Weil et al [2] found that 24.9% of adults with disability were obese compared with 15.1% of adults without disabilities. Problems with lower limb mobility conferred the greatest risk. Obesity generally is measured by body mass index (BMI), defined as mass divided by the square of height (kg/m^2). Obesity is defined as a BMI greater than 30.

Because of reduced muscle mass, individuals with NMDs and other disabilities may need to have BMI categories redefined; otherwise, the prevalence of obesity is likely to be underestimated. In individuals with spinal cord injury, BMI is a much poorer predictor of fat mass than in able-bodied individuals and is inconsistently related to risk of coronary heart disease [3]. In determining the importance of body composition to vascular disease and diabetes, it may be more beneficial to look at measures of body composition other than BMI. Regardless of composition, excessive weight increases muscular demand for movement, causing a muscle to exert at a higher percentage of its maximal capacity.

Dual-energy x-ray absorptiometry has been used to assess whole-body composition in individuals with slowly progressive NMDs [4]. Using this technique, the body mass can be divided into regional and total-body bone mineral, fat tissue, and lean soft tissue masses. The major portion of lean soft tissue is skeletal muscle; determination of lean soft tissue mass by dual-energy x-ray absorptiometry provides a relatively accurate measurement of skeletal muscle mass. Using this technique in slowly progressive NMDs, Kanda et al [4] found that subjects with myogenic atrophy had significantly higher fat-to-lean soft tissue ratios than did subjects with neurogenic atrophy, even though the BMI was similar in all subjects. The slope of the regression in subjects with myogenic muscular atrophy was comparable to controls; this was not the case for subjects with neurogenic atrophy. The authors concluded that fat infiltration into the muscles of subjects with myogenic atrophy is reflected by their increased fat-to-lean soft tissue ratio.

Another new technology for determining body composition has emerged that is ideally suited for NMD subjects because it requires little effort for the subject and the technician, and the measurement procedure is relatively brief. This method, air displacement plethysmography, uses Boyle's law to determine fat mass and fat-free mass [5]. Using this new technology, McCrory et al [6] found significantly increased body fat and fat mass in individuals with NMDs compared with an able-bodied control group, despite no differences in BMI. A more recent study confirmed the same findings in another group with a variety of NMDs [7] and a study limited to individuals with myotonic muscular dystrophy [8]. Another more recent study showed a significant reduction in body fat with a 6-month exercise and dietary intervention in individuals with NMDs [9].

In the absence of highly technical equipment such as dual-energy x-ray absorptiometry, a simple anthropometric technique, such as skin-fold calipers, can be used to estimate body composition [10]. Body fat prediction using four skin-fold measurements (subscapular, suprailiac, midthigh, triceps) has been shown to be precise and accurate relative to a four-compartment model [11].

Physical activity and energy expenditure in neuromuscular diseases

Obesity may result from excessive energy stores secondary to either excessive energy intake or reduced energy expenditure. Total energy expenditure is the sum of resting energy expenditure (or basal metabolic rate, used interchangeably in this article), dietary-induced thermogenesis, and energy expenditure in physical activity. Although clinicians presume that individuals with NMDs are likely to be more sedentary than able-bodied individuals, until more recently there was no evidence to support this. One reason is the challenge of measuring physical activity and energy expenditure. The crudest method is self-report, which has questionable accuracy. A more elegant method is to estimate total energy expenditure by determining a heart rate–oxygen consumption relationship at various ambulation levels, then using heart rate monitoring during awake hours and resting energy expenditure to estimate energy expenditure during sleep. Using this methodology, McCrory et al [6] found that total energy expenditure was significantly reduced in ambulatory individuals with NMDs compared with controls, and they spent fewer minutes each day in physical activity. Adiposity was associated with the low level of physical activity.

A study found that NMD subjects spent an average of 144 min/day in physical activity compared with 214 min/day in controls [7]. The notion that muscular weakness increases the likelihood of a sedentary lifestyle has some support in the literature for this population. One contributing factor may be the increased energy cost of physical activity [6]. This increased cost may lead to a spiral of inactivity and disuse, as the person gradually becomes more and more sedentary to avoid exhaustion with even routine activities. Another factor may be fear of physical activity secondary to concern of overworking muscles.

A simple method to measure physical activity is the pedometer. A typical step count for a moderately active person is 7000 steps/day, with a goal of

10,000 steps/day to help control weight and prevent cardiovascular disease in able-bodied individuals [12]. A reduced number of steps (<5500 steps/ day) is typical for individuals with disabilities and has been associated with components of the metabolic syndrome [13].

Using a simple activity prescription to increase steps by 25% per day, individuals with NMDs were shown to increase step counts by 27% over a 6-month period (approximately 4500–5800 steps/day) [9]. There were no untoward effects, and the intervention was home-based, making it practical for a disabled but ambulatory population.

Nutritional aspects of neuromuscular diseases

NMDs in adults are associated with loss of skeletal muscle, gain of excess body fat, and changes in energy metabolism and physical activity over time. A wide variety of techniques for nutritional measurement have been applied in monitoring the nutritional status of these individuals as the diseases progress.

Individuals with NMDs may be at risk for nutritional inadequacy secondary to impaired mobility, dysphagia, limited ability to shop for food, and socioeconomic issues related to employment. In a study in adults with myotonic muscular dystrophy and other NMDs, 62% of patients with myotonic muscular dystrophy and 82% of patients with other NMDs did not meet their daily energy needs, whereas 10% of patients with myotonic muscular dystrophy and 5% of patients with other NMDs did not meet the dietary reference intake for daily protein intake. About 55% of the myotonic muscular dystrophy subjects and 86% of the other NMD subjects had a fat intake greater than the suggested acceptable macronutrients distribution range [14].

A progressive loss of skeletal muscle contractile proteins is a characteristic of individuals with NMDs and is ultimately due to an imbalance between muscle protein synthesis and protein degradation. Although a reduction in protein synthesis seems to be the main factor contributing to a net negative protein balance in patients with NMDs, nutritional inadequacy has been shown to be associated with impaired muscle strength and pulmonary function [14], and high fat intake is associated with a high incidence of obesity and high risk of metabolic syndrome. Strategies such as energy and protein (including branched-chain amino acids) supplementation in NMDs have yielded promising but inconclusive results [15,16].

Metabolic syndrome

Metabolic syndrome (also called *syndrome X, insulin resistance syndrome,* and *dysmetabolic syndrome*) is a constellation of conditions that increases the risks for coronary artery disease and type 2 diabetes mellitus. The definition of metabolic syndrome varies according to different groups. The World Health Organization definition [17] is better suited as a research tool, whereas the National Cholesterol Education Program's Adult Treatment Panel III definition [18] is more useful for clinical practice. These definitions agree on the essential components, including glucose intolerance, obesity, hypertension, and dyslipidemia, but differ in the cutoff points for criteria for each component and the way of combining them to define the syndrome (Box 1). Because several definitions of the syndrome are in use, it is difficult to compare prevalence and impact among different countries. Ultimately, combined efforts among different organizations will result in a unified definition of the metabolic syndrome that is suitable for use worldwide.

Since the 1980s, a striking increase in the number of people with metabolic syndrome worldwide has occurred. Prevalence of metabolic syndrome in the United States is estimated at 24% among adults and is much more common in adults in their 60s (44%) than adults in their 20s (7%) [19]. The increased prevalence of metabolic syndrome is associated closely with the global epidemic of obesity in adults and children [20,21]. In the past, metabolic syndrome has been regarded as a disease of adults. With increasing rates of obesity in young people, the metabolic syndrome is seen among

---

Box 1. Comparison of definitions of metabolic syndrome

World Health Organization criteria:
Diabetes or impaired fasting glucose or impaired glucose tolerance or insulin resistance, plus ≥2 of the following:
1. Obesity: BMI >30 kg/m^2, or waist-to-hip ratio >0.90 (male) or >0.85 (female)
2. Dyslipidemia: triglycerides ≥1.7 mmol/L or HDL cholesterol <0.90 mmol/L (male) or <1 mmol/L (female)
3. Hypertension: blood pressure ≥140/90 mm Hg (or treated hypertension)
4. Microalbuminuria: albumin excretion >20 μg/min

Adult Treatment Panel III criteria:
Any ≥3 of the following:
1. Central obesity: waist circumference >120 cm (male) or >88 cm (female)
2. Hypertriglyceridemia: triglycerides ≥1.7 mmol/L
3. Low HDL cholesterol: HDL cholesterol <1 mmol/L (male) or <1.16 mmol/L (female)
4. Hypertension: blood pressure ≥130/85 mm Hg (or treated hypertension)
5. Fasting plasma glucose ≥6.1 mmol/L

different ages in all ethnic groups and already is evident in early childhood [21–23]. More importantly, the prevalence is significantly higher in obese children and adolescents, and it increases with severity of obesity, reaching 50% in severely obese youngsters [21].

Data are limited regarding the prevalence of metabolic syndrome in individuals with disabilities and the impact of disability on the syndrome. It is logical that individuals with physical disabilities are at higher risk for the development of metabolic syndrome secondary to decreased physical mobility and caloric expenditure, poor dietary choices, and possibly reduced accessibility to healthier food. A pilot study in individuals with slowly progressive NMDs showed increased adiposity; reduced physical activity; and multiple cardiovascular and metabolic risk factors, including low high-density lipoprotein (HDL) cholesterol and high glucose, triglyceride, and blood pressure in this population [7]. The study showed 55% of NMD subjects met the criteria for metabolic syndrome, which was significantly higher compared with an age-matched, able-bodied control group. Similar findings also are seen in individuals with a variety of other disabilities. Individuals with spinal cord injury had higher rates of insulin resistance with hyperinsulinemia and increased adiposity and lower HDL cholesterol levels compared with an age-matched control population [24–26]. In a long-term study, in individuals with traumatic lower limb amputation, higher rates of insulin resistance and mortality rates from cardiovascular disease were reported compared with a matched control group [27,28].

Metabolic syndrome is associated with an increased risk of type 2 diabetes mellitus and coronary artery disease. Several studies have indicated that metabolic syndrome predicts future type 2 diabetes mellitus. The overall hazard ratios for all-cause and cardiovascular disease mortality in individuals with metabolic syndrome compared with individuals without it were 1.44 and 2.26 in men and 1.38 and 2.78 in women after adjustment for age, blood cholesterol concentrations, and smoking [29].

Affecting metabolic syndrome risk factors in neuromuscular diseases

The epidemic of metabolic syndrome in the able-bodied population is proving to be a challenge to prevent and treat because of Americans' food choices, portion sizes, and inactivity associated with a sedentary lifestyle. A combination of appropriate diet with greater physical activity will be the mainstay of prevention and treatment in the future. There has been minimal research in individuals with disabilities to determine if increasing physical activity lowers the rate of secondary complications, particularly those associated with metabolic syndrome. Some indirect evidence exists. Slawta et al [30] showed that women with multiple sclerosis who participated in low to moderate leisure time physical activity had less abdominal fat accumulation, lower levels of triglycerides, and lower levels of glucose compared with inactive women with multiple sclerosis. In subjects with spinal cord injury, reduced activity level and increased BMI were associated with higher lipid levels and unfavorable lipoprotein profile [31]. One small study of five men with paraplegia showed a 26% reduction of low-density lipoprotein cholesterol and 10% elevation of HDL cholesterol with a 3-month upper limb resistance/endurance exercise regimen [32].

Addressing obesity, cardiovascular risk factors, and metabolic syndrome in patients with NMDs is even more challenging, given the additional issues faced by many individuals with these diseases, including the following:

- Less experience and confidence with exercise programs
- Exercise programs not designed for individuals with disabilities
- Decreased ability to exercise to a level sufficient for weight control
- Concern about overworking muscle
- Less access to comprehensive medical care
- Fewer financial resources available for diets and exercise programs

Many individuals with physical disabilities lack the confidence to be physically active, which serves as a barrier to involvement in an exercise program [33]. A program that is simple, such as a home walking program with quantitative feedback from pedometry, may be a good first step. It is unlikely that adults with NMDs would access typical venues for exercise, such as health clubs, given the known barriers for individuals with physical disabilities to access these types of facilities [34]. These issues are compounded if an individual with NMD becomes wheelchair dependent. Significant energy expenditure through exercise would be exceedingly difficult. In these cases, careful dietary modification may be the only way to have an impact on obesity and metabolic syndrome risk factors.

Access to comprehensive preventive care is a major issue in disabled populations because of lack of transportation, limited financial resources, difficulty in finding a physician, inaccessible equipment in health care facilities, and inadequate knowledge and poor attitudes from health care professionals [35,36]. These societal and health care issues must be addressed to improve the prevention and treatment of secondary conditions such as metabolic syndrome associated with physical disabilities.

Another difference between typical populations and individuals with NMDs is the ability to affect food intake and choices. In studies of able-bodied individuals with components of metabolic syndrome, dietary interventions successfully diminish body mass and metabolic risk factors [37–39]. The protocols are intensive and expensive, however, with significant personal costs. This type of program is impractical for many individuals with NMDs. Previous research has shown the poor diet choices made by these individuals [6], possibly partially related to limited income [40]. Obesity is associated with poverty, and inexpensive energy-dense foods with high sugar and fat are difficult to avoid [41]. An example is the drive-through fast-food phenomenon, which may be highly tempting to a person with limited ambulation ability or primarily using a wheelchair for mobility.

Abdominal obesity is the body fat parameter most closely associated with metabolic syndrome. Weight reduction is best achieved by behavioral change to reduce energy intake and by physical activity to enhance energy expenditure. Caloric intake should be reduced by 500 to 1000 calories/day to produce a weight loss of 0.5 to 1 kg/wk. The goal is to reduce body weight by about 7% to 10% over 6 to 12 months, followed by long-term behavior modification and maintenance of increased physical activity.

The general recommended diet for individuals with metabolic syndrome includes low intakes of saturated fats, *trans*-fatty acids, and cholesterol; reduced consumption of simple sugars; and increased intake of fruits, vegetables, and whole grains [18]. A reduction in the daily caloric intake to promote weight loss is the most important component of the dietary recommendation. Weight loss usually is associated directly with longer duration of dietary discretion and restriction of caloric intake. Given the difficulties in obtaining sufficient caloric expenditure to control weight as a result of fewer exercise options and limited access to exercise venues, dietary control has added importance in the prevention of metabolic syndrome in disabled populations. Healthy dietary modifications are notoriously difficult to maintain. Development of an effective, practical, sustainable dietary intervention program remains a major goal in able-bodied and disabled populations.

One simple intervention to affect nutrition in NMDs focused on a single meeting with a nutritional consultant to identify the most problematic area in each person's diet [9]. In addition, participants were educated about proper serving sizes. For individuals who ate no vegetables, 1 to 2 servings/day were suggested rather than trying to meet US Dietary Guidelines of 5 daily servings. This incremental approach was thought to give a greater chance at success, and participants did reduce caloric intake more than 300 kcal/day. This reduction did not lead to significant changes in most metabolic syndrome risk factors, however. This study is an encouraging first step, but a more aggressive approach may be necessary to reduce significantly secondary conditions associated with obesity in NMDs.

Given the additional challenges to affect the morbidity associated with obesity and physical inactivity in individuals with NMDs, a great amount of creativity is required to formulate practical recommendations with a reasonable chance of success. It is incumbent on clinicians caring for patients with NMDs to understand the importance of prevention and identification of diseases associated with obesity and physical inactivity and to encourage methods of prevention and treatment within the abilities and resources of each patient with NMD.

Summary

There is now preliminary evidence that with greater life span in individuals with NMDs, complications of obesity and reduced physical activity will gain increasing importance in reducing quality of life. Preventing and treating cardiovascular disease and type 2 diabetes mellitus and their precursor, metabolic syndrome, is even more challenging than in able-bodied individuals. Understanding the physical, emotional, and socioeconomic issues affecting many individuals with NMDs and other physical disabilities is the first step in finding a solution.

References

[1] Weil E, Wachterman M, McCarthy EP, et al. Obesity among adults with disabling conditions. JAMA 2002;288:1265–8.
[2] Brown DR, Yore MM, Ham SA, et al. Physical activity among adults > 50 yr with and without disabilities, BRFSS 2001. Med Sci Sports Exerc 2005;37:620–9.
[3] Buchholz AC, Bugaresti JM. A review of body mass index and waist circumference as markers of obesity and coronary heart disease risk in persons with chronic spinal cord injury. Spinal Cord 2005;43:513–8.
[4] Kanda F, Fujii Y, Takahashi K. Dual-energy x-ray absorptiometry in neuromuscular diseases. Muscle Nerve 1994;17:431–5.
[5] Dempster P, Aitkens S. A new air displacement method for the determination of human body composition. Med Sci Sports Exerc 1995;27:1692–7.
[6] McCrory MA. Him HR, Wright NC, et al. Energy expenditure, physical activity, and body composition of ambulatory adults with hereditary neuromuscular disease. Am J Clin Nutr 1998;67:1162–9.
[7] Aitkens S, Kilmer DD, Wright NC, et al. Metabolic syndrome in neuromuscular disease. Arch Phys Med Rehabil 2005;86:1030–6.
[8] Perseghin G, Comola M, Scifo P, et al. Postaborptive and insulin-stimulated energy and protein metabolism in patients with myotonic dystrophy type 1. Am J Clin Nutr 2004;80: 357–64.
[9] Kilmer DD, Wright NC, Aitkens S. Impact of a home-based activity and dietary intervention in persons with slowly progressive neuromuscular diseases. Am Phys Med Rehabil, in press.
[10] Lohman TG, Roche AF, Martorell R. Anthropometric standardization reference manual. Champaign (IL): Human Kinetics; 1988.
[11] Peterson MJ, Czerwinski SA, Siervogel RM. Development and validation of skinfold-thickness prediction equations with a 4-compartment model. Am J Clin Nutr 2003;77:1186–91.
[12] Tudor-Locke CE, Myers AM. Methodological considerations for researchers and practitioners using pedometers to measure physical (ambulatory) activity. Res Q Exerc Sport 2001;72:1–12.
[13] Chan CB, Spangler E, Valcour J, et al. Cross-sectional relationship of pedometer-determined ambulatory activity to indicators of health. Obes Res 2003;11:1563–70.
[14] Motlagh B, MacDonald JR, Tarnopolsky RA. Nutritional inadequacy in adults with muscular dystrophy. Muscle Nerve 2005;31:713–8.
[15] Goldstein M, Meyer S, Freund HR. Effects of overfeeding children with muscle dystrophies. J Parenter Enteral Nutr 1989;13:603–7.
[16] Stewart PM, Walser M, Drachman DB. Branched-chain ketoacids reduce muscle protein degradation in Duchenne muscular dystrophy. Muscle Nerve 1982;5:197–201.
[17] Alberti KG, Zimmet PZ. Definition, diagnosis and classification of diabetes mellitus and its complications: Part 1. Diagnosis and classification of diabetes mellitus, provisional report of a WHO consulatation. Diabet Med 1998;15:539–53.
[18] Executive summary of the third report of the National Cholesterol Education Program (NCEP) expert panel on detection, evaluation, and treatment of high blood cholesterol in adults (Adult Treatment Panel III). JAMA 2001;285:2486–97.

[19] Ford ES, Giles WH, Dietz WH. Prevalence of the metabolic syndrome among US adults: findings from the third National Health and Nutrition Examination Survey. JAMA 2002; 287:356–9.

[20] Zimmet P, Alberti KG, Shaw J. Global and societal implications of the diabetes epidemic. Nature 2001;414:782–7.

[21] Weiss R, Dziura J, Burgert TS, et al. Obesity and the metabolic syndrome in children and adolescents. N Engl J Med 2004;350:2362–74.

[22] Sinha R, Fisch G, Teague B, et al. Prevalence of impaired glucose tolerance among children and adolescents with marked obesity. N Engl J Med 2002;346:802–10.

[23] Wei JN, Sung FC, Lin CC, et al. National surveillance for type 2 diabetes mellitus in Taiwanese children. JAMA 2003;290:1345–50.

[24] Bauman WA, Spungen AM. Metabolic changes in persons after spinal cord injury. Phys Med Rehabil Clin N Am 2000;11:109–40.

[25] Zlotolow SP, Levy E, Bauman WA. The serum lipoprotein profile in veterans with paraplegia: the relationship to nutritional factors and body mass index. J Am Paraplegia Soc 1992; 15:158–62.

[26] Bauman WA, Adkins RH, Spungen AM, et al. The effect of residual neurological deficit on serum lipoproteins in individuals with chronic spinal cord injury. Spinal Cord 1998;36:13–7.

[27] Peles E, Akselrod S, Goldstein DS, et al. Insulin resistance and autonomic function in traumatic lower limb amputees. Clin Auton Res 1995;5:279–88.

[28] Modan M, Peles E, Halkin H, et al. Increased cardiovascular disease mortality rates in traumatic lower limb amputees. Am J Cardiol 1998;82:1242–7.

[29] Hu G, Qiao Q, Tuomilehto J, et al. Prevalence of the metabolic syndrome and its relation to all-cause and cardiovascular mortality in nondiabetic European men and women. Arch Intern Med 2004;164:1066–76.

[30] Slawta JN, McCubbin JA, Wilcox AR, et al. Coronary heart disease risk between active and inactive women with multiple sclerosis. Med Sci Sports Exerc 2002;34:905–12.

[31] Janssen TW, van Oers CA, van Kamp GJ, et al. Coronary heart disease risk indicators, aerobic power, and physical activity in men with spinal cord injuries. Arch Phys Med Rehabil 1997;78:697–705.

[32] Nash MS, Jacobs PL, Mendez AJ, et al. Circuit resistance training improves the atherogenic lipid profiles of persons with chronic paraplegia. J Spinal Cord Med 2001;24:2–9.

[33] Eyler AA. Correlates of physical activity: who's active and who's not? Arthritis Rheum 2003; 49:136–40.

[34] Rimmer JH, Riley B, Wang E, et al. Physical activity participation among persons with disabilities: barriers and facilitators. Am J Prev Med 2004;26:419–25.

[35] Iezzoni LI, McCarthy EP, Davis RB, et al. Mobility impairments and use of screening and preventive services. Am J Public Health 2000;90:955–61.

[36] Jha A, Patrick DL, MacLehose RF, et al. Dissatisfaction with medical services among Medicare beneficiaries with disabilities. Arch Phys Med Rehabil 2002;83:1335–41.

[37] Christ M, Iannello C, Iannello PG, et al. Effects of a weight reduction program with and without aerobic exercise in the metabolic syndrome. Int J Cardiol 2004;97:115–22.

[38] Diabetes Prevention Program Research Group. Reduction in the incidence of type 2 diabetes with lifestyle intervention or metformin. N Engl J Med 2002;346:393–403.

[39] Watkins LL, Sherwood A, Feinglos M, et al. Effects of exercise and weight loss on cardiac risk factors associated with syndrome X. Arch Intern Med 2003;163:1889–95.

[40] Fowler WM Jr, Abresch RT, Koch TR, et al. Employment profiles in neuromuscular diseases. Arch Phys Med Rehabil 1997;76:26–37.

[41] Drewnowski A, Specter SE. Poverty and obesity: the role of energy density and energy costs. Am J Clin Nutr 2004;79:6–16.

ELSEVIER
SAUNDERS

Phys Med Rehabil Clin N Am
16 (2005) 1063–1079

PHYSICAL MEDICINE
AND REHABILITATION
CLINICS OF
NORTH AMERICA

Approaching Fatigue in Neuromuscular Diseases

Jau-Shin Lou, MD, PhD

*MDA Clinic, ALS Center of Oregon, EMG Laboratory, and Department of Neurology,
CR120, Oregon Health & Science University, 3181 SW Sam Jackson Park Road,
Portland, OR 97234, USA*

Fatigue is common in many neurologic and nonneurologic conditions, such as neuromuscular diseases, multiple sclerosis, depression, renal failure, pulmonary diseases, cardiovascular diseases, and cancer. Fatigue also is common in healthy subjects. In one study, 18% of normal healthy controls complained of fatigue. Physicians and patients often use the term *fatigue* without defining it, however. There are no medical criteria for fatigue. The term *fatigue*, when used by physicians or patients, may have a meaning ranging from mental depression to neuromuscular weakness. Physicians cannot make progress or help patients to solve their problems with fatigue until they can scrutinize the various meanings of fatigue and correlate them with an organic or psychological disease state.

Since the 1990s, investigators have pursued research in seriously ill subjects (eg, amyotrophic lateral sclerosis [ALS] or other advanced neuromuscular diseases that cause immobility) that might lead to better palliation of disabling symptoms, including fatigue, pain, and dyspnea, and improve quality of life until the end of life [1]. Fatigue is highly prevalent in many serious medical conditions, including cancer, AIDS, and neurologic disorders such as multiple sclerosis and Parkinson's disease, and has deleterious effects on quality of life. Researchers in palliative care have focused on developing valid and reliable measures of fatigue; measuring the prevalence, incidence, and daily variation of this symptom; clarifying the relationship of fatigue to other symptoms and morbid outcomes; and testing interventions to treat fatigue.

Studies were supported by grants from the Medical Research Foundation of Oregon, Parkinson Disease Foundation, and National Institutes of Health.

E-mail address: Louja@ohsu.edu

Fatigue in neuromuscular disease

Fatigue is underinvestigated as a clinical problem in neuromuscular diseases and often is overlooked by clinicians who care for neuromuscular patients. Textbooks in neurology rarely mention fatigue as a clinical symptom. Fatigue as a symptom has not been studied systematically. ALS is a prime example. Except for one pilot study, no investigations characterize fatigue in ALS, examine the most valid and reliable manner in which to measure this symptom, explore potential pathophysiologic correlates, or examine the relationship of fatigue to quality of life. In patients with ALS, it is unclear if fatigue remains an independent symptom that is treatable after treating other symptoms or simply reflects other easily measured symptoms, such as sleep problems, dyspnea, or depression.

Approaches to fatigue in cancer, multiple sclerosis, and Parkinson's disease

Approaches to understanding and treating fatigue in other diseases merit review because they serve as potential models for investigation of fatigue in neuromuscular diseases. Fatigue in cancer has drawn researchers' attention since the early 1980s. Efforts to understand and treat fatigue in patients undergoing cancer treatment received little attention until the early 1990s [2,3]. Fatigue accompanying cancer treatment was not the same as the fatigue experienced by healthy people. Fatigue in cancer could occur in the absence of activity or exertion, was more severe than fatigue experienced before the illness, and was not fully relieved by sleep or rest. These observations prompted speculation about mechanisms of cancer treatment–related fatigue. Most studies of fatigue in cancer focus on developing new instruments for measuring fatigue, describing the incidence and prevalence of fatigue, defining the impact of fatigue on various components of quality of life, and examining correlates of fatigue. Correcting chemotherapy-induced anemia is the only mechanism-based intervention that has been studied. The other intervention that has accumulated significant research support is engaging aerobic exercise during cancer treatment to minimize fatigue [4]. Other interventions that now have preliminary evidence of effectiveness are the use of psychostimulants in selected populations and using a structured energy conservation intervention to plan and schedule activity [5,6]. The works on fatigue in cancer shed light on future studies of fatigue in neuromuscular diseases by suggesting that the approach of comparing existing instruments would yield the most useful information. This is especially true if the approach was conducted in a way that allowed investigators to make selected comparisons between known groups, examine change over time in subjects with neuromuscular diseases, and describe the relationship between fatigue and a set of clinical outcomes relevant to a variety of neuromuscular diseases [7].

Fatigue is increasingly recognized as a disabling symptom in neurologic diseases, such as multiple sclerosis (MS) [8] and Parkinson's disease (PD)

[9]. Fatigue in MS is well studied. Investigators have measured the prevalence of fatigue in MS [10], validated fatigue questionnaires such as Fatigue Severity Scale (FSS) [11], investigated underlying mechanisms [12,13], and conducted clinical trials to treat fatigue [14,15]. More than 75% of MS patients report fatigue, and more than half of MS patients believe that fatigue limits their ability to perform activities of daily living [10]. Fatigue in MS differs from acute fatigue localized to specific muscle groups because it is persistent, it is global, and it does not subside with rest [16]. The cause and pathogenesis of fatigue in MS are not well understood, but seem to be related directly to the disease process. The severity of fatigue in MS is correlated with depression, but is independent of neurologic disability [13]. Studies using MRI have shown a consistent lack of association between MS fatigue and brain atrophy or lesion load on T1-weighted or T2-weighted images [12,17]. Potential contributing factors to fatigue in MS include medications, infections, hot weather, sleep disturbance, spasticity, and depression [8]. Several medications have been tested in the treatment of fatigue in MS, including the dopaminergic agent amantadine and the amphetamine-related stimulant pemoline [14]. Modafinil, which was approved by the US Food and Drug Administration for the treatment of narcolepsy, also is effective for fatigue in MS [15]. These treatments may be tested in ALS patients if it can be shown that fatigue is a valid, independent clinical entity in ALS.

The author's laboratory has conducted a series of studies to characterize fatigue in patients with PD [9,18,19]. In the first study of fatigue in PD [9], investigators characterized fatigue in 39 PD patients and 32 age-matched normal controls using the Multidimensional Fatigue Inventory (MFI), which measures five dimensions of fatigue independently: general fatigue, physical fatigue, reduced motivation, reduced activity, and mental fatigue. The results showed that PD patients scored higher than normal controls in all five dimensions of fatigue in the MFI. The severity of physical fatigue did not correlate with that of mental fatigue. Disease severity, as measured by modified Hoehn and Yahr staging, did not correlate with any of the measures. In a second study [18], investigators quantitatively investigated the effect of carbidopa/levodopa (25/100) on physical fatigue during finger tapping and force generation in a double-blind, placebo-controlled cross-over study. Levodopa improves physical fatigue in finger tapping and force generation. In a third study [19], investigators used transcranial magnetic stimulation (TMS) to show that physical fatigue in PD is associated with abnormal cortical motor neuron excitability, and that levodopa normalizes exercise-related cortical motor neuron excitability. Garber and Friedman [20] showed that fatigue in PD is associated with negative effects, such as a decrease in physical activity and a loss of interests in social activity leading to feelings of loneliness and isolation and further decrease in activity. The author's laboratory currently is conducting a double-blind, placebo-controlled study testing effects of modafinil on fatigue and quality of life in PD patients.

Fatigue in a variety of neuromuscular diseases is likely to share common characteristics with fatigue in cancer, MS, and PD. Characterizing fatigue in these neuromuscular diseases would lead to better symptom management. Fatigue can be subjective or objective (Fig. 1). Subjective fatigue is fatigue as a sensation or feeling as assessed by patients themselves. Subjective fatigue is best measured by questionnaires. Objective fatigue is fatigue measured by quantitative physiologic methods in a laboratory setting. Different types of exercise protocols can measure physical fatigue.

Questionnaires used to characterize subjective fatigue

Most current fatigue questionnaires were developed for patients with nonneurologic diseases, and there are no data on which of these instruments are best suited to measuring fatigue in neuromuscular diseases. Neuromuscular diseases are characterized by profound muscle weakness and immobility. A primary issue in conceptualizing subjective fatigue in neuromuscular diseases is the degree to which fatigue differs from patients' perceptions of weakness and immobility or efforts to overcome weakness or immobility.

Questionnaires available to assess subjective fatigue can be one-dimensional or multidimensional. One-dimensional instruments, such as the

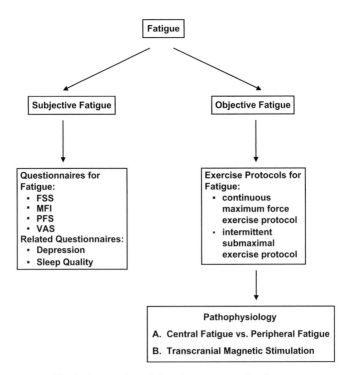

Fig. 1. Approach to fatigue in neuromuscular diseases.

Visual Analogue Scale (VAS) [21] and nine-item FSS [11], give a single score to indicate the severity of fatigue. The VAS is a simple, 10-cm-long horizontal line representing the severity of fatigue ranging from 0% to 100%. Subjects make a mark on the line to indicate how much fatigue they are experiencing. Multidimensional fatigue instruments contain several subscales usually based on a factor analysis [22]. The MFI has 20 items that are divided into five dimensions: general fatigue, physical fatigue, reduced motivation, reduced activity, and mental fatigue. Another multidimensional fatigue instrument, the Piper Fatigue Scale (PFS) [23], consists of 41 VAS representing the temporal, intensity, affective, and sensory dimensions of fatigue. The following four one-dimensional (the VAS and the FSS) and two multidimensional fatigue instruments (the MFI and the PFS) have been used in other neurologic or neuromuscular diseases, such as MS [11], PD [9], ALS [24], and postpolio syndrome [25].

Fatigue Severity Scale

Krupp et al [11] developed the FSS, a one-dimensional, nine-item fatigue inventory, and validated its internal consistency, sensitivity, and test-retest reliability. The 9-item FSS was selected from a 28-item questionnaire. These authors administered the 28-item questionnaire to 25 patients with MS, 29 patients with systematic lupus erythematosus, and 20 normal controls. They asked subjects to read each statement of the questionnaire and choose the number between 1 and 7 that best described their degree of agreement with each statement: *1* indicated strongly disagree and *7* strongly agree. Using factor analysis, item analysis, and theoretical considerations, they chose nine items from this questionnaire to form the FSS. The FSS was found to have good internal consistency (with a Cronbach α of 0.89 for MS, 0.81 for systemic lupus erythromatosus, and 0.88 for normal controls). They also examined sensitivity of the scale (ie, the ability of the scale to detect clinically appropriate and predicted changes in fatigue) by administering the scale to six patients with Lyme disease before and after antibiotic treatment and two MS patients before and after treatment with pemoline, a stimulant. In all of these subjects, clinical improvement was associated with reduced scores. In addition, Krupp et al [11] examined the test-retest reliability of the FSS by administering the scale to subjects in whom there was no clinical reason to expect changes in their fatigue state. The subjects were tested at two points of time separated by 5 to 33 weeks. As hypothesized, no significant changes in the scores were noted.

Mutidimensional Fatigue Inventory

The MFI is a 20-item self-report instrument designed to measure fatigue [22]. The 20 items cover five dimensions of fatigue: general fatigue, physical fatigue, mental fatigue, reduced motivation, and reduced activity. Smets et al [22] tested the psychometric properties of the MFI in 111 cancer patients receiving radiotherapy, 395 patients with chronic fatigue syndrome, 481 psychology students, 158 medical students, 46 junior physicians, 160 army recruits during their stay in the barracks, and 156 army recruits in the second week of intensive training. They showed that the MFI was well accepted in general and clinical populations. Of the respondents, 96% completed the MFI without omitting items. The investigators determined the five-dimensional structure using confirmatory factor analysis and showed that the five-factor model fit the data in all samples tested. The instrument had good internal consistency with a Cronbach α of 0.84. They also established the construct validity of the instrument by comparing groups, assuming differences in fatigue based on differences in circumstances or activity level. Patients with chronic fatigue syndrome scored higher than students and army recruits in barracks. Army recruits scored higher during intensive training than when they were in barracks.

Researchers have used the MFI to assess fatigue in cancer [3,26] and chronic obstructive pulmonary disease [27,28] patients. In a study of patients with chronic obstructive pulmonary disease, Breslin et al [27] measured pulmonary function, fatigue using the MFI, and depression using the Center of Epidemiological Study Depression Scale. They showed that depression correlated with general fatigue and mental fatigue, but not with physical fatigue in the MFI. In contrast, the severity of the pulmonary function impairment correlated with physical fatigue and reduced activity, but not with mental fatigue. Other investigators have shown this separation between physical fatigue and mental fatigue as well [26,28].

Piper Fatigue Scale

The PFS is a multidimensional questionnaire that includes 22 characteristics of fatigue in four different dimensions: behavioral/severity, affective meaning, sensory, and cognitive/mood [29]. The validity and reliability of the PFS have been well established in patients with cancer [23,30], myocardial infarction [31], and HIV [32]. The PFS has been validated in postpolio syndrome [25], a lower motor neuron disease. Strohschein et al [25] administered the PFS to 64 patients with postpolio syndrome and 25 healthy controls. They showed that the instrument has a high internal consistency with a Cronbach α coefficient of 0.98 and strong test-retest reliability with an intraclass correlation coefficient of 0.98. The convergent validity of the instrument was shown with a strong positive correlation between the PFS and Chalder Fatigue Questionnaire [33].

Visual Analogue Scale of fatigue

The VAS of fatigue is a 100-mm horizontal line representing the severity of fatigue ranging from 0% (right) to 100% (left). The subjects mark a point on the line that best represents the severity of their fatigue. The distance from the right is scored from 0 to 1. The scores in the VAS of fatigue correlated significantly with the multi-item fatigue subscale of the Profile of Mood States in subjects receiving long-term hemodialysis [34].

Not all of these questionnaires are suitable for all neuromuscular diseases. To choose a suitable questionnaire for a particular neuromuscular disease, researchers need to determine the reliability, ease of use, and construct validity of the fatigue questionnaire for measuring fatigue in that particular disease [7]. In addition, scores of a questionnaire should predict quality of life independently when adjusted for severity of associated conditions, such as immobility, depression, sleepiness, pulmonary function, and pain.

Depression, poor pulmonary function, and poor quality of sleep

In several studies, a significant positive correlation between depression and fatigue was reported in MS, cancer, and Alzheimer's disease patients [29]. In PD patients, the severity of depression correlated with mental fatigue [9]. The strong association between depression and fatigue leads to the speculation that fatigue and depression may share a common etiology. A study showed that paroxetine improved depression, but not fatigue in cancer patients who were receiving chemotherapy, suggesting that fatigue and depression do not share a common mechanism [35].

Poor pulmonary function, a common culprit for neuromuscular diseases, might cause fatigue through a variety of mechanisms, including insomnia, hypersomnia, and exercise intolerance. ALS patients often have central sleep apnea, obstructive sleep apnea, upper airway resistance, and hypoventilation disorders during sleep [36,37]. The overall quality of sleep in ALS patients is worse compared with normal controls. ALS patients had reduced total sleep time, reduced sleep efficiency, and increased apneas and hypopneas compared with normal controls [38]. Standard pulmonary function testing is useful in assessing the progression of muscle weakness in neuromuscular diseases. Forced vital capacity is indicative of inspiratory and expiratory muscle strength. Peak inspiratory pressures are more specific for diaphragmatic function, which correlate with a subject's ability to ventilate and are inversely correlated with the frequency and degree of sleep-disordered breathing.

Whether specific aspects of sleep affect fatigue in patients with neuromuscular diseases is unknown. Poor quality of sleep and excessive daytime somnolence are postulated as potential factors. The Pittsburgh Sleep Quality Index [39] and the Epworth Sleepiness Scale (ESS) [40] are widely used and have been validated. The Pittsburgh Sleep Quality Index and the ESS would be useful in assessing the relationship of quality of sleep and fatigue.

Objective physical fatigue measured in a laboratory setting

Physical fatigue, defined as the inability to maintain the desired force during sustained or repeated exercise, can be assessed objectively in a laboratory setting. The two most commonly used exercise protocols are the continuous maximal force exercise protocol and an intermittent submaximal exercise protocol.

In the maximal force exercise protocol, the subject generates a sustained maximal voluntary contraction (MVC). The MVC is defined as the contraction generated with feedback and encouragement, when the subject believes it is a maximal effort. During a sustained MVC, force declines steadily and fatigue develops over a short time (<60 seconds). The maximal force protocol mimics activities such as lifting heavy objects.

In the maximal force exercise protocol, subjects perform a continuous, maximal contraction of a muscle (eg, the extensor carpi radialis) for a period of time (eg, 30 seconds) The force level is recorded continuously (Fig. 2). The area under the force-time curve (AUC) is calculated by a computer. Fatigue is measured by the decay of the maximal force during continuous exercise. Fatigue index, a quantitative measure of the physical fatigue, is calculated as the difference between the measured AUC and the hypothetical AUC (ie, what would have been measured if maximal force were maintained without fatigue throughout muscle activation). The following formula was used (see Fig. 2):

$$\text{Fatigue index} = [1 - AUC/(\text{peak force} \cdot \text{time})]$$

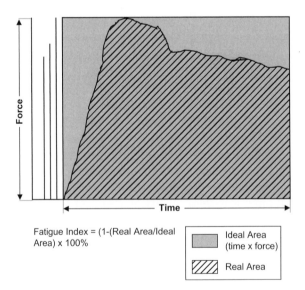

Fatigue Index = (1-(Real Area/Ideal Area) x 100%

Ideal Area (time x force)

Real Area

Fig. 2. Continuous maximal force exercise protocol. At the beginning of the trial, the subjects are encouraged to generate as much force as possible (maximal voluntary force). They make three attempts. The final maximal voluntary force is the highest value of the three attempts. Subjects then try to maintain the muscle contraction at the maximal force for a period of time (eg, 30 seconds). The force (*curved line*) declines owing to the development of fatigue. The higher the fatigue index, the more fatigue.

In the submaximal force protocol, subjects generate submaximal contraction intermittently (usually 50% of MVC with three to five repetitions every minute), and performance can be maintained at the target intensity for a long time (10 to 30 minutes). The submaximal force protocol mimics activities such as walking or cycling.

In an intermittent submaximal exercise protocol, we first measure the baseline MVC of muscles of interest, such as wrist extensors (Fig. 3). Baseline MVC is the contraction of the greatest force in three trials in which a subject performs MVC. The authors encourage the subject to increase the force from the previous maximum to minimize motivational error. When the baseline MVC is determined, the subject sustains a contraction of 50% MVC for 7 seconds and rests for 3 seconds repeatedly (ie, duty cycle was 70%). The subject attempts to perform an interval MVC after every three cycles. This series was repeated until the subject was unable to generate an interval MVC greater than 60% of the MVC. The authors use the slope of the interval MVC to measure the development of physical fatigue.

Twitch interpolation and transcranial magnetic stimulation to assess central and peripheral fatigue

Voluntary force generation in the maximal or submaximal exercise protocol results from a sequence of events, and each of these is a potential site for developing fatigue [41]. These events include all central nervous system processes influencing excitation and activation of the upper motor

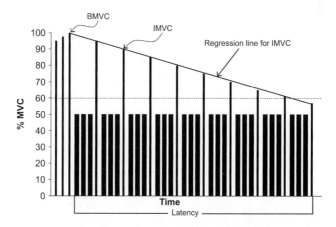

Fig. 3. Intermittent submaximal force exercise paradigm. After the baseline maximal voluntary contraction (BMVC) is determined, the subject performs an interval maximal voluntary contraction (IMVC) after every three cycles. Each cycle lasts 10 seconds with 7 seconds of muscle contraction at 50% of BMVC and 3 seconds of rest. This continues until the subject develops fatigue. Fatigue is defined as the inability of the subject to generate an IMVC greater than 60% of BMVC.

neurons, including motivational factors and integration of sensory information, the conduction along the pyramidal tract, the activation of lower motor neurons in the anterior horn of the spinal cord, and the signal transfer along the lower motor neuron and across the neuromuscular junction [41]. In addition, events occurring in the muscle during exercise can cause fatigue. Central fatigue refers to reduced force generation caused by events at or proximal to the anterior horn cells. Peripheral fatigue refers to the failure at or beyond the neuromuscular junction.

The relative roles of these processes in causing fatigue differ when different exercise protocols are used [41]. In the maximal force exercise protocol, the blood supply to the muscle is occluded completely during sustained MVC. As a result, there is extracellular accumulation of K^+ ion and other metabolites in the muscle within seconds that causes peripheral fatigue. When contraction is performed intermittently, as during low force exercise protocol, blood supply may be hindered during the contractions. Hyperemia between contractions still may provide the muscle with enough blood and oxygen, however, to prevent local accumulation of metabolites and causes less peripheral fatigue. The submaximal force exercise protocol is more relevant in studying fatigue because it mimics activities of daily living, such as walking, running, or bicycling. The low force exercise model is used widely in studying central fatigue.

The technique of twitch interpolation is a useful tool for studying fatigue [41]. In this technique, an electrical stimulus is delivered to the muscle or nerve to evoke a maximal evokable force. The maximal evokable force is the force generated by a muscle when additional electrical stimulation does not increase force. Based on this technique, central fatigue can be defined as any exercise-induced reduction in MVC force that is not accompanied by the same reduction in maximal evokable force. On the contrary, there is a parallel decrease in MVC and maximal evokable force in peripheral fatigue. The technique of twitch interpolation has been proved to be a useful tool in studying the mechanism of fatigue.

As mentioned earlier, central fatigue is the fatigue caused by any process proximal to or at the lower motor neurons. Some of these processes occurring at the brain cortex, such as motivation and sensory integration, ultimately affect the excitability of cortical motor neurons. A change of the excitability of cortical motor neurons associated with central fatigue would imply that processes proximal to upper motor neurons most likely cause central fatigue. As a result of recent development in TMS, a powerful technique is now available to study the excitability of the upper motor neurons. During TMS, a magnetic coil stimulator is placed over the motor cortex area. A changing magnetic field delivered by the stimulator induces an electric field in the motor cortex and excites the cortical motor neurons. The signals travel down the spinal cord and activate the lower motor neurons, which activate muscles. The results are the motor-evoked potentials (MEPs), which are the compound muscle action potentials recorded from the muscles of interest, such as limb muscles or trunk muscles. The excitability of the cortical motor neurons can be assessed either by comparing the amplitudes of MEPs by a given stimulus intensity or by calculating the probability of MEPs by stimulation at the threshold levels.

Samii et al [42] used TMS to investigate the change in cortical excitability–associated physical fatigue in normal subjects. Subjects performed intermittent, 30-second periods of isometric exercise of the extensor carpi radialis muscle at half-maximal force until fatigue (the inability to maintain half-maximal force). The amplitudes of the MEP from the rest muscle after each exercise period were measured. The investigators found that the size of MEPs before fatigue occurred were on average twice that of the pre-exercise MEPs, a phenomenon they called *postexercise facilitation*. After fatigue occurred, the MEP amplitudes were approximately 60% of the pre-exercise value, a phenomenon they called *postexercise depression*. There was a gradual recovery of the depressed MEPs to pre-exercise value over several minutes of rest. Postexercise facilitation during nonfatiguing exercise also decayed to baseline over several minutes after the end of exercise. Samii et al [42] also showed that there was no postexercise facilitation to transcranial electrical stimulation. A fundamental difference between transcranial electrical stimulation and TMS is that electrical stimulation depolarizes cortical motor neurons directly, whereas magnetic stimulation indirectly depolarizes cortical motor neurons by activating their afferents. They hypothesized that postexercise MEP facilitation and depression are due to intracortical mechanisms. Their findings suggest that postexercise depression that develops after fatiguing exercise may play a role in central fatigue.

The author's laboratory used TMS to investigate the physiologic mechanisms of objective physical fatigue in PD and showed that the increased objective physical fatigue in PD is associated with increased cortical excitability. Increased objective physical fatigue and increased cortical excitability respond to levodopa [19].

Using the techniques of twitch interpolation and TMS, Gandevia et al [43] investigated the mechanisms of central fatigue and showed that a reduced output from the motor cortex may cause central fatigue. During the experiment, eight normal subjects performed 100% MVC of the biceps muscle. Subjects initially performed brief MVCs of 2 to 3 seconds' duration, and TMS stimulation was given during contraction. Subjects then performed a sustained, fatiguing MVC of 1.5 to 2 minutes' duration. TMS stimuli were delivered every 10 to 15 seconds. Additional brief MVCs with superimposed stimuli were performed during the recovery period. Gandevia et al [43] found that the increment in force produced by TMS was initially small (1%), but increased to 9.8% during sustained MVCs with the development of fatigue. To examine if peripheral fatigue (fatigue at the neuromuscular junction or muscle) played a role, they placed a sphygmomanometer cuff around the upper arm to block the blood supply to the biceps. They found that neither maximal voluntary force nor voluntary activation recovered during ischemia. Fatigue-induced changes in electro-myography responses to TMS recovered rapidly, however, despite maintained ischemia. The investigators concluded that reduced output from the motor cortex was associated with fatigue. The physiologic techniques of twitch interpolation and TMS allow researchers to investigate the mechanisms of physical fatigue in neuromuscular diseases. Understanding the mechanisms of physical fatigue is the first step in developing effective treatments.

Fatigue in neuromuscular diseases

Research of fatigue in neuromuscular diseases is still at its embryonic stage. Several studies have been performed in understanding fatigue in ALS and postpolio syndrome. Much more work needs to be done, however, before investigators can develop treatment of fatigue in neuromuscular diseases.

Amyotrophic lateral sclerosis

ALS patients have more pronounced subjective fatigue than normal controls. The author's group conducted a pilot study to examine if ALS patients have excessive subjective fatigue and if fatigue affects the quality of life in these subjects [24]. The investigators used the MFI questionnaire to assess subjective fatigue, the Center of Epidemiological Study Depression Scale to assess depression, the ESS to assess sleepiness, and the multidimensional McGill Quality of Life (MQOL) questionnaire to assess quality of life. They used the ALS Functional Rating Scale to evaluate the severity of ALS. ALS patients reported more subjective fatigue, specifically physical fatigue, than normal controls. Of ALS patients, 44% reported abnormal depression. The severity of general fatigue contributed significantly to a lower physical symptoms subscale in the MQOL. The severity of depression contributed significantly to a lower psychological well-being subscale in the MQOL. Muscle strength, physical function, and disease duration did not correlate with fatigue and depression. The investigators concluded that subjective fatigue and depression are independent of disease severity in ALS patients, and they are associated with poorer quality of life in ALS patients. Treatment of fatigue and depression may improve quality of life in ALS patients. The MFI has not been validated in the ALS population, and no studies have shown whether the MFI is superior to other questionnaires, such as the FSS, PFS, and VAS. Further studies are needed to evaluate which of these questionnaires are more suitable to assess fatigue in ALS patients.

ALS patients have excessive objective physical fatigue compared with normal controls, who have peripheral and central components. Using an intermittent submaximal isometric contraction protocol, Sharma et al [44] showed that maximal voluntary force and tetanic force induced by electrical stimulation decline more in ALS patients than normal controls, suggesting that ALS patients have more subjective physical fatigue. The similar decline in voluntary force and tetanic force indicated that most physical fatigue was peripheral in origin at a site distal to lower motor neurons. Sharma et al [44] showed that evoked compound muscle action potential amplitude did not decline, indicating no neuromuscular transmission failure. Despite greater fatigability, changes during exercise in energy metabolites and proton signal intensity tended to be less in ALS patients compared with controls, suggesting impaired muscular activation. The authors concluded that the greater muscle fatigue in ALS patients results from activation impairment, owing in part to alterations distal to the muscle membrane [43].

Sharma and Miller [45] subsequently showed that increased muscle fatigability in ALS patients is partly due to dissociation between electrical and mechanical muscle properties. They compared motor unit potentials, muscle force, and muscle fatigability in patients with ALS and controls using low-intensity to moderate-intensity voluntary contraction. The enlarged motor units in patients correlated negatively to the muscle force and positively to muscle fatigability. After an average 9-month follow-up, the deterioration in force decline was greater than the decline in the amplitude of the compound muscle action potential, suggesting a relative dissociation between electrical and mechanical properties. The authors concluded that increased fatigue in ALS patients is associated with enlarged motor units that are mechanically less efficient and fatigue relatively more than normal muscles.

Central fatigue also plays a role in increased objective physical fatigue in ALS patients. Kent-Braun and Miller [46] used the technique of twitch interpolation and compared voluntary and electrically stimulated force, central and peripheral indices of muscle activation, and intramuscular energy metabolism before and during intermittent submaximal isometric ankle dorsiflexion in seven ALS patients and six normal controls. They showed that at the end of fatiguing exercise, only the ALS group had an increase in the added force in response to a stimulus train imposed during maximal voluntary contraction, indicating significant central fatigue in ALS.

Carter et al [47] have taken the first step to treat subjective fatigue in ALS patients. Fifteen ALS patients took 200 mg or 400 mg of modafinil in an open-label fashion for 2 weeks. After treatment, mean scores on the FSS decreased from 51.3 ± 9.2 to 42.8 ± 10.2. On the ESS, mean scores decreased from 8.2 ± 2 to 4.5 ± 2.4. Reductions in the FSS and the ESS were significant at $P < .001$. Mean scores on the self-report version of the Functional Independence Measure increased from 115.2 ± 5.6 to 118.1 ± 5.4 ($P < .01$). No patients dropped out because of side effects, which included diarrhea, headache, nervousness, and insomnia. This pilot study suggests that modafinil is well tolerated and may reduce symptoms of fatigue in ALS patients. Further blinded, controlled studies of modafinil in larger numbers of ALS patients are warranted.

Postpolio syndrome

Postpolio patients reported more subjective fatigue in a study designed to evaluate the applicability, validity, and reliability of the PFS in postpolio patients [25]. During the interview, 64 postpolio patients and 25 normal controls completed the PFS, the Beck Depression Inventory, and the Chalder Fatigue questionnaires. The study showed that postpolio patients had higher scores in the PFS than normal controls. The study proved that the PFS has good face and content validity, good convergent validity and reliability, and good test-retest reliability in postpolio patients. The authors concluded that the PFS might be useful in studying postpolio fatigue, including studies gauging the effectiveness of treatments.

Postpolio patients also have excessive objective physical fatigue that has central and peripheral components. Allen et al [48] investigated maximal voluntary activation without fatigue and peripheral and central components of muscle fatigue during exercise in 21 subjects with a history of poliomyelitis and 20 healthy, age-matched control subjects. Voluntary activation and strength of the elbow flexors were quantified using twitch interpolation during maximal isometric voluntary contractions at rest and during fatigue induced by 45 minutes of repeated isometric contractions. Compared with the control subjects, patients with prior polio had impaired voluntary activation when the elbow flexors were not fatigued and during fatiguing submaximal exercise. During exercise, polio patients also had lower twitch amplitudes and increased subjective fatigue. Central and peripheral fatigue was more marked in patients with postpolio syndrome. Another study observed only peripheral fatigue in postpolio patients, however, possibly owing to the differences in techniques used [49].

Summary

Fatigue is a complex phenomenon that is understudied. Fatigue may affect quality of life in patients with neuromuscular diseases. It is crucial for physicians to assess subjective fatigue and objective fatigue simultaneously. Questionnaires are useful in assessing the severity of subjective fatigue, and exercise protocols are useful in assessing objective physical fatigue. Validation studies need to be conducted to investigate which questionnaires are suitable for each individual neuromuscular disease. Physiologic techniques are now available for researchers to measure central and peripheral physical fatigue.

It is unclear how subjective fatigue (as measured by questionnaires) correlates with objective physical fatigue (as measured by exercise protocols). The author's study in PD [18] showed that objective physical fatigue did not correlate with the symptom of fatigue that many PD patients report. This lack of correlation can be explained by the fact that the MFI measures chronic physical fatigue over weeks, whereas intermittent exercise measures acute physical fatigue over minutes. In the MFI instructions used in the author's study, subjects were told that investigators were attempting to discern "how they have been feeling lately." The force generation administered to subjects lasts no more than a few minutes, however. It also is possible that the physical fatigue as estimated by the MFI is on a global scale that does not distinguish mental effort, the ability to sustain repetitive muscular action, or the strength of muscle contraction. These findings suggest the MFI measures different aspects of physical fatigue compared with those measured by force generation. All three measurements may be useful in future studies. It would be of interest in future studies to administer a questionnaire to measure instantaneous fatigue (with questions such as "How do you feel this instant?") and to correlate it with the physical fatigue measured by finger tapping and force generation. Studying the severity of fatigue and its underlying pathophysiology would help physicians to develop effective symptomatic treatments and improve quality of life in patients with neuromuscular diseases.

References

[1] Field MJ, Cassel CK. Approaching death: improving care at the end of life. Washington (DC): National Academy Press; 1997.

[2] Winningham ML, Nail LM, Burke MB, et al. Fatigue and the cancer experience: the state of the knowledge. Oncol Nurs Forum 1994;21:23–36.

[3] Smets EM, Garssen B, Schuster-Uitterhoeve AL, et al. Fatigue in cancer patients. Br J Cancer 1993;68:220–4.

[4] Nail LM. Fatigue in patients with cancer. Oncol Nurs Forum 2002;29:537–44.

[5] Schwartz AL, Mori M, Gao R, Nail LM, King ME. Exercise reduces daily fatigue in women with breast cancer receiving chemotherapy. Med Sci Sports Exerc 2001;33:718–23.

[6] Barsevick AM, Dudley W, Beck S, et al. A randomized clinical trial of energy conservation for patients with cancer-related fatigue. Cancer 2004;100:1302–10.

[7] Meek PM, Nail LM, Barsevick A, et al. Psychometric testing of fatigue instruments for use with cancer patients. Nurs Res 2000;49:181–90.

[8] Bakshi R. Fatigue associated with multiple sclerosis: diagnosis, impact and management. Mult Scler 2003;9:219–27.

[9] Lou JS, Kearns G, Oken B, et al. Exacerbated physical fatigue and mental fatigue in Parkinson's disease. Mov Disord 2001;16:190–6.

[10] Freal JE, Kraft GH, Coryell JK. Symptomatic fatigue in multiple sclerosis. Arch Phys Med Rehabil 1984;65:135–8.

[11] Krupp LB, LaRocca NG, Muir-Nash J, et al. The fatigue severity scale: application to patients with multiple sclerosis and systemic lupus erythematosus. Arch Neurol 1989;46: 1121–3.

[12] Bakshi R, Miletich RS, Hanschel K, et al. Fatigue in multiple sclerosis: cross-sectional correlation with brain MRI findings in 71 patients. Neurology 1999;53:1151–3.

[13] Bakshi R, Shaikh ZA, Miletich RS, et al. Fatigue in multiple sclerosis and its relationship to depression and neurologic disability. Mult Scler 2000;6:181–5.

[14] Krupp LB, Coyle PK, Dascher C, et al. Fatigue therapy in multiple sclerosis: results of a double-blind, randomized, parallel trial of amatidine, pemoline, and placebo. Neurology 1995;45:1956–61.

[15] Rammohan KW, Rosenberg JH, Lynn DJ, et al. Efficacy and safety of modafinil for the treatment of fatigue in multiple sclerosis: a two-center phase 2 study. J Neurol Neurosurg Psychiatry 2002;72:179–83.

[16] Janardhan V, Bakshi R. Quality of life in patients with multiple sclerosis: the impact of fatigue and depression. J Neurol Sci 2002;205:51–8.

[17] Mainero C, Faroni J, Casperini C, et al. Fatigue and magnetic resonance imaging activity in multiple sclerosis. J Neurol 1999;246:454–8.

[18] Lou JS, Kearns G, Benice T, et al. Levodopa improves physical fatigue in Parkinson's disease—a double blind, placebo-controlled crossover study. Mov Disord 2003;18:1108–14.

[19] Lou JS, Benice T, Sexton G, et al. Levodopa normalizes exercise related cortico-motoneuron excitability abnormalities in Parkinson's disease. Clin Neurophysiol 2003;114:930–7.

[20] Garber CE, Friedman JH. Effects of fatigue on physical activity and function in patients with Parkinson's disease. Neurology 2003;60:1119–24.

[21] Krupp LB, Avarez LA, Larocca NG, et al. Fatigue in multiple sclerosis. Arch Neurol 1988; 45:435–7.

[22] Smets EMA, Grassen B, Bonke B, et al. The Multidimensional Fatigue Inventory (MFI) psychometric qualities of an instrument to assess fatigue. J Psychosom Res 1995;39:315–25.

[23] Piper PF, Dibble SL, Dodd MJ, et al. The revised Piper Fatigue Scale: psychometric evaluation in women with breast cancer. Oncol Nurs Forum 1998;25:677–84.

[24] Lou JS, Reeves A, Benice T, et al. Fatigue and depression are associated with poor quality of life in ALS. Neurology 2003;60:122–3.

[25] Strohschein FJ, Kelly CG, Clarke AG, et al. Applicability, validity, and reliability of the Piper Fatigue Scale in postpolio patients. Am J Phys Med Rehabil 2003;82:122–9.

[26] Schneider RA. Reliability and validity of the Multidimensional Fatigue Inventory (MFI-20) and the Rhoten Fatigue Scale among rural cancer outpatients. Cancer Nurs 1998;21:370–3.

[27] Breslin E, van der Schans C, Breukink S, et al. Perception of fatigue and quality of life in patients with COPD. Chest 1998;114:958–64.

[28] Breukink SO, Strijbos JH, Koorn M, et al. Relationship between subjective fatigue and physiological variables in patients with chronic obstructive pulmonary disease. Respir Med 1998; 92:676–82.

[29] Piper PF, Lindsey AM, Dodd MJ, et al. The development of an instrument to measure the subjective dimension of fatigue. In: Funk SG, Tornquist EM, Champagne MT, et al, editors. Key aspects of comfort: management of pain, fatigue, and nausea. New York: Springer; 1989. p. 199–208.

[30] Dean GE, Spears L, Ferrell BR, et al. Fatigue in patients with cancer receiving interferon alpha. Cancer Pract 1995;3:164–72.

[31] Varvaro FF, Sereika SM, Zullo TG, et al. Fatigue in women with myocardial infarction. Health Care Women Int 1996;17:593–602.

[32] Grady C, Anderson R, Chase GA. Fatigue in HIV-infected men receiving investigational interleukin-2. Nurs Res 1998;47:227–34.

[33] Chalder T, Berelowitz G, Pawlikowska T, et al. Development of a fatigue scale. J Psychosom Res 1993;37:147–53.

[34] Brunier G, Graydon J. A comparison of two methods of measuring fatigue in patients on chronic haemodialysis: visual analogue vs Likert scale. Int J Nurs Stud 1996;33:338–48.

[35] Morrow GR, Hickok JT, Roscoe JA, et al. Differential effects of paroxetine on fatigue and depression: a randomized, double-blind trial from the University of Rochester Cancer Center Community Clinical Oncology Program. J Clin Oncol 2003;21:4635–41.

[36] Gay PC, Westbrook PR, Daube JR, et al. Effects of alterations in pulmonary function and sleep variables on survival in patients with amyotrophic lateral sclerosis. Mayo Clin Proc 1991;66:686–94.

[37] Barthlen GM, Lange DJ. Unexpectedly severe sleep and respiratory pathology in patients with amyotrophic lateral sclerosis. Eur J Neurol 2000;7:299–302.

[38] Ferguson KA, Strong MJ, Ahmad D, George CF. Sleep-disordered breathing in amyotrophic lateral sclerosis. Chest 1996;110:664–9.

[39] Buysse DJ, Reynolds CF III, et al. The Pittsburgh Sleep Quality Index: a new instrument for psychiatric practice and research. Psychiatry Res 1989;28:193–213.

[40] Jones MW. A new method for measuring daytime sleepiness: the Epworth sleepiness scale. Sleep 1991;14:540–5.

[41] Vollestad NK. Measurement of human muscle fatigue. J Neurosci Methods 1997;74:219–27.

[42] Samii A, Wassermann EM, Ikoma K, et al. Characterization of postexercise facilitation and depression of motor evoked potentials to transcranial magnetic stimulation. Neurology 1996;46:1376–82.

[43] Gandevia SC, Allen GM, Butler JE, Taylor JL. Supraspinal factors in human muscle fatigue: evidence for suboptimal output from the motor cortex. J Physiol 1996;490:529–36.

[44] Sharma KR, Kent-Braun JA, Majumdar S, et al. Physiology of fatigue in amyotrophic lateral sclerosis. Neurology 1995;45:733–40.

[45] Sharma KR, Miller RG. Electrical and mechanical properties of skeletal muscle underlying increased fatigue in patients with amyotrophic lateral sclerosis. Muscle Nerve 1996;19:1391–400.

[46] Kent-Braun J, Miller RG. Central fatigue during isometric exercise in amyotrophic lateral sclerosis. Muscle Nerve 2000;23:909–14.

[47] Carter GT, Weiss MD, Lou JS, et al. Modafinil to treat fatigue in amyotrophic lateral sclerosis: an open label pilot study. Am J Hospice Palliat Care 2005;22:55–9.

[48] Allen GM, Gandevia SC, Neering IR, et al. Muscle performance, voluntary activation and perceived effort in normal subjects and patients with prior poliomyelitis. Brain 1994;117:661–70.

[49] Sharma KR, Kent-Braun JA, Mynhier MA, et al. Excessive muscular fatigue in the post-polio syndrome. Neurology 1994;44:642–6.

PHYSICAL MEDICINE
AND REHABILITATION
CLINICS OF
NORTH AMERICA

ELSEVIER
SAUNDERS

Phys Med Rehabil Clin N Am
16 (2005) 1081–1090

The Role of Microglial Cells in Amyotrophic Lateral Sclerosis

Patrick Weydt, MD[a,*], Thomas Möller, PhD[b,c]

[a]Department of Laboratory Medicine, University of Washington, 1959 NE Pacific Street,
Seattle, WA 98195, USA
[b]Department of Neurology, University of Washington, 1959 NE Pacific Street, Seattle,
WA 98195, USA
[c]Center for Neurogenetics and Neurotherapeutics, University of Washington,
1959 NE Pacific Street, Seattle, WA 98195, USA

Amyotrophic lateral sclerosis (ALS) is the most common adult-onset motor neuron disease [1,2]. Patients typically present with clinical evidence of corticospinal (upper) and anterior horn cell (lower) motor neuron weakness [3]. While continuously losing their muscle strength, patients typically remain cognitively intact and completely aware of their progressive disability. The prevalence of ALS is approximately 5 to 7/100,000 worldwide [3]. ALS strikes adults of any age, and most patients die within 3 to 5 years after onset of symptoms. Among the major neurodegenerative disorders, such as Alzheimer's, Parkinson's, and Huntington's disease, ALS is clearly the most rapidly progressive. Most cases of ALS are sporadic and probably acquired; however, approximately 10% of cases of ALS are familial, usually inherited in an autosomal dominant pattern. ALS pathology is characterized by neuronal atrophy and degeneration limited almost exclusively to upper and lower motor neurons. Tragically, available treatment is limited and does not prevent disease progression and death.

The cause of sporadic ALS and most familial cases is still unknown. Most likely, ALS represents a heterogeneous group of disorders with environmental and genetic causes, which all lead to a common final pathway of selective motor neuron degeneration [1]. Several pathogenetic mechanisms have been suggested, including (1) oxidative stress, (2) glutamate toxicity, (3) neurofilament

This article was supported by the Muscular Dystrophy Association, ALS Association, ALS-TDF, DA Leopoldina, Project ALS, and Royalty Research Fund of the University of Washington.

* Corresponding author.
E-mail address: weydt@u.washington.edu (P. Weydt).

accumulation, (4) exogenous factors (eg, toxins, viruses), and (5) neuroinflammation [1,2,4]. These hypotheses are not mutually exclusive, however, and may individually or together cause motor neuron loss [2].

The study of the rare hereditary forms of ALS has triggered important advances in our understanding of motor neuron degeneration. In 10% to 20% of patients with familial ALS, the gene encoding for Cu/Zn superoxide dismutase (SOD1) is carrying missense mutations [5]. The normal function of SOD1 is to protect cells from oxidative injury by converting superoxide to hydrogen peroxide. Detailed studies of mutant SOD1 (mtSOD1) have shown that motor neuron degeneration is caused by an as yet unknown toxic gain-of-function rather than by diminished mtSOD1 activity [6]. This insight led to increasing interest in familial ALS, because it is believed to have a similar pathogenesis to sporadic ALS and allows for genetic approaches [4,7]. Most significantly, the discovery of this first ALS-linked gene has led to the generation of useful rodent models of ALS [8–12]. Transgenic mice and rats that overexpress human mtSOD1 develop a motor neuron disease remarkably similar to that seen in patients with ALS [1,4,7]. In addition to being useful tools for preclinical validation of potential therapies, the mtSOD1 transgenic animals have been highly instructive toward understanding the pathophysiology of motor neuron degeneration.

Microglia as mediators of neuroinflammation

Microglia, which resemble peripheral tissue macrophages, are the resident immune cells of the central nervous system (CNS) and are the primary mediators of neuroinflammation [13]. The last two decades have brought overwhelming evidence that microglia are important determinants of the microenvironment of the brain, involved in many acute and chronic neurologic diseases [13,14]. In the unperturbed adult brain, microglia exist as so-called "resting" microglia, which typically have a small cell body with fine, ramified processes and minimal expression of surface antigens. They are believed to virtually patrol the brain tissue [15–17]. In the event of CNS injury, these cells are swiftly activated and contribute to the pathogenesis of neurologic disorders. Microglia secrete various inflammatory molecules, including interleukin-1β, tumor necrosis factor-α, and nitric oxide [18]. Death of other CNS cells activates microglia further and they transform into phagocytes [13]. It is generally believed that substances released from injured cells within the CNS trigger microglial activation, which consequently leads to the long-term changes of gene expression and reorganization of the cell phenotype [13,14].

Microglial effects on neurons and macroglia (astrocytes and oligodendrocytes) are mediated by the release of toxic substances, such as nitric oxide, oxygen radicals, glutamate, proteases, and neurotoxic cytokines, and protective agents, such as plasminogen, plasminogen activator, growth factors, and neuroprotective cytokines [18]. These effects are modulated by cytokines and neurotransmitters released from astrocytes and neurons, which gives rise to complex interactions among microglia, neurons, and astrocytes.

Microglial cells are intimately involved in the pathogenesis of multiple sclerosis and HIV-associated dementia [19,20]. In addition to inflammatory and infectious diseases, there is overwhelming evidence that microglia play a major role in the pathogenesis of neurodegenerative diseases [21]. For example, in Alzheimer's disease, activated microglia are found near amyloid plaques and neurofibrillary tangles, abnormalities that are central to the pathogenesis of the disease [13,14,22,23]. Additional support for a prominent role of microglia and neuroinflammation in Alzheimer's disease has come from studies that demonstrate that anti-inflammatory medications, known to attenuate microglia activation, reduce the risk of Alzheimer's disease [23]. Recent evidence also suggests that microglial activation is detrimental for the generation of endogenous stem cells in the brain [24].

Neuroinflammation and amyotrophic lateral sclerosis

The main mediators of neuroinflammation are soluble proinflammatory molecules, such as cytokines, prostaglandins, and nitric oxide. Several studies showed that the expression of proinflammatory mediators (eg, tumor necrosis factor-α, interleukin-1β, inducible nitric oxide synthase [iNOS] or cyclooxygenase [COX-2]) is an early event in murine ALS, even preceding the development of clinical signs [25–31]. The profile of proinflammatory molecules was distinctly microglia- and macrophage-like. The cellular localization of these factors was not investigated. In contrast to other neurodegenerative diseases, such as multiple sclerosis or Alzheimer's disease, influx of peripheral immune cells, such as lymphocytes or neutrophils, is a rare event in ALS and only associated with end-stage disease [1,32–34]. As a result, neuroinflammation in ALS is caused solely by the interaction of microglia, neurons, and macroglia. In this vicious circle, astrocytes are target and the source of neuroinflammation [35]. Mediators released from microglia downregulate the expression of neurotrophic factors in astrocytes and lead to the release of additional inflammatory mediators, which in turn further microglial activation [13,18]. The participation of neurons in this process is not well understood [36].

Microglia and amyotrophic lateral sclerosis

Although implicated in nearly all disorders of the CNS, the role of microglia in ALS is only beginning to be explored [37–41]. Histologic studies provided clear evidence of microglial activation and proliferation in regions of motor neuron loss, such as the primary motor cortex, brain stem motor nuclei, corticospinal tracts, and the ventral horns of the spinal cord [34,42]. In familial and sporadic ALS, postmortem studies revealed that activated microglia are found not only in areas of severe motor neuron loss but also in regions in which there was (clinically and morphologically) only mild motor neuron injury [42]. This hints toward early microglial activation in the pathogenesis of human ALS, either detecting earliest neuronal stress or actually triggering the process. Positron emission tomography that detected microglial activation in humans in vivo confirmed the presence of neuroinflammation in sporadic ALS [43]. Recent evidence suggests that this inflammatory response is not limited to the CNS but is also detectable systemically [44]. This evidence is remarkably similar to recent reports regarding Alzheimer's disease [45]. Results from transgenic animals also implicate microglia in the early pathogenesis of ALS. Investigations of disease course and genetic manipulations have been especially revealing. Studies in asymptomatic ALS transgenic mice uncovered evidence that microglial activation starts before the motor symptoms become apparent [32,38].

An important series of studies revealed—rather unexpectedly—that SOD1 mutations can exert their neurodegenerative effects in a non-cell autonomous fashion. This is to say that other nonneuronal cells are critically involved in the mtSOD1-mediated demise of motor neurons. For example, it was shown that neither neuronal nor astrocytic expression of the mtSOD1 transgene is sufficient to produce motor neuron degeneration in mice [46–48]. In a groundbreaking report, Clement and colleagues [49] showed that in mtSOD1 chimeric mice (ie, mice with mosaic expression of the mtSOD1 transgene), the severity of the ALS phenotype depended on the proportion of CNS cells expressing the mutant transgene but not on the cell type (ie, neurons versus nonneurons). Individual motor neurons that expressed mtSOD1 but were surrounded by nontransgenic glia remained healthy, whereas nontransgenic neurons neighbored by glia that expressed mtSOD1 degenerated. This occurrence established that mtSOD1 expression in motor neurons is neither sufficient nor necessary to produce motor neuron degeneration and raises the intriguing question as to which other cell type or combination of cell types mediates the motor neuron–specific toxicity of mtSOD1. To date the ALS-causing mutations have been shown to have cell autonomous effects on neurons, astrocytes, and microglia. In neurons, SOD1 mutations confer an increased susceptibility to nitric oxide and tumor necrosis factor-α–induced cell death [50]. Trotti and colleagues [51] demonstrated that mutated SOD1 can significantly impair the activity of the astrocytic glutamate transporter GLT-1 (or EAAT2), which would add to the excitotoxic stress that motor neurons are thought to experience in ALS. Finally our group has shown that compared with wild-type controls, microglia from adult but not newborn ALS transgenic mice release significantly more tumor necrosis factor-α in response to inflammatory stimuli [41]. Microglia seem to be an integral part of a vicious cycle that culminates in rapid and selective motor neuron degeneration. This scenario is further supported by data presented at the Annual Society for Neuroscience meeting in 2004 in which D.W. Cleveland reported that in a cell-specific knockdown of mtSOD1, mice that selectively lacked expression of mtSOD1 in microglia/macrophages showed a substantial slowing of disease progression and a significant increase in survival [52]. Of note, Wang and colleagues [53] showed that expression of mutated SOD1 limited to neurons, astrocytes, and muscle and not microglia/macrophages is sufficient to produce the full ALS phenotype in mice. This fact argues against microglia being the actual trigger of motor neuron degeneration. The implications of this study for the role of skeletal muscle in ALS pathogenesis are discussed elsewhere in this issue (see the article by Abmayr and Weydt elsewhere in this issue).

These data suggest that microglia are critical propagators but not instigators of motor neuron degeneration in ALS. It still remains unclear how microglial cells exert their detrimental effects and what renders motor neurons selectively vulnerable. Increasing evidence challenges the simplistic concept of microglial activation being uniformly deleterious for neurons [13,21]. Resting and activated microglia release growth factors, remove glutamate from the extracellular space, and actively participate in tissue repair [13,18,54,55]. Besides a direct neurotoxic activation, a failure of mtSOD1 microglia to participate appropriately in tissue repair might contribute significantly to ALS pathology (Fig. 1).

Anti-inflammatory amyotrophic lateral sclerosis therapy

Gaining increasing acceptance, the hypothesis of neuroinflammation as an contributor to disease progression in ALS has led to a series of successful animal trials testing the efficacy of immunomodulating therapies in ALS [1,40]. The most promising and most widely studied anti-inflammatory compounds to date are celecoxib and minocycline.

Celecoxib is an inhibitor of the inflammatory regulator cyclo-oxygenase 2. It was widely used as an improved therapy for rheumatoid arthritis, but because of serious cardiovascular safety concerns with this class of drugs its use is greatly restricted [56]. In mtSOD1 mice, celecoxib prolonged survival and reduced microglial activation as assessed by immunohistochemistry [57–59]. It is currently pursued as a therapeutic approach in neurodegenerative disease, including ALS, but preliminary results do not seem to fulfill high expectations currently [57,59–61].

Minocycline, a semisynthetic second-generation tetracycline antibiotic, is also a potent inhibitor of microglial activation [62–64]. It has been shown to be neuroprotective in models of ischemia, Parkinson's disease, and spinal cord injury at least in part via inhibition of microglial activation [65] In mtSOD1 mice, minocycline significantly slowed disease onset and progression and reduced microglial activation [66–68]. Based on these data, phase I/II trials are currently underway for the use of minocycline in ALS [69]. Despite these encouraging results, the molecular mechanisms underlying these effects are still unclear. Proposed actions of minocycline are p38 MAP kinase inhibition and inhibition of mitochondrial cytochrome c release [65].

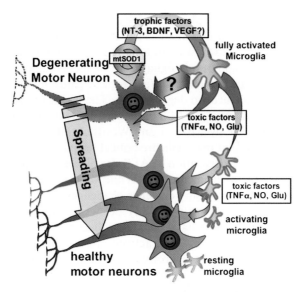

Fig. 1. Microglial activation accelerates and facilitates disease spreading in the ALS spinal cord (simplification): Via not yet defined signals (*purple arrow*), microglia (*red*) sense when an individual motor neuron (*blue*) starts to degenerate. Microglial activation leads to the release of neurotoxic mediators, such as nitric oxide (NO), tumor necrosis factor-α (TNFα) and glutamate (glu) (*red arrows*), and neuroprotective mediators (*green arrows*), such as neurotrophin-3 (NT-3), brain-derived neurotrophic factor (BNDF), and vascular-endothelial growth factor (VEGF). mtSOD1-expressing microglia might show a particularly unbalanced inflammatory response. The proinflammatory mediators hasten the demise of the stressed motor neuron and recruit more microglia to the disease focus. The inflammatory mediators and the newly recruited microglia spill over to neighboring motor neurons and the disease process begins to spread. Other cell types, such as astrocytes, oligodendrocytes, and muscle cells, were omitted in this figure but also play an important role.

Summary

Neuroinflammation is a significant pathogenic factor in ALS. Anti-inflammatory agents that are in clinical use significantly slow disease progression in ALS transgenic mice. The current data suggest that microglial activation is detrimental for motor neurons and might be a driving force in the rapid progression of the disease. As our understanding of neuroinflammation in general and in ALS in particular advances, however, it is becoming clear that in addition to the well-established deleterious consequences, microglial activation also might have considerable beneficial effects. The emerging data on the detrimental impact of neuroinflammation on the generation of endogenous stem cells raises the possibility that control of microglial activation in ALS might be critical for implementing stem cell therapies. It is of utmost importance to understand better the interactions between activated microglia and ailing motor neurons. Co-culture systems and tissue-specific expression of ALS-relevant transgenes are the most promising approaches toward this goal. Once better understood, interfering with the microglia-mediated inflammatory process might contain the spread of the disease and help pave the way for regenerative therapies.

Acknowledgments

The authors would like to thank Anke Witting, PhD, for invaluable help with the artwork in this article.

References

[1] Brujin LI, Miller TM, Cleveland DW. Unraveling the mechanisms involved in motor neuron degeneration in ALS. Annu Rev Neurosci 2004;27:723.

[2] Strong MJ. The basic aspects of therapeutics in amyotrophic lateral sclerosis. Pharmacol Ther 2003;98:379.

[3] Rowland LP, Shneider NA. Amyotrophic lateral sclerosis. N Engl J Med 2001;344:1688.

[4] Brown RH, Meininger V, Swash M. Amyotrophic lateral sclerosis. In: Brown RH, Meininger V, Swash M, editors. Amyotrophic lateral sclerosis. London: Martin Dunitz; 2000.

[5] Rosen DR, Siddique T, Patterson D, et al. Mutations in Cu/Zn superoxide dismutase gene are associated with familial amyotrophic lateral sclerosis. Nature 1993;362:59.

[6] Subramaniam JR, Lyons WE, Liu J, et al. Mutant SOD1 causes motor neuron disease independent of copper chaperone-mediated copper loading. Nat Neurosci 2002;5:301.

[7] Cleveland DW, Rothstein JD. From Charcot to Lou Gehrig: deciphering selective motor neuron death in ALS. Nat Rev Neurosci 2001;2:806.

[8] Brujin LI, Becher MW, Lee MK, et al. ALS-linked SOD1 mutant G85R mediates damage to astrocytes and promotes rapidly progressive disease with SOD1-containing inclusions. Neuron 1997;18:327.

[9] Gurney ME. Transgenic animal models of amyotrophic lateral sclerosis. In: Brown RH, Meininger V, Swash M, editors. Amyotrophic lateral sclerosis. London: Martin Dunitz; 2000. p. 251.

[10] Gurney ME, Pu H, Chiu AY, et al. Motor neuron degeneration in mice that express a human Cu, Zn superoxide dismutase mutation. Science 1994;264:1772.

[11] Howland DS, Liu J, She Y, et al. Focal loss of the glutamate transporter EAAT2 in a transgenic rat model of SOD1mutant-mediated amyotrophic lateral sclerosis (ALS). Proc Natl Acad Sci U S A 2002;99:1604.

[12] Nagai M, Aoki M, Miyoshi I, et al. Rats expressing human cytosolic copper-zinc superoxide dismutase transgenes with amyotrophic lateral sclerosis: associated mutations develop motor neuron disease. J Neurosci 2001;21:9246.

[13] Streit WJ. Microglia as neuroprotecitve, immunocompetent cells of the CNS. Glia 2002;40:133.

[14] Kreutzberg GW. Microglia: a sensor for pathological events in the CNS. Trends Neurosci 1996;19:312.

[15] Davalos D, Grutzendler J, Yang G, et al. ATP mediates rapid microglial response to local brain injury in vivo. Nat Neurosci 2005;8:752.

[16] Fetler L, Amigorena S. Neuroscience: brain under surveillance. The microglia patrol. Science 2005;309:392.

[17] Nimmerjahn A, Kirchhoff F, Helmchen F. Resting microglial cells are highly dynamic surveillants of brain parenchyma in vivo. Science 2005;308:1314.

[18] Hanisch UK. Microglia as a source and target of cytokines. Glia 2002;40:140.

[19] Carson MJ. Microglia as liaisons between the immune and central nervous system: functional implications in multiple sclerosis. Glia 2002;40:218.

[20] Garden GA. Microglia in human immunodeficiency virus-associated neurodegeneration. Glia 2002;40:240.

[21] Wyss-Coray T, Mucke L. Inflammation in neurodegenerative disease: a double-edged sword. Neuron 2002;35:419.

[22] Eikelenboom P, Bate C, Van Gool WA, et al. Neuroinflammation in Alzheimer's disease and prion disease. Glia 2002;40:232.

[23] McGeer EG, McGeer PL. Brain inflammation in Alzheimer disease and the therapeutic implications. Curr Pharm Des 1999;5:821.

[24] Monje ML, Toda H, Palmer TD. Inflammatory blockade restores adult hippocampal neurogenesis. Science 2003;302:1760.

[25] Almer G, Guegan C, Teismann P, et al. Increased expression of the pro-inflammatory enzyme cyclooxygenase-2 in amyotrophic lateral sclerosis. Ann Neurol 2001;49:176.

[26] Elliott JL. Cytokine upregulation in a murine model of familial amyotrophic lateral sclerosis. Brain Res Mol Brain Res 2001;95:172.

[27] Hensley K, Floyd RA, Gordon B, et al. Temporal patterns of cytokine and apoptosis-related gene expression in spinal cords of the G93A–SOD1 mouse model of amyotrophic lateral sclerosis. J Neurochem 2002;82:365.

[28] Nguyen MD, Julien JP, Rivest S. Induction of proinflammatory molecules in mice with amyotrophic lateral sclerosis: no requirement for proapoptotic interleukin-1beta in neurodegeneration. Ann Neurol 2001;50:630.

[29] Olsen MK, Roberds SL, Ellerbrock BR, et al. Disease mechanisms revealed by transcription profiling in SOD1–G93A transgenic mouse spinal cord. Ann Neurol 2001;50:730.

[30] Xie Y, Weydt P, Howland DS, et al. Inflammatory mediators and growth factors in the spinal cord of G93A SOD1 rats. Neuroreport 2004;15:2513.

[31] Yoshihara T, Ishigaki S, Yamamoto M, et al. Differential expression of inflammation- and apoptosis-related genes in spinal cords of a mutant SOD1 transgenic mouse model of familial amyotrophic lateral sclerosis. J Neurochem 2002;80:158.

[32] Alexianu ME, Kozovska M, Appel SH. Immune reactivity in a mouse model of familial ALS correlates with disease progression. Neurology 2001;57:1282.

[33] Engelhardt JI, Tajti J, Appel SH. Lymphocytic infiltrates in the spinal cord in amyotrophic lateral sclerosis. Arch Neurol 1993;50:30.

[34] Kawamata T, Akiyama H, Yamada T, et al. Immunologic reactions in amyotrophic lateral sclerosis brain and spinal cord tissue. Am J Pathol 1992;140:691.

[35] Dong Y, Benveniste EN. Immune function of astrocytes. Glia 2001;36:180.

[36] Neumann H. Control of glial immune function by neurons. Glia 2001;36:191.

[37] Almer G, Vukosavic S, Romero N, et al. Inducible nitric oxide synthase upregulation in a transgenic model of familial amyotrophic lateral sclerosis. J Neurochem 1999;72:2415.

[38] Hall ED, Oostveen JA, Gurney ME. Relationship of microglial and astrocytic activation to disease onset and progression in a transgenic model of familial ALS. Glia 1998;23:249.

[39] Mariotti R, Bentivoglio M. Activation and response to axotomy of microglia in the facial motor nuclei of G93A superoxide dismutase transgenic mice. Neurosci Lett 2000;285:87.

[40] Weydt P, Weiss MD, Moller T, et al. Neuro-inflammation as a therapeutic target in amyotrophic lateral sclerosis. Curr Opin Investig Drugs 2002;3:1720.

[41] Weydt P, Yuen EC, Ransom BR, et al. Increased cytotoxic potential of microglia from ALS-transgenic mice. Glia 2004;48:179.

[42] Ince PG, Shaw PJ, Slade JY, et al. Familial amyotrophic lateral sclerosis with a mutation in exon 4 of the Cu/Zn superoxide dismutase gene: pathological and immunocytochemical changes. Acta Neuropathol (Berl) 1996;92:395.

[43] Turner MR, Cagnin A, Turkheimer FE, et al. Evidence of widespread cerebral microglial activation in amyotrophic lateral sclerosis: an [11C](R)-PK11195 positron emission tomography study. Neurobiol Dis 2004;15:601.

[44] Zhang R, Gascon R, Miller RG, et al. Evidence for systemic immune system alterations in sporadic amyotrophic lateral sclerosis (sALS). J Neuroimmunol 2005;159:215.

[45] Fiala M, Liu QN, Sayre J, et al. Cyclooxygenase-2-positive macrophages infiltrate the Alzheimer's disease brain and damage the blood-brain barrier. Eur J Clin Invest 2002;32:360.

[46] Gong YH, Parsadanian AS, Andreeva A, et al. Restricted expression of G86R Cu/Zn superoxide dismutase in astrocytes results in astrocytosis but does not cause motoneuron degeneration. J Neurosci 2000;20:660.

[47] Lino MM, Schneider C, Caroni P. Accumulation of SOD1 mutants in postnatal motoneurons does not cause motoneuron pathology or motoneuron disease. J Neurosci 2002; 22:4825.

[48] Pramatarova A, Laganiere J, Roussel J, et al. Neuron-specific expression of mutant superoxide dismutase 1 in transgenic mice does not lead to motor impairment. J Neurosci 2001; 21:3369.

[49] Clement AM, Nguyen MD, Roberts EA, et al. Wild-type nonneuronal cells extend survival of SOD1 mutant motor neurons in ALS mice. Science 2003;302:113.

[50] Raoul C, Estevez AG, Nishimune H, et al. Motoneuron death triggered by a specific pathway downstream of Fas potentiation by ALS-linked SOD1 mutations. Neuron 2002;35: 1067.

[51] Trotti D, Rolfs A, Danbolt NC, et al. SOD1 mutants linked to amyotrophic lateral sclerosis selectively inactivate a glial glutamate transporter. Nat Neurosci 1999;2:427. [Erratum appears in Nat Neurosci 1999;2(9):848.]

[52] Cleveland DW. Presidential symposium: from Charcot to Lou Gehrig. Motor neuron growth and death. Presented at the 34th Annual Meeting of the Society for Neuroscience. San Diego, October 24, 2004.

[53] Wang J, Xu G, Slunt HH, et al. Coincident thresholds of mutant protein for paralytic disease and protein aggregation caused by restrictively expressed superoxide dismutase cDNA. Neurobiol Dis 2005; in press.

[54] Lopez-Redondo F, Nakajima K, Honda S, et al. Glutamate transporter GLT-1 is highly expressed in activated microglia following facial nerve axotomy. Brain Res Mol Brain Res 2000;76:429.

[55] Plate KH, Beck H, Danner S, et al. Cell type specific upregulation of vascular endothelial growth factor in an MCA-occlusion model of cerebral infarct. J Neuropathol Exp Neurol 1999;58:654.

[56] Drazen JM. COX-2 inhibitors: a lesson in unexpected problems. N Engl J Med 2005;352: 1131.

[57] Drachman DB, Frank K, Dykes-Hoberg M, et al. Cyclooxygenase 2 inhibition protects motor neurons and prolongs survival in a transgenic mouse model of ALS. Ann Neurol 2002;52:771.

[58] Kiaei M, Kipiani K, Petri S, et al. Integrative role of cPLA with COX-2 and the effect of nonsteroidal anti-inflammatory drugs in a transgenic mouse model of amyotrophic lateral sclerosis. J Neurochem 2005;93:403.

[59] Klivenyi P, Gardian G, Calingasan NY, et al. Additive neuroprotective effects of creatine and a cyclooxygenase 2 inhibitor against dopamine depletion in the 1-methyl-4-phenyl-1,2,3,6-tetrahydropyridine (MPTP) mouse model of Parkinson's disease. J Mol Neurosci 2003;21:191.

[60] Consilvio C, Vincent AM, Feldman EL. Neuroinflammation, COX-2, and ALS: a dual role? Exp Neurol 2004;187:1.

[61] Pompl PN, Ho L, Bianchi M, et al. A therapeutic role for cyclooxygenase-2 inhibitors in a transgenic mouse model of amyotrophic lateral sclerosis. FASEB J 2003;17:725.

[62] Tikka T, Fiebich BL, Goldsteins G, et al. Minocycline, a tetracycline derivative, is neuroprotective against excitotoxicity by inhibiting activation and proliferation of microglia. J Neurosci 2001;21:2580.

[63] Tikka T, Usenius T, Tenhunen M, et al. Tetracycline derivatives and ceftriaxone, a cephalosporin antibiotic, protect neurons against apoptosis induced by ionizing radiation. J Neurochem 2001;78:1409.

[64] Tikka TM, Koistinaho JE. Minocycline provides neuroprotection against N-methyl-D-aspartate neurotoxicity by inhibiting microglia. J Immunol 2001;166:7527.

[65] Domercq M, Matute C. Neuroprotection by tetracyclines. Trends Pharmacol Sci 2004;25: 609.

[66] Kriz J, Nguyen M, Julien J. Minocycline slows disease progression in a mouse model of amyotrophic lateral sclerosis. Neurobiol Dis 2002;10:268.

[67] Van Den Bosch L, Tilkin P, Lemmens G, et al. Minocycline delays disease onset and mortality in a transgenic model of ALS. Neuroreport 2002;13:1067.

[68] Zhu S, Stavrovskaya IG, Drozda M, et al. Minocycline inhibits cytochrome c release and delays progression of amyotrophic lateral sclerosis in mice. Nature 2002;417:74.

[69] Gordon PH, Moore DH, Gelinas DF, et al. Placebo-controlled phase I/II studies of minocycline in amyotrophic lateral sclerosis. Neurology 2004;62:1845.

ELSEVIER
SAUNDERS

Phys Med Rehabil Clin N Am
16 (2005) 1091–1097

PHYSICAL MEDICINE
AND REHABILITATION
CLINICS OF
NORTH AMERICA

Skeletal Muscle in Amyotrophic Lateral Sclerosis: Emerging Concepts and Therapeutic Implications

Simone Abmayr, PhD[a], Patrick Weydt, MD[b],*

[a]Department of Neurology, University of Washington,
1959 NE Pacific Street Seattle, WA-98195, USA
[b]Department of Laboratory Medicine, University of Washington,
1959 NE Pacific Street Seattle, WA-98195, USA

Amyotrophic lateral sclerosis (ALS) is the most common adult-onset motor neuron disorder [1]. It is invariably fatal, and despite enormous research efforts, the therapeutic options remain limited. Muscle wasting (ie, amyotrophy) and weakness are the most prominent symptoms of ALS, yet its pathogenesis and its relation to motor neuron degeneration is only incompletely understood. Selective degeneration of the motor neurons in the prefrontal cortex, brainstem, and anterior horns of the spinal cord are the classic pathological hallmarks of the disease, but focal weakness and subtle, asymmetric muscle atrophy at the distal limbs or in the bulbar region are typically the earliest symptoms noted by patients [1–3]. In the advanced disease stages, ALS patients experience severe generalized muscle wasting and substantial weight loss of more than 15% [4–6]. The most incapacitating ALS symptoms—such as loss of mobility and increasing dependence on caregivers for activities of daily living, as well as terminal respiratory failure—are direct manifestations of muscle weakness.

Traditionally, muscle weakness and wasting has been attributed to a combination of muscle denervation resulting from motor neuron degeneration and malnutrition due to dysphagia [7]. As a result, therapeutic strategies have focused on pharmacologic protection of the degenerating motor neurons on the one hand and assuring adequate caloric intake on the other hand. We summarize recent insights emerging from clinical studies and

Patrick Weydt is the recipient of a Career Development Award from the Muscular Dystrophy Association (MDA3981).
* Corresponding author.
E-mail address: weydt@u.washington.edu (P. Weydt).

pmr.theclinics.com

transgenic animal research, which suggest that skeletal muscle is more autonomously involved in the pathogenesis of ALS than previously thought. The implications of this new perspective for developing innovative therapies directly targeted at the muscle are discussed.

Clinical clues

There is increasing awareness that amyotrophic lateral sclerosis is not just a "motor neuron disease" but is in fact a multisystem disorder whose most prominent manifestation is degeneration of the motor neurons [3].

Kasarskis and colleagues were the first to notice that the measured energy expenditure of some ALS patients significantly exceeds the predicted value [5]. They concluded that ALS patients are in an apparent "paradoxical hypermetabolic state." Although this was initially interpreted as a manifestation of the increased respiratory effort, a follow-up study found the increased metabolic rate not to be associated with reduction in respiratory function suggesting other causes, including mitochondrial and muscle abnormalities [6,7].

There are no generally accepted exogenous risk factors for sporadic ALS [8]. However, athleticism, epitomized by American sports icon and ALS victim Lou Gehrig, has been implicated repeatedly as a risk factor, most recently in a retrospective study on incidence of ALS among professional soccer players [9–11]. It is less well recognized that Lou Gehrig is also a striking example of the dramatic and rapid weight loss that often accompanies motor symptom progression in ALS patients: in the final days of his disease at age 37, Gehrig weighed a mere 56 kg (125 lbs), down from an athletic 102 kg (225 lbs) less than 3 years earlier, before he was diagnosed [12].

Insights from transgenic models of ALS

Rational ALS therapy development was boosted enormously by the advent of transgenic animal models of the disease. The identification of mutations in the ubiquitously and abundantly expressed superoxide dismutase 1 (SOD1) gene as the cause for some of the rare hereditary forms of ALS was a landmark discovery and rapidly led to the development of several transgenic mouse models [13–16]. These animals are genetically engineered to express the human mutated SOD1 gene and recapitulate the basic clinical and pathological characteristics of the human disease with striking accuracy [17]. The G93A-SOD1 high expressing line (G93A-SOD1h) has the most rapid disease progression as it shows symptom onset around 90 days of age and has a life expectancy of only 120 to 140 days [13]. Therefore, G93A-SOD1h mice have become by far the most widely used screening tools for evaluating the therapeutic potential of novel compounds and interventions against ALS (for a continuously updated list of completed animal trials, refer to http://www.als.net/research/studies/animalStudyList.asp). The close similarities between familial and sporadic human ALS with the paralytic disease phenotype of the SOD1 transgenic mouse models, namely the adult onset of symptoms, the selective and progressive motor neuron degeneration, and the greatly reduced life span, have inspired the hope that "hits" from the mouse screenings would be beneficial in humans as well. However, with now over a decade of experience using these models, the high expectations have so far proven overly optimistic, and the role of animal studies in guiding clinical trials is being critically re-evaluated [18].

To date, studies using transgenic mice still do not adequately predict the outcomes of human trials; however, they have shed important new light on the cellular basis of motor neuron degeneration in ALS [18–20]. For one, transgenic mice allow for the analysis of the critical presymptomatic stages of the disease process, which cannot realistically be studied in patients. As discussed elsewhere in this issue, this has (among other things) led to the realization that neuroinflammation plays an important role in ALS pathogenesis and represents a promising therapeutic target [21].

Another fundamental insight from the study of transgenic mouse models is that the demise of motor neurons in ALS can be non–cell autonomous; that is, cell types other than motor neurons themselves can be critically involved in the degenerative process. Neurons depend on and intimately interact with their tissue environment, which is composed of astrocytes, oligodendrocytes, microglia, and, in the special case of motor neurons, muscle cells (Fig. 1).

The first indication that mutant SOD1 toxicity is non–cell autonomous came when targeted expression of the mutant SOD1 transgene in neurons failed to produce a phenotype [22,23]. Because previous work had shown that transgene expression limited to astrocytes also failed to elicit motor neuron degeneration [24], it was immediately speculated whether still other cellular compartments of the central nervous system are involved or whether the mutant SOD1 mutations have to be expressed in a combination of cell populations. To address this issue, a consortium of researchers led by Don Cleveland generated several independent lines of chimeric mice that are random mixtures of normal and mutant SOD1-expressing cells [25]. Through clever labeling strategies, they were able to differentiate between normal and SOD1 transgenic cells in situ. Their analysis showed that (1) disease severity depended directly on the percentage of SOD1 transgenic/nontransgenic cells in the spinal cord and (2) even nontransgenic motor neurons (and only motor neurons) degenerate in the tissue context of mutant SOD1 chimeric mice. This landmark study established that the ALS causing SOD1 mutations can act non–cell autonomously; that is, they can produce degeneration of nontransgenic motor neurons. In the analysis of their data, the authors chose to focus on the role of astrocytes and microglia and did not further address the possible contribution of skeletal muscle to the disease process.

Transgenic mice have also helped understand the generalized metabolic abnormalities reported by clinicians as described above [26]. For instance, we noticed that weight loss, not motor symptoms, is the first objectively measurable abnormality of the G93A-SOD1h transgenic mice [27]. In an

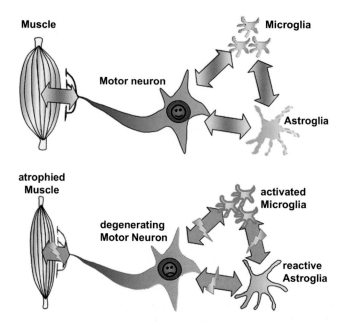

Fig. 1. Simplified model of the microenvironment of a lower motor neuron in the spinal cord: Under normal conditions the motor neuron (blue) interfaces with astrocytes (green), microglia (red), oligodendrocytes/Schwann cells (not shown) and skeletal muscle. The motor neuron interacts with and is vitally dependent on each of these cell types (grey arrows). Non-cell autonomous motor neuron degeneration occurs when disruptions (red flashes) in non-neuronal cells result in the death of a healthy motor neuron. It is not known whether the different non-neuronal cells have to conspire or whether a single hit suffices to kill a motor neuron.

intriguing study, Dupuis and colleagues [28] demonstrated that ALS mice experience a hypermetabolic state, as has been suggested for ALS patients, and that this abnormality well precedes motor onset and is most likely of muscular origin. Remarkably, compensation of the metabolic deficit with a high caloric diet significantly extended the life span of these mice.

Finally, a timely study by Wang and colleagues [29] just now demonstrated that expression of the mutant SOD1 transgene restricted to neurons, astrocytes, and muscle—notably excluding microglia and oligodendrocytes—is sufficient to evoke the full ALS phenotype in mice. In the context of three other studies showing that neuronal and astrocytic expression of the transgene does not result in motor neuron degeneration, this strongly suggests that skeletal muscle is indeed critical for disease development at least in the SOD1 linked variants of ALS [22–24].

Therapeutic implications

The possibility that skeletal muscle may be a critical player in motor neuron degeneration has inspiring implications for devising therapy strategies against ALS. Although the concept of treating the muscle to treat ALS is not new—in fact, one of the earliest modern therapy trials in ALS explicitly targeted the muscle [30]—recent trials have almost entirely focused on direct neuroprotection and anti-inflammation [3,31].

The most powerful survival effects in preclinical trials have been achieved with gene therapeutic delivery of two specific growth factors: insulin-like growth factor 1 (IGF-1) and vascular endothelial growth factor (VEGF) [32,33]. The IGF-1 approach was pioneered by Kaspar and colleagues [33], who also showed that intramuscularly injected adeno-associated virus (serotype 2) (AAV2) expressing IGF-1 under the cytomegalovirus (CMV) promoter is taken up by motor neurons and retrogradely transported into the spinal cord. Using a different gene vector, EIAV, and a similar intramuscular injections route, Azzouz and colleagues [32] subsequently demonstrated that VEGF is at least equally as potent as IGF-1 in ALS mice.

Recently, for the first time, a SOD1 mouse study successfully deviated from the central nervous system–centric delivery paradigms and found that muscle-specific overexpression of insulin-like growth factor 1 (IGF-1) is sufficient to also substantially prolong survival of G93A-SOD1 transgenic mice [34]. This finding stimulated the ALS research community to take a fresh look at the data reported in the Kaspar and Azzouz studies. It turns out that only a very small fraction (<2%) of the intramuscularly injected virus particles are taken up by the motor neurons—the rest remains in the muscle. Because in both studies ubiquitously active promoters were used, viral vector remaining in the injected muscle also produce substantial quantities of growth factors and—especially with the results of Dobrowolny [34] in mind—this raises the possibility that muscle-produced rather than neuron-produced growth factors are responsible for the therapeutic effect. Settling the questions about the extent of skeletal muscle involvement in the therapeutic effects of the IGF-1 and VEGF studies will be helpful in designing the optimal gene delivery strategy in human trials. On the one hand, both VEGF and IGF-1 are pleitropic factors with potentially severe side effects (eg, tumor development), so precise targeting is imperative to attain an acceptable safety profile. On the other hand, there is much progress being made in targeting gene therapies to the musculature in other diseases, and this experience could be exploited for ALS treatments [35,36].

Finally, it is critical to effectively reach specific vital regions of the motor system, namely the respiratory apparatus, including the diaphragm and the bulbar nerves and musculature. Unfortunately, these regions are especially difficult to access safely with conventional injection techniques. However, a recent breakthrough in gene delivery offers a possible answer to this challenge. Gregorevic and colleagues have used systemically delivered adeno-associated virus serotype 6 (AAV6) to adult mice in order to achieve virtually body-wide transduction of skeletal muscle with a therapeutic gene [35,36]. This method therefore represents also a promising approach for muscle gene therapy in ALS. In addition, there is reason to suggest that AAV6 is also efficiently taken up and retrogradely transported by motor neurons.

Summary

We have briefly summarized the emerging evidence that skeletal muscle might be an active player in ALS pathogenesis: (1) clinical studies and animal experiments suggest that a significant subpopulation of ALS patients experience a hypermetabolic state of the musculature; (2) the non–cell autonomous nature of mutant SOD1 toxicity and the new ALS mouse model from the Borchelt laboratory raises the possibility that skeletal muscle is the critical cell compartment in mediating selective motor neuron degeneration in the transgenic mouse model; and (3) circumstances of the two most successful preclinical gene therapy trials in ALS indicate that targeting skeletal muscle rather than motor neurons with growth factor therapy might be beneficial. This would also mean that the ALS community can greatly benefit from the progress made in designing gene therapy strategies for many other neuromuscular disorders.

References

[1] Brown RHJ. Amyotrophic lateral sclerosis. In: Kasper DL, Braunwald E, Fauci AS, et al, editors. Harrison's principles of internal medicine. 16th edition. New York: McGraw-Hill; 2005.

[2] Rowland LP, Shneider NA. Amyotrophic lateral sclerosis. N Engl J Med 2001;344: 1688–700.

[3] Strong MJ. Amyotrophic lateral sclerosis: contemporary concepts in etiopathogenesis and pharmacotherapy. Expert Opin Investig Drugs 2004;13:1593–614.

[4] Mazzini L, Corra T, Zaccala M, et al. Percutaneous endoscopic gastrostomy and enteral nutrition in amyotrophic lateral sclerosis. J Neurol 1995;242:695–8.

[5] Kasarskis EJ, Berryman S, Vanderleest JG, et al. Nutritional status of patients with amyotrophic lateral sclerosis: relation to the proximity of death. Am J Clin Nutr 1996;63:130–7.

[6] Desport JC, Preux PM, Truong TC, et al. Nutritional status is a prognostic factor for survival in ALS patients. Neurology 1999;53:1059–63.

[7] Cameron A, Rosenfeld J. Nutritional issues and supplements in amyotrophic lateral sclerosis and other neurodegenerative disorders. Curr Opin Clin Nutr Metab Care 2002;5:631–43.

[8] Armon C. An evidence-based medicine approach to the evaluation of the role of exogenous risk factors in sporadic amyotrophic lateral sclerosis. Neuroepidemiology 2003;22:217–28.

[9] Kurtzke JF, Beebe GW. Epidemiology of amyotrophic lateral sclerosis: 1. A case-control comparison based on ALS deaths. Neurology 1980;30:453–62.

[10] Scarmeas N, Shih T, Stern Y, et al. Premorbid weight, body mass, and varsity athletics in ALS. Neurology 2002;59:773–5.

[11] Chio A, Benzi G, Dossena M, et al. Severely increased risk of amyotrophic lateral sclerosis among Italian professional football players. Brain 2005;128:472–6.

[12] Eig J. Luckiest man—the life and death of Lou Gehrig. New York: Simon & Schuster; 2005.

[13] Gurney ME, Pu H, Chiu AY, et al. Motor neuron degeneration in mice that express a human Cu, Zn superoxide dismutase mutation. Science 1994;264:1772–5.

[14] Bruijn LI, Becher MW, Lee MK, et al. ALS-linked SOD1 mutant G85R mediates damage to astrocytes and promotes rapidly progressive disease with SOD1-containing inclusions. Neuron 1997;18:327–38.

[15] Wong PC, Pardo CA, Borchelt DR, et al. An adverse property of a familial ALS-linked SOD1 mutation causes motor neuron disease characterized by vacuolar degeneration of mitochondria. Neuron 1995;14:1105–16.

[16] Rosen DR, Siddique T, Patterson D, et al. Mutations in Cu/Zn superoxide dismutase gene are associated with familial amyotrophic lateral sclerosis. Nature 1993;362:59–62.

[17] Cleveland DW, Rothstein JD. From Charcot to Lou Gehrig: deciphering selective motor neuron death in ALS. Nat Rev Neurosci 2001;2:806–19.

[18] Rothstein JD. Preclinical studies: how much can we rely on? Amyotroph Lateral Scler Other Motor Neuron Disord 2004;5(Suppl 1):22–5.

[19] Rothstein JD. Of mice and men: reconciling preclinical ALS mouse studies and human clinical trials. Ann Neurol 2003;53:423–6.

[20] Brujin LI, Miller TM, Cleveland DW. Unraveling the mechanisms involved in motor neuron degeneration in ALS. Annu Rev Neurosci 2004;27:723–49.

[21] Weydt P, Weiss MD, Moller T, et al. Neuro-inflammation as a therapeutic target in amyotrophic lateral sclerosis. Curr Opin Investig Drugs 2002;3:1720–4.

[22] Lino MM, Schneider C, Caroni P. Accumulation of SOD1 mutants in postnatal motoneurons does not cause motoneuron pathology or motoneuron disease. J Neurosci 2002;22: 4825–32.

[23] Pramatarova A, Laganiere J, Roussel J, et al. Neuron-specific expression of mutant superoxide dismutase 1 in transgenic mice does not lead to motor impairment. J Neurosci 2001; 21:3369–74.

[24] Gong YH, Parsadanian AS, Andreeva A, et al. Restricted expression of G86R Cu/Zn superoxide dismutase in astrocytes results in astrocytosis but does not cause motoneuron degeneration. J Neurosci 2000;20:660–5.

[25] Clement AM, Nguyen MD, Roberts EA, et al. Wild-type nonneuronal cells extend survival of SOD1 mutant motor neurons in ALS mice. Science 2003;302:113–7.

[26] Gonzalez de Aguilar JL, Dupuis L, Oudart H, et al. The metabolic hypothesis in amyotrophic lateral sclerosis: insights from mutant Cu/Zn-superoxide dismutase mice. Biomed Pharmacother 2005;59:190–6.

[27] Weydt P, Hong SY, Kliot M, et al. Assessing disease onset and progression in the SOD1 mouse model of ALS. Neuroreport 2003;14:1051–4.

[28] Dupuis L, Oudart H, Rene F, et al. Evidence for defective energy homeostasis in amyotrophic lateral sclerosis: benefit of a high-energy diet in a transgenic mouse model. Proc Natl Acad Sci U S A 2004;101(30):11159–64.

[29] Wang J, Xu G, Slunt HH, et al. Coincident thresholds of mutant protein for paralytic disease and protein aggregation caused by restrictively expressed superoxide dismutase cDNA. Neurobiol Dis, in press.

[30] Liversedge LA. Glycocyamine and betaine in motor-neurone disease. Lancet 1956;271: 1136–8.

[31] Weiss MD, Weydt P, Carter GT. Current pharmacological management of amyotropic lateral sclerosis and a role for rational polypharmacy. Expert Opin Pharmacother 2004;5: 735–46.

[32] Azzouz M, Ralph GS, Storkebaum E, et al. VEGF delivery with retrogradely transported lentivector prolongs survival in a mouse ALS model. Nature 2004;429:413–7.

[33] Kaspar BK, Llado J, Sherkat N, et al. Retrograde viral delivery of IGF-1 prolongs survival in a mouse ALS model. Science 2003;301:839–42.

[34] Dobrowolny G, Giacinti C, Pelosi L, et al. Muscle expression of a local Igf-1 isoform protects motor neurons in an ALS mouse model. J Cell Biol 2005;168:193–9.

[35] Abmayr S, Gregorevic P, Allen JM, et al. Phenotypic improvement of dystrophic muscles by rAAV/microdystrophin vectors is augmented by Igf1 codelivery. Mol Ther 2005;12:441.

[36] Gregorevic P, Blankinship MJ, Allen JM, et al. Systemic delivery of genes to striated muscles using adeno-associated viral vectors. Nat Med 2004;10:828.

PHYSICAL MEDICINE
AND REHABILITATION
CLINICS OF
NORTH AMERICA

ELSEVIER
SAUNDERS

Phys Med Rehabil Clin N Am
16 (2005) 1099–1112

Chronic Pain in Persons with Neuromuscular Disease

Amy J. Hoffman, MPH[a], Mark P. Jensen, PhD[a,b],
R. Ted Abresch, MS[c], Gregory T. Carter, MD[a,*]

[a]Department of Rehabilitation Medicine, Box 356490,
University of Washington School of Medicine, Seattle, WA 98195-6490, USA
[b]Multidisciplinary Pain Center, University of Washington Medical Center–Roosevelt,
4245 Roosevelt Way Northeast, Seattle, WA 98105-6920, USA
[c]Department of Physical Medicine and Rehabilitation, PM&R TB 191,
University of California, Davis, CA 95616, USA

Pain historically has not been a focus of clinicians and researchers who study neuromuscular diseases (NMDs). The available literature on NMDs gives scant mention to pain as a component of these disorders. In the authors' clinical experience, chronic pain seems to be a serious problem for many persons with NMDs. To help determine the accuracy of this opinion based initially on clinical experience, the authors' group began a multicenter program of research to study the nature and scope of chronic pain and its impact on functioning in patients with NMDs.

Nature and scope of pain in persons with neuromuscular diseases

Research conducted by the authors and others suggests that chronic pain is a significant problem for many individuals with NMDs [1–6]. One of the first studies that examined this issue was a prospective longitudinal study of 55 patients with Guillain-Barré syndrome [1]. Pain was reported by 49 patients (89.1%); they reported an average pain intensity of 4.7 (SD = 3.3) on a 0-to-10 Visual Analogue Scale. Severe pain was reported by 26 patients

This article was supported by grant PO1 HD33988 from the National Institutes of Health, National Institute of Child Health and Human Development, National Center for Medical Rehabilitation Research, and grant H133B03118 from the National Institute on Disability and Rehabilitation Research Training Center.

* Corresponding author. 1809 Cooks Hill Road, Centralia, WA 98531, USA.
E-mail address: gtcarter@u.washington.edu (G.T. Carter).

(47.3%) (average 7; SD = 2); they described their pain as "distressing," "horrible," or "excruciating." Back and leg pain of a moderate-to-severe nature was a presenting symptom in more than half (61.8%) of the study patients [1]. Other pain sites reported included the extremities (49.1% dyesthetic extremity pain, 34.5% myalgic-rheumatic extremity pain) and pelvis or rectal area (20%). Half of the patients (50.9%) used analgesics or anti-inflammatories; 41 patients (74.5%) required oral or parenteral opioids at some point during treatment.

A case report of four patients with facioscapulohumeral muscular dystrophy described pain characteristics, persistence, severity, frequency, site, and precipitating and relieving factors [2]. Each of the four patients identified pain as their most disabling symptom and complained of three to seven separate pain complaints. None had more than 1 pain-free day per month, and all complained of disturbed sleep. The description of pain seemed to vary as a functioning of pain site, with forearm and thigh pains most often described as having a "sharp" or "stabbing" nature [2]. Response to conventional first-line pain treatments (eg, analgesics or anti-inflammatories) was poor. One patient responded well to morphine during a particularly long and severe pain episode, and three patients reported considerable benefit from swimming or hydrotherapy.

A large survey of patients with Charcot-Marie-Tooth (CMT) disease reported on pain intensity, description, location, and treatments [3]. Of 617 CMT patients, 440 (71%) reported having pain; these patients were significantly younger than the patients reporting no pain. Chronic pain was described as "dull" (15%) or "burning" (8%), whereas intermittent or breakthrough pain was described as "sharp" (18%), "stabbing" (12%), "burning" (3%), "hot" (2%), or "cold" (2%). The most frequent pain sites were low back (70%), knees (53%), ankles (50%), toes (46%), and feet (44%). Most patients (64%) reported using medication to manage pain, with 38% using non-narcotic medications (analgesics and anti-inflammatories) and 22% using narcotic medications.

Another survey studied health-related quality of life in slowly progressive NMDs [4]. The investigators found that 83% of 811 participants reported having at least some pain. Many of these participants (54%) reported that their pain was moderate to very severe. The frequency and severity of pain in this population were significantly greater than levels of pain reported by the general US population, with the noted exception of participants with spinal muscular atrophy. Because this study was a secondary analysis of a quality-of-life survey, the investigators did not report on pain locations or pain treatments.

A more recent study compared 24 patients with myotonic dystrophy type 2, also known as proximal myotonic myopathy, and 24 age-matched and sex-matched patients with other chronic noninflammatory muscle disorders using the McGill Pain Questionnaire [5]. Most participants in this study reported experiencing musculoskeletal pain (96% of patients with myotonic dystrophy type 2 and 75% of patients with other chronic noninflammatory muscle disorders). Participants with myotonic dystrophy type 2 described their pain as significantly more "dull," "stabbing," and "tender" than participants with other chronic noninflammatory muscle disorders. They also described their pain as lasting significantly longer (average 10 hours) than patients with other disorders (average 5 hours).

A more recent study examined the nature and scope of pain in persons with NMDs [6]. The investigators surveyed 193 individuals with NMDs about pain intensity, quality, interference, location, treatment, and general quality of life. Of the sample, 73% reported pain; 27% reported severe pain. Pain was described most frequently as "deep," "tiring," "sharp," and "dull." Pain interfered with daily activities the most in patients with myotonic muscular dystrophy (myotonic muscular dystrophy types 1 and 2) and amyotrophic lateral sclerosis (ALS) and the least in patients with CMT disease. The most frequent pain sites were the back (49%), leg (47%), shoulder (43%), and neck (40%). Over-the-counter (OTC) medications were used most often for pain relief (ibuprofen/aspirin 61%, acetaminophen 47%), followed by physical therapy (43%) and narcotic analgesics (35%). Respondents with severe pain (average pain ≥ 7 on 0–10 scale) reported using narcotics (50%), followed by ibuprofen/aspirin (47%) and acetaminophen (37%). These participants also reported on the effectiveness of treatments for pain. Treatments reported as giving the most pain relief were chiropractic manipulation and nerve blocks, but only a few participants reported trying these treatments. Finally, quality of life was measured using the SF-36. The respondents reported significantly greater dysfunction than other persons without health problems on many of the SF-36 scales. Although no significant differences were found in emotional or mental health scales, there was significant impairment in other domains of quality of life. Table 1 outlines the dimensions that are most important in determining quality of life.

Few studies have examined the nature and scope of pain in persons with NMDs. Of the six studies that were identified, each one reported chronic pain in 60% or more of their samples of persons with NMDs, and this pain was reported as severe (eg, rated as ≥ 7 on 0–10 intensity scales) in significant subgroups of patients with NMDs, indicating that chronic pain is a serious problem for many of these patients. Preliminary evidence suggests that pain problems occur more frequently and at a higher severity in some NMD populations than others. Jensen et al [6] found that frequency and intensity of pain varied by diagnostic group, ranging from 60% (among patients with ALS) to 100% (among patients with postpolio syndrome). Average pain also varied among diagnostic groups, ranging from 4 to 6.28 (on 0–10 scales of pain intensity) with relatively large SDs. Further support for the variability of pain severity among different NMD diagnostic groups was reported by Abresch et al [4], who studied patients with slowly progressive NMDs, including CMT disease, facioscapulohumeral muscular

Table 1
Dimensions that are most important in determining quality of life

Physical and material well-being	Material well-being and financial security
	Health and personal safety
Relations with other people	Relations with spouse
	Having and rearing children
	Relations with parents, siblings, or other relatives
	Relations with friends
Social, community, civic activities	Helping and encouraging others
	Participating in local and governmental affairs
Personal development, fulfillment	Intellectual development
	Understanding and planning
	Occupational role career
	Creativity and personal expression
Recreation	Socializing with others
	Passive and observational recreational activities
	Participating in active recreation

dystrophy, limb-girdle muscular dystrophy, myotonic muscular dystrophy types 1 and 2, spinal muscular atrophy, and postpolio syndrome. These investigators found that patients with spinal muscular atrophy reported no more frequency of pain than the general population, whereas patients with muscular dystrophies (facioscapulohumeral muscular dystrophy, limb-girdle muscular dystrophy, myotonic muscular dystrophy types 1 and 2) reported greater frequency of pain [4]. Patients with CMT disease and postpolio syndrome reported the highest pain severity among diagnostic groups.

Preliminary evidence suggests that pain sites also might vary as a function of NMD diagnosis. The most common pain sites for patients with CMT disease were the low back, legs, and feet, which is consistent with the disease, which affects the legs and feet sooner and more severely than other parts of the body [3,6]. Patients with facioscapulohumeral muscular dystrophy reported pain more often in their back and shoulders, which is consistent with the disease, which usually encompasses severe lumbar lordosis and shoulder girdle instability [2,6].

Finally, evidence suggests the possibility that pain can have a negative impact on functioning in persons with NMDs. Abresch et al [4] found a significant correlation between increased pain and lower levels of general health, vitality, social function, and physical role in each of the NMD groups. They also found that sleep disturbance was a problem in 68% of their sample and was associated with pain. Jensen et al [6] found a greater impact of pain on mobility, normal work, enjoyment of life, and recreational activities. They also found that persons with NMD reported significantly greater dysfunction than healthy populations, as measured by physical functioning, physical role, bodily pain, general health, vitality, and social functioning. Table 2 shows the World Health Organization's definitions of impairment, disability, and handicap. With regards to pain, this would represent part of the disability.

Causes of pain in persons with neuromuscular diseases

Possible causes of pain in patients with NMDs depend primarily on the type of disease (neuropathic versus myopathic) and the degree of mobility the person has (ie, ambulatory versus wheelchair dependent). In primary neuropathies, such as the family of hereditary neuropathies, there is likely neuropathic pain stemming directly from damaged, demyelinated nerves; this would include, as noted earlier, CMT disease. As prior studies showed, patients with CMT disease reported pain descriptors that matched well with other painful neuropathies [3]. CMT-related pain may be generated from ectopic impulses propagated from the site of injury and the adjacent dorsal root ganglia. Other mechanisms contributing to pain in this setting include abnormal involvement of the sympathetic nervous system and neuroplastic changes within the central nervous system [7,8]. This is the "pain memory" that many people with chronic neuropathic pain develop.

Table 2
World Health Organization definitions of impairment, disability, handicap

Organ	Impairment (usually progressive)	Disability	Handicap
Skeletal muscle	↓ Strength and endurance	↓ Motor performance	↓ Quality of life
		↓ Mobility	
		↓ Upper extremity function	↓ Educational opportunities
		↑ Fatigue	
		Muscle spasm and cramps	↓ Employment opportunities
			↑ Dependency and disadvantage
Bone and joint	Joint contractures	↓ Function	
	Spine deformity	Pain and deformity	
Lungs	↓ Pulmonary function	Restrictive lung disease	
		↑ Fatigue	
Heart	Cardiomyopathy	↓ Cardiopulmonary adaptations	
	Conduction defects	↑ Fatigue	
Central nervous system	↓ Intellectual capacity	↓ Learning ability	
		↓ Psychosocial adjustment	

In the broader category of NMDs in general, there are likely many other significant pain generators, including the musculoskeletal system. Impaired mobility is expected with disease progression and often causes pain. Even in CMT patients, there are significant mobility and joint instability issues. The French neurologist Charcot, who was cocredited with first describing the disease, first described the *neuropathic joint,* also referred to as a *Charcot joint* [8]. This entity occurs as a result of joint instability secondary to muscle weakness, coupled with impaired proprioception, leading to joint destruction from abnormal biomechanics. Charcot first described this problem in tabes dorsalis (tertiary neurosyphilis), but the same problem and mechanism occur in CMT disesase. CMT patients show significant muscle weakness, producing 20% to 40% lower force than normal controls using quantitative strength measurements in prior studies [9–11]. This muscle weakness also occurs, to varying degrees, in all other NMDs. This weakness may place a higher stress on the musculoskeletal system and contribute to pain generation. This weakness also results in significant functional problems. All of the major NMDs have significant prolongation of timed motor performance tasks (Box 1), which also may be influenced by pain.

Prior studies in patients with NMDs have shown marked reduction in functional aerobic capacity during exercise testing, even in patients with normal or relatively normal pre-exercise pulmonary function and exercise heart rate, blood pressure, and maximum ventilation [12–25]. This reduction implies that patients with NMDs, as a whole, may be deconditioned and at high risk for the development of metabolic syndrome (obesity, elevated blood glucose with insulin resistance, and hyperlipidemia) [26]. Deconditioned states also usually are associated with a decreased pain tolerance

---

Box 1. Timed motor performance tasks

Time to perform is measured in seconds with a stopwatch. Failure is considered inability to complete the task by a time limit of 120 seconds.
1. Standing from lying supine
2. Climbing 4 standard stairs (beginning and ending standing with arms at sides)
3. Running or walking 30 ft (as fast as is compatible with safety)
4. Standing from sitting on chair (chair height should allow feet to touch floor)
5. Propelling a wheelchair 30 ft
6. Putting on a T-shirt (sitting in chair; see instructions)
7. Cutting a 3 inch × 3 inch premarked square from a piece of paper with safety scissors (lines do not need to be followed precisely)

[27]. This decreased tolerance is likely a major factor that negatively affects quality of life for persons with NMDs because numerous secondary painful musculoskeletal syndromes can arise [27].

Muscle weakness also may be accompanied by spasticity in some NMDs, such as ALS. This combination, along with progressive loss of mobility, places a high stress on the musculoskeletal system, contributing to pain generation. Patients with NMDs are at high risk for developing progressive loss of range of motion, particularly in the shoulders. If left untreated, a patient can develop a joint contracture. In the case of frozen shoulder (adhesive capsulitis), this can be extremely painful. Loss of range of motion not only can result in a painful frozen shoulder, but also has been reported to cause complex regional pain syndrome in some patients with NMDs [28]. Because of immobility and neck and trunk muscle weakness leading to poor spinal support, many NMD patients experience some degree of back and neck pain. Spinal bracing may be used to improve sitting posture and balance. This bracing would not prevent neuromuscular scoliosis, however, which can be treated only with spinal fusion; this also may be a pain-generating issue (see the article on pain in pediatric NMDs by Engel and colleagues elsewhere in this issue). Severe neck flexor and extensor weakness can lead to a "floppy head" associated with severe neck pain and tightness; this is a particular problem in ALS.

Treatment of pain in persons with neuromuscular diseases

Any treatment strategy should begin with an initial diagnostic workup to determine if there is a modifiable pathophysiologic process that might underlie the pain. When examining possible treatments, the clinician also should consider all the ways in which a person is affected by chronic pain. This consideration includes measurements of pain intensity, the emotional impact of pain, limitations in the individual's ability to engage in daily activities because of pain, and limitations in participation in important social roles, such as employment [29,30]. Next, it is important to establish identifiable treatment goals and measurable markers of pain relief. The clinician should consider self-reported pain reduction and other indicators (eg, a return to work or spousal reports) as indicators of improvement. Finally, the clinician should monitor the progress made and reassess as needed [31].

Pharmacologic measures

Research into the treatment of pain in NMDs has been limited to reports on the different kinds of treatments persons with NMDs have tried. No clinical trials evaluating treatments for NMD-related pain have been identified. Health care providers seeking to help patients with NMDs experiencing significant pain must depend on clinical experience and on research evaluating pain treatments in other populations when making treatment decisions. Further research is needed to clarify the nature, scope, and, perhaps most importantly, treatment of pain in persons with NMDs, and this is the intent of the authors' research group. It is hoped, however, that this article encourages others to undertake investigation in this area of research.

Some knowledge is available of what persons with NMDs have reported using to treat their pain. The most common pain treatments seem to be OTC analgesics. Prior studies found that most patients with NMDs used ibuprofen, aspirin, or acetaminophen for pain, but that these OTC analgesics provide only moderate relief on average [1,3,6]. Four facioscapulohumeral muscular dystrophy patients in Bushby's study [2] also reported a poor response to OTC medications. Many patients with NMDs resort to opioid analgesics for relief of severe pain, but they also report that these are not effective long-term treatments [1–3,6].

Given that no clinical trials have been reported in treating chronic pain in persons with NMDs, there is an obvious lack of evidence-based clinical standards for the treatment in this area. Clinicians can turn to the broader pain treatment literature, however, for ideas on treating pain in this population. One approach that has been suggested is to try one reasonable pain treatment at a time until a treatment regimen that maximizes pain relief but minimizes side effects and costs is found for an individual patient. Beyond OTC medications, tricyclic antidepressants and antiepileptic drugs are often helpful, particularly for neuropathic pain [7,32]. The antiepileptic drug gabapentin also has the added benefit of reducing spasticity via glutamate and γ-aminobutyric acid pathways. Cannabinoids, the active ingredients in marijuana (cannabis), have numerous pharmacologic properties that may be applicable to the management of NMDs [33,34], including analgesia, muscle relaxation, bronchodilation, saliva reduction, appetite stimulation, and sleep induction. In addition, cannabinoids have strong antioxidative and neuroprotective effects, which may prolong neuronal cell survival [33,34]. The authors performed an anonymous survey of 131 patients with ALS, who reported that cannabis was effective at reducing symptoms of appetite loss, depression, pain, spasticity, drooling, and weakness [35]. The cannabis was reported as being extremely well tolerated; the biggest reported factor limiting its use was lack of access. Further investigation into the usefulness of cannabinoids for treating NMD-related pain is warranted. Opioids may be necessary for refractory pain. If required, it is best to administer opioids on a regular dosing schedule and titrate to the point of comfort. When considering the use of long-term opiate therapy, it is important to use a contract that outlines the ground rules and consequences.

Some NMDs, most notably ALS, produce spasticity. Many drugs may be used with good effect in treating spasticity in ALS [36]. The γ-aminobutyric acid analogue baclofen acts to facilitate motor neuron inhibition at spinal levels and is the agent of choice. In primary lateral sclerosis, a purely upper motor neuron variant of ALS, an intrathecal baclofen pump may be beneficial [36]. Tizanidine, an α_2-agonist similar to clonidine, inhibits excitatory interneurons and may be helpful. Baclofen and tizanidine can be used effectively together, as long as side effects, particularly increasing weakness and hypotension, are monitored. Benzodiazepines also may be helpful in a small subset of patients, but can cause respiratory depression and somnolence and should be used with extreme caution. Although effective at reducing muscle tone, dantrolene blocks Ca^{++} release in the sarcoplasmic reticulum and causes too much generalized muscle weakness to be useful in NMD patients. Slow (30 seconds sustained), static muscle stretching may be helpful, particularly in more symptomatic muscle groups, such as the gastrocnemius, and may be done in bed. Positional splinting also is a helpful adjunctive modality, but skin must be monitored frequently for pressure areas.

Rehabilitation modalities to treat pain: exercise paradigms to prevent deconditioning

With respect to secondary painful musculoskeletal syndromes, the best management is proactively preventing their development, and this approach is most effective when started in the early stages of the disease. As mentioned earlier, muscle weakness, with or without spasticity, and progressive loss of mobility place a higher stress on the musculoskeletal system, contributing to pain generation. This pain generation is enhanced by a reduction in overall functional conditioning, including reduced aerobic capacity and pulmonary function. As any NMD progresses, patients are at high risk of becoming deconditioned. The generalized loss of cardiopulmonary fitness or "deconditioning" can lower pain tolerance and contribute to depression. Aerobic exercise helps maintain cardiorespiratory fitness and has a beneficial effect on mood, psychological well-being, appetite, and sleep.

Fatigue in NMDs is likely multifactorial and due in part to impaired muscular activation—neurogenic, myogenic, or a combination thereof. In some NMDs, particularly ALS, fatigue can be severe. The authors performed an open-label trial of modafinil (Provigil) to determine whether this drug would be effective in treating fatigue in ALS. Fifteen ALS patients were treated for 2 weeks with either 200 mg or 400 mg of modafinil [37]. Side effects of the medication were mild and included diarrhea, headache, nervousness, and insomnia; side effects did not result in any study dropouts. Average scores on the Fatigue Severity Scale and Epworth Sleepiness Scale decreased by 6.8 (SD 3.4) and 3.4 (SD 1.4; $P < .001$ for both scales). Average scores on the self-report version of the Functional Independence Measure increased 2.3 (SD 1.9; $P < .001$). This pilot study indicated that modafinil may reduce symptoms of fatigue in ALS, although further investigation is warranted. There is evidence that modafanil also helps with fatigue in myotonic muscular dystrophy type 1 [38–40].

Deconditioning and loss of mobility undoubtedly play a significant role. Submaximal, low-impact aerobic exercise (walking, swimming, stationary bicycling) improves symptoms of fatigue via enhancement of cardiovascular performance and increases muscle oxygen and substrate use [16,41,42]. Aerobic exercise also helps achieve and maintain ideal body weight [15].

Maintaining flexibility and range of motion

Just as exercise may help proactively with maintaining mobility and preventing the development of secondary deconditioning, a good stretching program may help prevent painful musculoskeletal syndromes, such as joint contracture or adhesive capsulitis. If a painful joint contracture develops, more aggressive treatment may be indicated [43,44]. This treatment would include radiographs to ensure the joint cartilage space is intact and there are no gross anatomic deformities. An intra-articular corticosteroid injection may help reduce inflammation. Inflammation also may be reduced with dexamethasone given via electrical current (iontophoresis), although this may be less effective in a deeper joint such as the shoulder. Topical heat and ice, given alone or sequentially (contrast therapy), may help reduce pain. If local treatment does not control the pain completely, oral pain medications should be used. Cooling and heating the joint and limb are short-term measures that may be effective. Cooling and heating must be done with physical therapy supervision to avoid thermal damage to the extremity. Aggressive manipulation, including manipulation under anesthesia, is contraindicated in NMDs because of the risk of significant joint damage.

Spinal deformities, such a scoliosis or kyphosis, are a manifestation of a joint contracture [45,46]. Because of immobility and neck and trunk muscle weakness leading to poor spinal support, most NMD patients experience some degree of back and neck pain, particularly if they are wheelchair dependent [47,48]. Spinal bracing may be used to improve sitting posture and balance, although this does not prevent or treat scoliosis. Neck pain and tightness may be helped by a cervical orthosis.

Given that impaired mobility is expected to contribute to pain, any mobility device must be fitted carefully. Wheelchairs should have adequate lumbar support and good cushioning (eg, Gelfoam). Wheelchairs and beds should be fitted properly with good pressure relief over all bony prominences to avoid pain and pressure ulcers [49,50]. If the patient cannot perform pressure relief maneuvers independently, a power tilt-in-space attachment to the wheelchair is crucial to protect the patient's skin. This device, which allows the patient to tilt back the entire seat on the wheelchair, also relieves pressure on the low back. Foam wedges should be used to facilitate proper positioning. Daily passive and active-assisted range of motion also is helpful in treating pain resulting from immobility [48].

Nutrition and weight control

Nutrition may be a significant problem in more severe NMDs, in which there is a tendency toward obesity shortly after the loss of functional ambulation. Evidence has shown that NMD patients are at high risk of developing metabolic syndrome [26]. Obesity is common in NMDs, particularly Duchenne muscular dystrophy, in which a prevalence of 54% has been reported. Weight control has its primary rationale in maintaining patient comfort and ease of transfers, skin care, decreasing postoperative complication risk, and decreasing risk of developing metabolic syndrome [26,51,52].

The incidence of obesity in NMD is unknown, but studies of body composition in Duchenne muscular dystrophy have shown a high ratio of fat to lean mass and bone mineral content [53]. One prior study showed weight reduction in Duchenne muscular dystrophy through rigorous, yet quite difficult, diet [30]. There is anecdotal evidence that topiramate, an antiepileptic agent with a side effect of inducing anorexia, is well tolerated and may be useful in helping patients with Duchenne muscular dystrophy lose weight [54]. There are untoward side effects, however, including somnolence, difficulty with mentation, and paresthesias. In the reported cases, weight loss did decrease pain and improve ease of transfers, skin care, and positioning. Obesity can be a significant, pain-inducing clinical problem in NMD patients, and further study is warranted.

Summary

The NMD literature provides strong evidence that chronic pain is a significant problem for many, but not all, persons with NMDs. The rates of pain have been found to vary in different studies and by NMD diagnosis. Less is known about specific details concerning the nature and impact of chronic pain in persons with NMDs. Additional research is urgently needed to understand NMD-related pain better, especially the effective treatment of NMD-related pain. This research ultimately should contribute to an overall increase in well-being and a decrease in suffering in persons with NMDs and chronic pain. In the meantime, clinicians should use the available, time-honored modalities to address and treat pain in persons with NMDs.

References

[1] Moulin DE, Hagen N, Feasby TE, Amireh R, Hahn A. Pain in Guillain-Barre syndrome. Neurology 1997;48:328–31.
[2] Bushby KMD, Pollitt C, Johnson MA, Rogers MT, Chinnery PF. Muscle pain as a prominent feature of facioscapulohumeral muscular dystrophy (FSHD): four illustrative case reports. Neuromusc Disord 1998;8:574–9.
[3] Carter GT, Jensen MP, Galer BS, et al. Neuropathic pain in Charcot-Marie-Tooth disease. Arch Phys Med Rehabil 1998;79:1560–4.
[4] Abresch RT, Carter GT, Jensen MP, Kilmer DD. Assessment of pain and health-related quality of life in slowly progressive neuromuscular disease. Am J Hosp Palliat Med 2002; 19:39–48.
[5] George A, Schneider-Gold C, Zier S, Reiners K, Sommer C. Musculoskeletal pain in patients with myotonic dystrophy type 2. Arch Neurol 2004;61:1938–42.

[6] Jensen MP, Abresch RT, Carter GT, McDonald CM. Chronic pain in persons with neuromuscular disease. Arch Phys Med Rehabil 2005;86:1155–63.

[7] Robinson J, Jensen MP. Chronic pain management in patients with a history of trauma. In: Robinson LR, editor. Trauma rehabilitation. Philadelphia: Lippincott Williams & Wilkins; 2005. p. 205–23.

[8] Carter GT, England JD, Chance PF. Charcot-Marie-Tooth disease: electrophysiology, molecular biology, and clinical management. Drugs 2004;7:151–9.

[9] Carter GT, Abresch RT, Fowler WM, Johnson ER, Kilmer DD, McDonald CM. Profiles of neuromuscular disease: hereditary motor and sensory neuropathy, types I and II. Am J Phys Med Rehabil 1995;74:S140–9.

[10] Chetlin RD, Gutmann L, Tarnopolsky M, Ullrich IH, Yeater RA. Resistance training effectiveness in patients with Charcot-Marie-Tooth disease: recommendations for exercise prescription. Arch Phys Med Rehabil 2004;85:1217–23.

[11] Chetlin RD, Gutmann L, Tarnopolsky MA, Ullrich IH, Yeater RA. Resistance training exercise and creatine in patients with Charcot-Marie-Tooth disease. Muscle Nerve 2004;30: 69–76.

[12] Carter GT, Abresch RT, Fowler WM, Johnson ER, Kilmer DD, McDonald CM. Profiles of neuromuscular disease: spinal muscular atrophy. Am J Phys Med Rehabil 1995; 74:S150–9.

[13] Johnson ER, Abresch RT, Carter GT, et al. Profiles of neuromuscular diseases: myotonic dystrophy. Am J Phys Med Rehabil 1995;74:S104–16.

[14] Kilmer D. Response to resistive strengthening exercise training in humans with neuromuscular disease. Am J Phys Med Rehabil 2002;81:S121–6.

[15] Kilmer DD. Response to aerobic exercise training in humans with neuromuscular disease. Am J Phys Med Rehabil 2002;81:S148–50.

[16] Kilmer DD. The role of exercise in neuromuscular disease. Phys Med Rehabil Clin N Am 1998;9:115–25.

[17] Kilmer DD, Abresch RT, McCrory MA, et al. Profiles of neuromuscular disease: facioscapulohumeral dystrophy. Am J Phys Med Rehabil 1995;74:S131–9.

[18] McCrory MA, Kim HR, Wright NC, Lovelady CA, Aitkens S, Kilmer DD. Energy expenditure, physical activity, and body composition of ambulatory adults with hereditary neuromuscular disease. Am J Clin Nutr 1998;67:1162–9.

[19] McDonald CM, Abresch RT, Carter GT, Fowler WM Jr, Johnson ER, Kilmer DD. Profiles of neuromuscular disease: Duchenne muscular dystrophy. Am J Phys Med Rehabil 1995;74: S70–92.

[20] McDonald CM, Abresch RT, Carter GT, Fowler WM Jr, Johnson ER, Kilmer DD. Profiles of neuromuscular disease: Becker muscular dystrophy. Am J Phys Med Rehabil 1995;74: S93–103.

[21] McDonald CM, Johnson ER, Abresch RT, et al. Profiles of neuromuscular disease: limb-girdle syndromes. Am J Phys Med Rehabil 1995;74:S117–30.

[22] McDonald CM, Widman LM, Walsh DD, Walsh SA, Abresch RT. Use of step activity monitoring for continuous physical activity assessment in boys with Duchenne muscular dystrophy. Arch Phys Med Rehabil 2005;86:802–8.

[23] Sockolov R, Irwin B, Dressendorfer RH, Bernauer EM. Exercise performance in 6- to 11-year old boys with Duchenne muscular dystrophy. Arch Phys Med Rehabil 1977;58: 195–201.

[24] Scott OM, Hyde SA, Goddard C, Dubowitz V. Quantitation of muscle function in children: a prospective study in Duchenne muscular dystrophy. Muscle Nerve 1982;5:291–301.

[25] Uchikawa K, Liu M, Hanayama K, Tsuji T, Fujiwara T, Chino N. Functional status and muscle strength in people with Duchenne muscular dystrophy living in the community. J Rehabil Med 2004;36:124–9.

[26] Aitkens S, Kilmer DD, Wright NC, McCrory MA. Metabolic syndrome in neuromuscular disease. Arch Phys Med Rehabil 2005;86:1030–6.

[27] Abresch RT, Jensen MP, Carter GT. Health-related quality of life in peripheral neuropathy. Phys Med Rehabil Clin N Am 2001;12:461–72.

[28] Shibata M, Abe K, Jimbo A, et al. Complex regional pain syndrome type I associated with amyotrophic lateral sclerosis. Clin J Pain 2003;19:69–70.

[29] Fowler WM Jr, Carter GT, Kraft GH. Role of physiatry in the management of neuromuscular disease. Phys Med Rehabil Clin N Am 1998;9:1–8.

[30] Jensen MP, Abresch RT, Carter GT. The reliability and validity of a self-reported version of the FIM instrument in persons with neuromuscular disease and chronic pain. Arch Phys Med Rehabil 2005;86:116–22.

[31] Carter GT, Galer BS. Advances in the management of neuropathic pain. Phys Med Rehabil Clin N Am 2001;12:447–59.

[32] Carter GT, Sullivan MD. Antidepressants in pain management. Curr Opin Invest Drugs 2002;3:454–8.

[33] Carter GT, Weydt P. Cannabis: old medicine with new promise for neurological disorders. Curr Opin Invest Drugs 2002;3:437–40.

[34] Carter GT, Rosen BS. Marijuana in the management of amyotrophic lateral sclerosis. Am J Hosp Palliat Care 2001;18:264–70.

[35] Amtmann D, Weydt P, Johnson KL, Jensen MP, Carter GT. Survey of cannabis use in patients with amyotrophic lateral sclerosis. Am J Hosp Palliat Care 2004;21:95–104.

[36] Carter GT, Krivckas LS, Weydt P, Weiss MD, Miller RG. Drug therapy for amyotrophic lateral sclerosis: where are we now? Drugs 2003;6:147–53.

[37] Carter GT, Weiss MD, Lou JS, et al. Modafinil to treat fatigue in amyotrophic lateral sclerosis: an open label pilot study. Am J Hosp Palliat Care 2005;22:55–9.

[38] Talbot K, Stradling J, Crosby J, Hilton-Jones D. Reduction in excess daytime sleepiness by modafinil in patients with myotonic dystrophy. Neuromuscul Disord 2003;13:357–64.

[39] MacDonald JR, Hill JD, Tarnopolsky MA. Modafinil reduces excessive somnolence and enhances mood in patients with myotonic dystrophy. Neurology 2002;59:1876–80.

[40] Damian MS, Gerlach A, Schmidt F, Lehmann E, Reichmann H. Modafinil for excessive daytime sleepiness in myotonic dystrophy. Neurology 2001;56:794–6.

[41] Aitkens SG, McCrory MA, Kilmer DD, Bernauer EM. Moderate resistance exercise program: its effect in slowly progressive neuromuscular disease. Arch Phys Med Rehab 1993;74:711–5.

[42] Eagle M. Report on the muscular dystrophy campaign workshop: exercise in neuromuscular diseases. Newcastle, January 2002. Neuromuscul Disord 2002;12:975–83.

[43] McDonald CM. Limb contractures in progressive neuromuscular disease and the role of stretching, orthotics, and surgery. Phys Med Rehabil Clin N Am 1998;9:187–211.

[44] Johnson ER, Fowler WM Jr, Lieberman JS. Contractures in neuromuscular disease. Arch Phys Med Rehabil 1992;73:807–10.

[45] Hart DA, McDonald CM. Spinal deformity in progressive neuromuscular disease: natural history and management. Phys Med Rehabil Clin N Am 1998;9:213–32.

[46] Lord J, Behrman B, Varzos N, Cooper D, Lieberman JS, Fowler WM. Scoliosis associated with Duchenne muscular dystrophy. Arch Phys Med Rehabil 1990;71:13–7.

[47] Liu M, Mineo K, Hanayama K, Fujiwara T, Chino N. Practical problems and management of seating through the clinical stages of Duchenne muscular dystrophy. Arch Phys Med Rehabil 2003;84:818–24.

[48] Scott OM, Hyde SA, Goddard C, Dubowitz V. Prevention of deformity in Duchenne muscular dystrophy: a prospective study of passive stretching and splintage. Physiotherapy 1981;67:177–80.

[49] Butler C, Okamoto G, McKay T. Motorized wheelchair driving by disabled children. Arch Phys Med Rehabil 1984;65:95–7.

[50] Butler C, Okamoto G, McKay T. Powered mobility for very young disabled children. Dev Med Child Neurol 1983;25:472–4.

[51] Edwards RJ, Round JM, Jackson MJ, Griffiths RJ, Lilburn MF. Weight reduction in boys with muscular dystrophy. Dev Med Child Neurol 1984;26:384–90.

[52] McCrory MA, Wright NC, Kilmer DD. Nutritional aspects of neuromuscular diseases. Phys Med Rehabil Clin N Am 1998;9:127–43.

[53] McDonald CM, Carter GT, Abresch RT, et al. Body composition and water compartment measurements in boys with Duchenne muscular dystrophy. Am J Phys Med Rehabil 2005;84: 483–91.

[54] Carter GT, Yudkowsky MP, Han JJ, McCrory MA. Topiramate for weight reduction in Duchenne muscular dystrophy. Muscle Nerve 2005;6:788–9.

ELSEVIER
SAUNDERS

Phys Med Rehabil Clin N Am
16 (2005) 1113–1124

PHYSICAL MEDICINE
AND REHABILITATION
CLINICS OF
NORTH AMERICA

Exploring Chronic Pain in Youths with Duchenne Muscular Dystrophy: A Model for Pediatric Neuromuscular Disease

Joyce M. Engel, OT, PhD[a],*,
Deborah Kartin, PT, PhD[a], Kenneth M. Jaffe, MD[b]

[a]Department of Rehabilitation Medicine, Box 356490, Division of Occupational Therapy,
University of Washington, Seattle, WA 98195-6490, USA
[b]Department of Rehabilitation Medicine, Box 359300, University of Washington,
Seattle, WA 98195-6490, USA

Chronic pain in children is drawing increasing attention from families, clinicians, and researchers. Its prevalence is conservatively estimated at 15% to 20% of the pediatric population [1]. There remains, however, a paucity of published research on chronic pain in children with neuromuscular disease (NMD) [2].

Neuromuscular disorders constitute a diverse spectrum of conditions that anatomically span the nerve (motor, sensory, or autonomic) and its supporting structures, the neuromuscular junction, and muscle—skeletal, smooth, and cardiac. Encompassed are a wide variety of clinical entities including anterior horn cell disorders, neuropathies, neuromuscular junction disorders, and myopathies and muscular dystrophies. Our understanding of chronic pain in this group of disorders is strikingly limited. Gaps in our knowledge include the nature and scope of the associated pain (its frequency, intensity, and quality); areas of the body most affected; the impact of pain on function and quality of life; and pain treatments and their effectiveness.

In order to explore the complexities of chronic pain in children with NMD, we will use Duchenne Muscular Dystrophy (DMD), the most common NMD of childhood, as an informative model [3]. The inherent

This article was supported by the Management of Chronic Pain in Rehabilitation grant, NIH HD 33988 Department of Rehabilitation Medicine.

* Corresponding author.

    E-mail address: knowles@u.washington.edu (J.M. Engel).

limitations of this approach are obvious, but posit that it serves as a useful starting point, particularly in a context constrained by a limited history of formal inquiry and agreed upon knowledge.

Duchenne muscular dystrophy: an overview

DMD is a congenital disorder caused by a mutation in the DMD gene located on the short arm of the X chromosome at the Xp21 locus. This gene, the largest one presently mapped in the human genome, produces a muscle wall structural protein called dystrophin. Categorized as a dystrophinopathy, DMD is part of a spectrum of muscle diseases caused by mutations in this gene. An almost complete absence of dystrophin is responsible for DMD's protean clinical features [4]. DMD is inherited in an X-linked recessive pattern. Its incidence is 1 per 3500 live male births [5]. All racial groups are affected.

DMD typically presents before the age of 5 years. Its characteristic clinical features include proximal muscle weakness; delayed motor milestones in sitting, standing, and walking independently; muscle pseudohypertrophy, particularly involving the calves and the tongue; a waddling gait with toe walking and decreased heel strike; a tendency to fatigue easily; inability to keep up in age-appropriate physical activities; difficulties with stair climbing; and frequent falls. The progression of the muscle weakness results in loss of ambulation between the ages of 8 to 13 years [6]. Soft tissue contractures of the arms and legs are frequently present during the first decade, and accelerate with the commencement of full-time wheelchair use [6,7].

Scoliosis is common, occurring in approximately 90% of affected boys [7]. Its onset coincides with adolescent growth and increased wheelchair use following the loss of ambulation. Restrictive pulmonary disease typically does not become clinically concerning until the second decade of life [8]. Respiratory complications are common after age 15, and usually are the cause of death in the late teenage years or the early 20s.

Cardiac and smooth muscle are affected by the dystrophin deficiency. Although electrocardiographic and echocardiographic changes are common, most boys are asymptomatic [9]. Gastrointestinal involvement includes difficulties in swallowing, acute gastric dilatation, and intestinal pseudo-obstruction [10–12]. A significant proportion of boys with DMD have neurobehavioral difficulties, including language delays and intellectual impairments that have implications for educational planning.

Pediatric pain assessment

Over the last decade, recognition of the importance of pain assessment and treatment has dramatically increased [1,13–16]. Irrespective of the treatment, effective pain management demands accurate diagnosis and continuous assessment using the best methods currently available. This requires the use of assessment tools that are standardized, valid, and reliable. The choice of assessment tools and treatment is based on the child's unique clinical circumstances [17] and the familial, cultural, and spiritual contexts [18]. Comprehensive and continuous assessment of pain intensity and how pain interferes in the daily life of the child and family enable practitioners to determine the effectiveness of treatments. The variability of pain expression and its effects on engagement in life's activities and social participation must be recognized.

The assessment of pain can be divided into three major categories: self-report or covert measures, behavioral observations or overt pain behaviors, and physiologic measures. Self-report or covert measures are the "gold standard" in pain assessment as pain is considered primarily a private subjective experience. The importance of listening to the child cannot be minimized. Self-report measures of nociception, pain, and suffering in youths must reflect the child's age, as well as language and cognitive development [19,20]. Clinical interviews and questionnaires, pain intensity scales, body outlines, adjective checklists, and pain diaries allow for information to be directly obtained from the youth. Clinical interviews and questionnaires focus on the characteristics of pain (eg, frequency, duration, sensorimotor components, exacerbating and relieving pain factors, pain interference). Verbal, facial, and visual rating scales are used to assess pain intensity. Youths as young as age 4 years are capable of identifying the location of their pain and using a pain numeric rating scale (eg, 0 = "no pain"; 10 = "strong pain") [21], or the Faces Pain Scale—Revised [22]. Other standardized valid and reliable evaluations with clinical utility such as the Pediatric Pain Questionnaire [23] and the Varni/Thompson Pediatric Pain Questionnaire (1987) can be used to gather information about the youth's pain experiences [24–26]. The youth's self-reports are best supplemented with the parents' assessments and health care practitioners' assessment of the child's pain.

Overt motor behaviors or observable pain responses (eg, crying, pain medication intake, avoidance of specific activities) are commonly targeted for assessment. Behavioral scales (eg, Observational Scale of Behavioral Distress) [27] are typically used in the assessment of pain in infants and youths who are nonverbal, severely distressed, or cognitively impaired. The assessment of pain behaviors in youths, however, may be problematic. As illustration, children experiencing pain of mild to moderate intensity often engage in routine daily activities including play [28].

Physiologic variables (eg, heart rate, vagal tone) are believed to be associated with pain [24]. Similar to pain behaviors, physiologic measures may reflect a generalized response to a stressor other than pain (eg, anxiety, fatigue) [29]. Over time, physiological pain responses demonstrate a process of adaptation and normalization [30]. They are, therefore, best used in conjunction with self-report and overt motor behaviors [29].

Duchenne muscular dystrophy and pain

Clinical experience teaches that over time boys with DMD increasingly experience pain, paralleling the disease's natural progression and concomitant increase in physical disability [3,31–33]. Recent studies suggest the incidence of pain in adults with NDM is relatively high ranging from nearly 40% to 75% [34,35].

Youths with physical disabilities can experience disruptions in their daily activities, participation, mood, and life satisfaction due to the nature of their impairments and secondary pain [36–40]. The longer pain persists, the greater the probability pain will interfere with an individual's participation in life activities [41].

The etiologies, probable, and possible factors contributing to pain in youths with DMD subsequently discussed are many and often interactive. It may be helpful to organize them relative to body systems (eg, musculoskeletal, gastrointestinal) and function (eg, mobility, overuse), and those that are iatrogenic.

Chronic pain in boys with DMD is most usefully categorized according to the organ system that is affected and the phase of evolution of this rapidly progressive condition—either the ambulatory or the wheelchair years.

Most impairments in DMD that can result in chronic pain are related to the musculoskeletal system. Mention is made in the literature of occasional localized calf pain, a problem that could be related the pathokinesiologic adaptation of prolonged daily toe walking (universally present during the late ambulatory years), an overuse syndrome (muscular sprain or strain) or muscular fatigue [42,43]. Overly zealous passive range of motion (ROM) to the gastrocnemius–soleus muscle complex could, conceivably, also lead to this complaint. Youths with DMD may interchangeably complain of pain, fatigue, cramps, stiffness, heaviness or tenderness—alone or in some combination—when, in fact, they may be describing the same sensation. Cramps are, however, typically related to a prolonged muscular contraction with resultant ischemia and can be particularly intense, a symptom not usually associated with DMD.

Contractures, a lack of full active or passive ROM, can be due to joint, muscle, or other soft tissue limitation, and are a cardinal feature of DMD. Contributory factors include fatty tissue infiltration and fibrosis of muscle; muscular weakness or a relative strength imbalance of agonist/antagonist muscles across a joint resulting in lack of full active ROM; or static prolonged positioning or immobilization. Clinically significant contractures are rare in DMD for all joints during the ambulatory years [6]. The reliance on full-time wheelchair use is strongly associated with the development and rapid progression of both upper and lower extremity contractures [6]. It is unlikely that soft tissue contractures are, of themselves, a source of pain at rest. Pain does occur, however, when joints and their capsules are deliberately, as part of passive ROM therapy, or incidentally pushed toward their end range. Positioning in bed or in a wheelchair, particularly of the lower extremities, can dramatically influence the degree of painful stretch on soft tissues. Nighttime can be particularly challenging for these youths and their families, as the combination of soft tissue contractures and weakness necessitate frequent passive repositioning to alleviate pain.

Progressive weakness and increased wheelchair dependency results in prolonged sitting and the inability to perform independent weight shifts or pressure relief. This causes ischemia over dependent bony surfaces such as the ischial tuberosities or sacrum while sitting, or the sacrum, trochanters, lateral malleoli, and heels while recumbent. For those youths who self-propel a manual wheelchair, an activity that typically does not go on for very long in DMD, painful muscular, ligamentous, or other soft tissue injury can occur, either acutely or subacutely as in an overuse syndrome. The other major potential source of chronic musculoskeletal pain in a progressive NMD such as DMD is spinal deformity. Spinal orthoses are ineffective, uncomfortable, and poorly tolerated by these children, and need to be avoided. Spinal deformities are frequently associated with pelvic obliquity (where body weight is disproportionately distributed over a single ischial tuberosity), unstable sitting balance, and difficulty with upright seating. Severe scoliosis and pelvic obliquity when left untreated can ultimately preclude comfortable upright wheelchair seating.

Fractures, an obvious source of pain, are not uncommon in DMD. They occur from falls during the ambulatory years, as a side effect of prednisone treatment to slow the rapid progression of muscular weakness, and from the development of osteoporosis associated with the loss of ambulation and wheelchair use [44]. The weakened pull of dystrophic muscle on fractured bone in DMD may contribute to reduced pain intensity and duration boys, particularly in those youths with nondisplaced fractures characteristic of the wheelchair years [45].

Another potential source of recurrent musculoskeletal pain is the poorly understood entity of growing pains, typically affecting the 6- to 10-year-old child [46]. This is a clinical diagnosis of exclusion with symmetric involvement of the thighs, knees, calves, or shins. It awakens the child once a night, as often as three to four times per month, sometimes on consecutive nights. Typically, there should be complete remission between attacks with pain-free intervals of days to months, and no physical examination findings [47]. Another entity, restless leg syndrome, has similar characteristics, including a desire to move the extremities, particularly in the evening or night, and worsening of symptoms at rest [48]. Unlike growing pains, children with this condition do not outgrow their symptoms.

The other potential source of pain in DMD is the gastrointestinal system, where involvement of visceral smooth muscle is frequently overlooked. Symptoms of upper gastrointestinal dysfunction, particularly gastroesophageal reflux disease, are statistically more common in boys with DMD than age-matched controls [10]. Compared with controls, more symptoms, most notably heartburn, occurred during the wheelchair than the ambulatory years. This suggests a direct or possibly causal relationship. Other entities associated with gastrointestinal pain in DMD include acute gastric dilatation, intestinal pseudoobstruction, and obstipation [11,12]. These various clinical entities may represent a clinical continuum with an analogous pathologic process in smooth muscle to that found in skeletal muscle.

Pain treatments

A multi-faceted comprehensive approach to pain management in boys with DMD should embrace a child- and family-centered standard of care, with the child and family central to the process of developing an appropriate plan of care. Attention must focus on the existing impairments and disabilities, as well as those that can be anticipated from knowledge of the disease's natural history. Coordination of care, competent communication, and education of the child and family about strategies for pain management are the underpinnings of success in developing a plan of care [49,50].

Recent pediatric pain textbooks and review articles make no specific mention of pain as a symptomatic component of childhood neuromuscular disease, reflecting the paucity of research on the effects of various pain interventions for children with DMD [51,52]. It is possible that these interventions may be beneficial. Pain interventions may be viewed along a continuum of care, with best practice suggesting they be applied from least to most invasive.

From our earlier discussion, however, it is apparent that the most common likely source of pain is the musculoskeletal system. This includes overuse syndromes, muscular fatigue, soft tissue contractures and stretch, spinal deformities, and fractures. Typical pharmacological options for these entities include first-line analgesics such as acetaminophen and nonsteroidal anti-inflammatory drugs (NSAID), followed by opioids as deemed clinically necessary. The World Health Organization's analgesic ladder represents a graduated and practical approach for routine types of pain management [53]. The route of medication administration should be the least invasive and tailored to the patient, and the source, frequency, and magnitude of the pain. All else being equal, the oral or nasogastric route of administration is preferable. Intramuscular injections, because of their added pain, the reduced muscle mass in children with neuromuscular disease, and frequent fears, are to be avoided.

Gastrointestinal side effects of NSAIDs, common in adult patients, appear less frequently in youths [54]. The side effects of systemic opioids include respiratory depression, altered bulbar reflexes, decreased gastric emptying, nausea, and constipation. Their use in youths with DMD, particularly those with clinically significant restrictive pulmonary disease and gastrointestinal symptoms, must be undertaken with caution.

With disease progression comes wheelchair dependence, contractures, spinal deformity, orthotic use, and the increasing likelihood of pain. There are a number of logical non-pharmacological considerations in rehabilitation for proactive pain management and prevention. These include the use of assistive devices, orthoses, and recommendations for positioning and mobility. All must address form, fit, function, and comfort, initially and over time. Ongoing monitoring is necessary, particularly as a child grows and becomes more physically dependent [55]. While decreased sensation is typically not a problem for children with DMD, both the child and family should be instructed in skin inspection for possible pressure areas related to these mechanical interventions.

Increasing pain and discomfort in sitting have been reported to be a function of severity of disease progression, including dependence on wheelchair mobility and presence of spinal deformity [55]. Relieving pressure points and frequent position change in general, initially actively performed by the child and later by caregivers, may help to maximize comfort. Pressure reducing mattresses (air and foam), the addition of foam mattress pads, and foam wedges are suggested for relieving pressure and improving positioning and comfort during sleep [3].

Careful selection of a dynamic seating and mobility system is important for the management/prevention of musculoskeletal pain. For example, a wheelchair with tilt-in-space features may be useful in relieving pressure in the seated position, recognizing, however, that functional abilities are often compromised while in the reclined position. If the addition of a foam seat cushion is not adequate for comfort in a more erect sitting posture, the use of a gel, fluid, or air filled seat cushion may provide a better alternative. These cushions modify seated posture through the redistribution of the air or fluid that may be "locked" into place and as comfort needs change, may be redistributed. Careful consideration of a dynamic seating/mobility system may provide flexible yet stable seating, maximizing comfort and function [55].

Exercise is increasingly being included as part of pain management programs in youths as a distraction from pain, stress reduction, and improved quality of life [20,56–58]. Given the susceptibility of dystrophin deficient muscles to exercise-induced injury [3,59,61] and muscle cramping [3], the use of exercise as a pain management strategy in youths with DMD needs to be approached with caution. Low-impact aerobic exercise from walking, swimming, and stationary cycling is advocated. In moderation, these activities may have a positive effect on not only cardiovascular functioning and fatigue, but on mental health, weight management, and pain management as well. If exercise is to be used as a pain management strategy for youths with DMD there are several cautionary guidelines [3,55]. It is essential that overexertion be avoided. As well, exercise(s) involving high-impact, heavy resistance, and training with eccentric (lengthening) muscle contraction should be avoided [3,59–62]. Youths and families need to be educated about the signs of overwork weakness including feeling weaker, as opposed to stronger, shortly after exercise; experiencing excessive delayed onset muscle soreness (24–48 hours postexercise); severe muscle cramping, heaviness in the limbs; or prolonged shortness of breath [3]. Exercises with high impact or heavy resistance and training with eccentric (lengthening) muscle contraction should be avoided because of potential risk for muscle damage [3,59,61].

Many modalities (eg, transcutaneous stimulation [TENS], ultrasound, superficial heat and cold), have been proposed as possible pain interventions for children [29]. There is, however, no empirical support for their use in children with DMD. Before considering using any modality for pain relief, the practitioner must be aware of the modalities contraindications and precautions and the child's unique clinical presentation. For example, ultrasound over the epiphyseal plates of growing bones in children is contraindicated [63]. In addition, caution is warranted in applying ultrasound over areas in which there are plastic or metal implants [63,64]. This has implications for boys with DMD who have back pain and whose spines have been instrumented. Finally, because superficial heat has systemic effects, it may be contraindicated in children with DMD and who have advanced cardiac involvement [64].

The child's cognitive level and the reliability with which they can communicate about their sensory experiences (ie, pain, temperature) suggests caution in the application of modalities for pain management [63]. It is essential that the child is able to reliably report pain in order to determine the child's tolerance for and effectiveness of the modality.

Cognitive behavioral interventions for pediatric pain control are becoming increasingly popular. Relaxation training, with or without biofeedback, distraction including virtual reality, cognitive restructuring, and hypnosis have been found effective in relieving some chronic pain complaints in children [29,65,66]. As illustration, Jones [67] used hypnosis with children undergoing spinal instrumentation for scoliosis management and found a reduced need for anesthesia. Pain behavior regulation (eg, contingency management, time out procedures) is used to modify socio-environmental factors that influence pain expression and rehabilitation to routine activities and participation. It has been used successfully to increase activity level with children experiencing pain [68–70]. The efficacy of these interventions for pain behavior regulation in children with DMD is unknown.

Summary

It is obvious through our exploration of pain associated with DMD, empirical research is needed to address the assessment and treatment of pain in children with all NMD. The initial research aim should be to determine the nature and scope of pain in children with NMD. Information is then needed on the frequency of pain in this population, pain severity, pain quality, pain location, the impact of pain on the daily activities, and quality of life for the child and his family. Pain treatment begins with the elimination of the causes of pain and exacerbating pain factors when ever feasible. Controlled trials of analgesics, therapeutic exercise, modalities, and cognitive behavioral interventions are warranted.

Given our current knowledge about pain in children with NMD we offer several basic clinical recommendations. First, all providers need to routinely assess pain in children with NMD, using standardized assessment tools that are valid and reliable for the age and cognitive abilities of the child. Pain is now considered the 5th Vital Sign [14]. Routinely assessing and addressing pain in all children needs to be the standard of care for all healthcare practitioners. With our increasing understanding of pain in the life experiences of children with DMD and the interplay of acute, chronic and recurrent pain through disease progression and management, this is particularly important. Second, a plan of care for pain management and prevention needs to be developed in collaboration with the interprofessional team, with the child and family at its center. Pain treatments must be carefully selected from among the logical options, with thoughtful consideration to the unique characteristics of the child and family and the specific precautions of a given intervention. Third, ongoing evaluation is essential to assess the effectiveness of pain treatments with respect to function and comfort of the child over time. Failure to do so will impact the quality of life of the child and family by dramatically altering meaningful engagement and social participation in life's activities.

References

[1] American Pain Society. Pediatric chronic pain: a position statement from he American Pain Society. Available at: http://www.ampainsoc.org/advicacy/pediatric.htm. Accessed July 25, 2005.

[2] Ehde D, Jensen M, Engel J, et al. Chronic pain secondary to disability: a review. Clin J Pain 2003;19:3–17.

[3] Carter G. Rehabilitation management in neuromuscular disease. J Neurol Rehabil 1997;11: 69–80.

[4] Hoffman EP, Fischbeck KH, Brown RH, et al. Characterization of dystrophin in muscle-biopsy specimens from patients with Duchenne's or Becker's muscular dystrophy. N Engl J Med 1988;318(21):1363–8.

[5] Emery AE. Population frequencies of inherited neuromuscular diseases—a world survey. Neuromuscul Disord 1991;1(1):19–29.

[6] McDonald CM, Abresch RT, Carter GT, et al. Profiles of neuromuscular diseases. Duchenne muscular dystrophy. Am J Phys Med Rehabil 1995;74(5 suppl):S70–92.

[7] Oda T, Shimizu N, Yonenobu K, et al. Longitudinal study of spinal deformity in Duchenne muscular dystrophy. J Pediatr Orthop 1993;13(4):478–88.

[8] American Thoracic Society. Respiratory care of the patient with Duchenne muscular dystrophy. Am J Respir Crit Care Med 2004;170:456–65.

[9] D'Orsogna L, O'Shea JP, Miller G. Cardiomyopathy of Duchenne muscular dystrophy. Pediatr Cardiol 1988;9(4):205–13.

[10] Jaffe KM, McDonald CM, Ingman E, et al. Symptoms of upper gastrointestinal dysfunction in Duchenne muscular dystrophy: case–control study. Arch Phys Med Rehabil 1990;71(10): 742–4.

[11] Leon SH, Schuffler MD, Kettler M, et al. Chronic intestinal pseudoobstruction as a complication of Duchenne's muscular dystrophy. Gastroenterology 1986;90(2):455–9.

[12] Bensen ES, Jaffe KM, Tarr PI. Acute gastric dilatation in Duchenne muscular dystrophy: a case report and review of the literature. Arch Phys Med Rehabil 1996;77(5):512–4.

[13] National Institutes of Health Pain Consortium. Pain instensity scales. Available at: http://painconsortium,nih.gov/pain_scales/index.html. Accessed: January 12, 2005.

[14] American Pain Society. Pain: the fifth vital sign. Available at: http://www.ampainsoc.org/advicacy.fifth.htm. Accessed: July 25, 2005.

[15] Agency for Health Care Policy and Research. Clinical practice guideline. Acute pain management. Operative or medical procedures and trauma. Management of post-operative and procedural pain in children. Washington (DC): AHCPR; 1992.

[16] Department of Health and Human Services. Healthy people 2010: understanding and improving health (Stock No. 017-001-00550-9). Available at: http://www.health.gov./healthypeople. Accessed: July 30, 2005.

[17] McGrath PA, Koster AL. Headache measures for children: a practical approach. In: McGrath PA, Hillier LM, editors. The child with headache: diagnosis and treatment. Seattle (WA): IASP Press; 2001. p. 29–56.

[18] Chapman CR, Tumer JA. Psychological and pyschosocial asects of acute pain. In: Bonica JJ, editor. The management of pain. 2nd edition. Philadelphia: Lea and Febiger; 1990. p. 122–32.

[19] McGrath PA, Seifert CE, Speechley KN, et al. A new analogue scale for assessing children's pain: an initial validation study. Pain 1996;64(3):435–43.

[20] Engel JM, Kartin D. Pain in youth: a primer for current practice. Crit Rev Phys Rehabil Med 2004;16(1):53–76.

[21] Ferraz MB, Quaresma MR, Aquino LR, et al. Reliability of pain scales in the assessment of literate and illiterate patients with rheumatoid arthritis. J Rheumatol 1990;17(8):1022–4.

[22] Bieri D, Reeve RA, Champion GD, et al. The Faces Pain Scale for the self-assessment of the severity of pain experienced by children: development, initial validation, and preliminary investigation for ratio scale properties. Pain 1990;41(2):139–50.

[23] Reid GJ, Gilbert CA, McGrath PJ. The Pain Coping Questionnaire: preliminary validation. Pain 1998;76:83–96.

[24] McGrath PA, Gillespie JM. Pain assessment in children and adolescents. In: Turk DC, Melzack R, editors. Handbook of pain assessment. New York: Guilford Press; 2001. p. 97–118.

[25] Gaffney A, McGrath PJ, Dick B. Measuring pain in children: developmental and instrument issues. In: Schechter NL, Berde CB, Yaster M, editors. Pain in infants, children, and adolescents. 2nd edition. Philadelphia (PA): Lippincott, Williams, and Wilkins; 2003. p. 128–41.

[26] Institute RNC. Clinical guidelines for the recognition ad assessment of acute pain in children. Recommendations. London: RCN Publishing; 1999.

[27] Jay SM, Elliott C. Behavioral observation scales for measuring children's distress: the effects of increased methodological rigor. J Consult Clin Psychol 1984;52(6):1106–7.

[28] Engel JM. Physical therapy and occupational therapy for pain management in children. Child Adolesc Psychiatr Clin N Am 1997;6(4):817–28.

[29] Engel J, Kartin D. Pain in youth: a primer for current practice. Crit Rev Phys Rehab Med 2004;16(1):53–76.

[30] Zeltzer LKM, Bush JP, Chen E, et al. A psychobilogic approach to pediatric pain: part I. History, physiology, and assessment strategies. Curr Probl Pediatr 1997;6:225–53.

[31] Bushby KM, Pollitt C, Johnson MA, et al. Muscle pain as a prominent feature of faciosca-pulohumeral muscular dystrophy (FSHD): four illustrative case reports. Neuromuscul Disord 1998;8(8):574–9.

[32] Carter GT, Jensen MP, Galer BS, et al. Neuropathic pain in Charcot-Marie-Tooth disease. Arch Phys Med Rehabil 1998;79(12):1560–4.

[33] Moulin DE, Hagen N, Feasby TE, et al. Pain in Guillain-Barre syndrome. Neurology 1997; 48(2):328–31.

[34] Rahbek J, Werge B, Madsen A, et al. Adult life with Duchenne muscular dystrophy: observations among an emerging and unforeseen patient population. Pediatr Rehabil 2005;8(1): 17–28.

[35] Jensen MP, Abresch RT, Carter GTA, et al. Chronic pain in persons with neuromuscular disease. Arch Phys Med Rehab 2005;86(6):1155–63.

[36] Carter B, Lambrenos K, Thursfield J. A pain workshop: an approach to eliciting the views of young people with chronic pain. J Clin Nurs 2002;11(6):753–62.

[37] Engel JM, Patrina T, Dudgeon B, et al. Youths with cerebral palsy and chronic pain: a descriptive study. Phys Occup Ther Pediatr. In press.

[38] Kashikar-Zuck S, Goldschneider KR, Powers SW, et al. Depression and functional disability in chronic pediatric pain. Clin J Pain 2001;17(4):341–9.

[39] Palermo TM, Witherspoon D, Valenzuela D, et al. Development and validation of the Child Activity Limitations Interview: a measure of pain-related functional impairment in school-age children and adolescents. Pain 2004;109(3):461–70.

[40] France RD. Chronic pain. Washington (DC): American Psychiatric Press; 1988.

[41] France RD, Ramakrishnan KR. Chronic pain. Washington, DC: American Psychiatric Press; 1988.

[42] Sutherland DH, Olshen R, Cooper L, et al. The pathomechanics of gait in Duchenne muscular dystrophy. Dev Med Child Neurol 1981;23(1):3–22.

[43] McDonald C. Clinical findings, measurement of ipairment, and naatural history of Duchenne's muscular dystrophy and spinal muscular atrophy. In AAEM Course D: updates in neuromuscular disease in children. Paper presented at the American Assoiation of Electrodiagnostic Medicine, 21st Annual Conntinuing Education Courses, Orlando, FL; 1998.

[44] Siegel IM. Fractures of long bones in Duchenne muscular dystrophy. J Trauma 1977;17(3): 219–22.

[45] Hsu JD. Extremity fractures in children with neuromuscular disease. Johns Hopkins Med J 1979;145(3):89–93.

[46] de Inocencio J. Musculoskeletal pain in primary pediatric care: analysis of 1000 consecutive general pediatric clinic visits. Pediatrics 1998;102(6):E63.

[47] Abu-Arafeh I, Russell G. Recurrent limb pain in school children. Arch Dis Child 1996;74(4): 336–9.

[48] Walters AS, Picchietti DL, Ehrenberg BL, et al. Restless legs syndrome in childhood and adolescence. Pediatr Neurol 1994;11(3):241–5.

[49] APTA. Guide to physical therapist practice. 2nd edition. Alexandria (VA): American Physical Therapy Association; 2003.

[50] Stuberg W. Muscular dystropy and spinal muscular atrophy. In: Campbell SK, Vander Linden DW, Palisano RJ, editors. Physical therapy for children. 2nd edition. Philadelphia (PA): W.B. Saunders; 2000. p. 339–69.

[51] Schechter N, Berde C, Yaster M, editors. Pain in infants, children, and adolescents. 2nd edition. Philadelphia: Lippincott Williams & Wilkins; 2003.

[52] Berde CB, Sethna NF. Analgesics for the treatment of pain in children. N Engl J Med 2002; 347(14):1094–103.

[53] World Health Organization. Cancer pain relief and palliative care: technical report series 804. Geneva: World Health Oganization; 1990.

[54] Dowd JE, Cimaz R, Fink CW. Nonsteroidal antiinflammatory drug-induced gastroduodenal injury in children. Arthritis Rheum 1995;38(9):1225–31.

[55] Liu M, Mineo K, Hanayama K, et al. Practical problems and management of seating through the clinical stages of Duchenne's muscular dystrophy. Arch Phys Med Rehabil 2003;84(6):818–24.

[56] McGrath PA. Pain in children nature, assessment, and treatment. New York: Guilford Press; 1990.

[57] Calvert P, Jureidini J. Restrained rehabilitation: an approach to children and adolescents with unexplained signs and symptoms. Arch Dis Child 2003;88(5):399–402.

[58] Long TM, Harp KA. Pain in Children. Orthop Phys Ther Clin North Am 1995;4(4): 503–17.
[59] Petrof BJ. The molecular basis of activity-induced muscle injury in Duchenne muscular dystrophy. Mol Cell Biochem 1998;179(1–2):111–23.
[60] Carter G, Abresch R, Fowler W. Adaptations to exercise training and contraction-induced muscle injury in animal models of muscular dystrophy. Am J Phys Med Rehabil 2002; 81(11 suppl):S151–61.
[61] Ansved T. Muscular dystrophies: influence of physical conditioning on the disease evolution. Curr Opin Clin Nutr Metab Care 2003;6(4):435–9.
[62] Urtizberea JA, Fan QS, Vroom E, et al. Looking under every rock: Duchenne muscular dystrophy and traditional Chinese medicine. Neuromuscul Disord 2003;13(9):705–7.
[63] Michlovitz SL, Nolan TP. Modalities for therapeutic intervention. 4th edition. Philadelphia: F.A. Davis; 2005.
[64] Bracciano AG. Physical agent modalities: theory and application for the occupational therapist. Thorofare (NJ): SLACK; 2000.
[65] Eccleston C, Malleson P, Clinch J, et al. Chronic pain in adolescents: evaluation of a programme of interdisciplinary cognitive behaviour therapy. Arch Dis Child 2003;88:881–5.
[66] Walco GA, Varni JW, Ilowite NT. Cognitive-behavioral pain management in children with juvenile rheumatoid arthritis. Pediatrics 1992;89(6 Pt 1):1075–9.
[67] Jones C. Hypnosis and spinal fusion by Harrington instrumentation. Am J Clin Hypn 1977; 19:155–7.
[68] Sank LI, Biglan A. Operant treatment of a case of recurrent abdominal pain in a 10 year old boy. Behav Ther 1974;5:677–81.
[69] Miller A, Kratochwill T. Reduction of frequent stomache complaints by time out. Behav Ther 1979;16:211–8.
[70] Varni JW, Bessman CA, Russo DC, et al. Behavioral management of chronic pain in children: case study. Arch Phys Med Rehabil 1980;61(8):375–9.

ELSEVIER
SAUNDERS

Phys Med Rehabil Clin N Am
16 (2005) 1125–1139

PHYSICAL MEDICINE
AND REHABILITATION
CLINICS OF
NORTH AMERICA

Respiratory Support of Individuals with Duchenne Muscular Dystrophy: Toward a Standard of Care

Joshua O. Benditt, MD*, Louis Boitano, RRT, MS

*Respiratory Care Services, University of Washington Medical Center,
1959 NE Pacific Street, Seattle, WA 98195, USA*

Effects of Duchenne muscular dystrophy on respiratory function

Pneumonia and respiratory failure represent the leading cause of death and a frequent cause of morbidity for patients with Duchenne muscular dystrophy (DMD) [1–5]. Respiratory muscle weakness is found in all individuals with DMD, although it may develop at varying rates [6]. Restrictive physiology is seen with reductions in lung volumes, including total lung capacity and vital capacity, resulting from muscle weakness and associated changes in the mechanical respiratory system. Vital capacity tends to increase in a normal pattern until age 10 years, after which a plateau phase and a more rapidly progressive decline is seen [6–9]. In addition to muscle weakness, the compliance of the respiratory system is reduced in DMD secondary to numerous causes, including concomitant scoliosis [10], fibrotic changes in the dystrophic chest wall muscles, stiffening of unstretched tissues [11], and microatelectatic changes [12]. Disorders in gas exchange as a result of respiratory muscle weakness often are seen first during sleep [13–16] for many reasons. First, during sleep and particularly during rapid-eye-movement sleep, neural output from the central nervous system is decreased, which when coupled with weak inspiratory muscles leads to an increase in carbon dioxide and central apnea. In addition, weakness in the upper airway muscles leads to upper airway instability and an increased likelihood of obstruction. Central and obstructive apneic events often are seen in individuals with DMD [14]. Prevention of sleep-disordered breathing is important because hypercarbia and hypoxemia may accelerate the progressive decline in respiratory and cardiac function [17].

---

* Corresponding author.
E-mail address: benditt@u.washington.edu (J.O. Benditt).

1047-9651/05/$ - see front matter © 2005 Elsevier Inc. All rights reserved.
doi:10.1016/j.pmr.2005.08.017

Expiratory muscle function also is impaired, and this contributes not only to the reduction in vital capacity, but also to an elevated residual volume because of the impaired ability of the individual to breath out below functional residual capacity. Adequate inspiratory and particularly expiratory muscle function is crucial for clearance of airway secretions through the normal cough mechanism. Reductions in the ability to generate cough flow during the cough maneuver increase the risk of retained secretions, atelectasis, and pneumonia [18]. Simple devices to measure peak expiratory cough flow are available and are described subsequently [19,20]. Expiratory muscles may be more affected than inspiratory muscles in DMD so that impairment of cough function may be present earlier in the disease than other evidence of respiratory muscle weakness [21]. Cough impairment may become apparent only during a viral respiratory tract infection, however, in which an increase in secretions places a substantial stress on the system. A worsening spiral of cough impairment followed by atelectasis and pneumonia can be seen resulting in frank respiratory failure, leading to intubation or death. Maintenance of adequate cough function is a prime concern for clinicians caring for individuals with DMD. Numerous methodologies are available for cough augmentation and are discussed subsequently.

Assessment of function in Duchenne muscular dystrophy

Respiratory muscle function assessment

The management of respiratory issues in DMD is aimed at preventing emergency situations and improving quality of and duration of life. Because the onset of respiratory muscle weakness, sleep-disordered breathing, and hypercapnia is insidious and often not experienced symptomatically by the patient until weakness is far advanced, routine monitoring of respiratory function is strongly advised. An American Thoracic Society (ATS) Consensus Statement by expert pediatric pulmonologists, nurses, and neurologists has been published [22]. Few data are available to guide the frequency or extent of diagnostic evaluations required for best practice; however, the ATS Consensus Panel has suggested that children should have at least one visit with a physician specializing in pediatric respiratory care early in the course of the disease, between 4 and 6 years of age and before confinement to a wheelchair. When the patient requires either ventilatory or cough augmentation therapy, the recommendation is visits with a respiratory specialist every 3 to 6 months.

The ATS panel also recommends that all patients with DMD undergo respiratory evaluation before any surgical procedure. The clinical evaluation at these visits should include a careful history, physical examination, and limited number of pulmonary function and gas exchange tests that are easily accomplished in the clinic. Questions in the history should include those related to hypoventilation, cough function, respiratory tract infections, and sleep-disordered breathing. Symptoms consistent with sleep-disordered breathing include more frequent nocturnal awakenings, nocturia, vivid nightmares, night sweats, and daytime hypersomnolence, morning headaches, depression, decreased concentration or school performance, and nausea. Assessment of pulmonary function should include tests of inspiratory and expiratory muscle function and resting gas exchange. The ATS panel has recommended routine measurements of forced vital capacity, forced expiratory volume in 1 second, maximum midexpiratory flow rate, maximum inspiratory and expiratory pressures, and peak cough flow rate (PCF). PCF can be measured easily with an asthma peak flowmeter connected to a facemask or mouthpiece (Fig. 1). Normal values range from 360 to 960 L/min [23], and it has been suggested that a value less than 160 L/min places individuals at high risk for cough insufficiency and ventilator dependence [24]. PCF is known to decrease substantially during respiratory tract infection, and a PCF of less than 270 L/min during a healthy period has been shown to correlate with a PCF less than 160 L/min during infection. Cough assistance is suggested for individuals with a PCF less than 160 L/min. Oximetry is accomplished easily with a portable oximeter, which should be available in almost all health care facilities. Low saturation of hemoglobin may be consistent with hypoventilation or atelectasis secondary to secretions or inadequate expansion of the lungs and is a simple and noninvasive way to follow respiratory status at home or in the clinic.

The ATS Consensus Panel has suggested that carbon dioxide levels be assessed annually. $Paco_2$ is the traditionally used measure of adequate ventilation; however, exhaled or end-tidal CO_2 ($PETco_2$), transcutaneous CO_2, and arterial blood or capillary gas sampling all are measurement options. Arterial blood gas sampling, although the most accurate, can be difficult and uncomfortable for the patient. $PETco_2$ measurement in individuals without intrinsic lung disease is an easy and apparently accurate method of estimating arterial blood CO_2 [25]. Transcutaneous CO_2 measurements

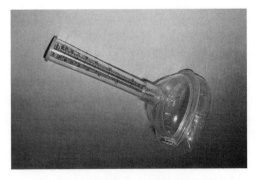

Fig. 1. Simple device for measurement of peak cough flow with facemask attached to asthma peak flowmeter.

have been accomplished successfully in children, and the technology to allow more widespread use is improving [26–28].

Sleep assessment in Duchenne muscular dystrophy

Often the first signs of hypoventilation occur at night. Symptoms of sleep-disordered breathing as noted earlier should be sought at each clinic visit. Polysomnography has been used to evaluate sleep in patients with DMD. The timing and necessity of diagnostic polysomnography have not been determined clearly, and because of the difficulty of the overnight stay in a sleep laboratory (eg, personal care attendant, position changes, toileting) for individuals with DMD, ensuring a high pretest probability before ordering a sleep study is important. Hukins and Hillman [29] found that an awake $Paco_2$ 45 mm Hg or greater and a base excess of 4 mEq or greater correlated with sleep hypoventilation. The authors order overnight polysomnography if there are symptoms of sleep-disordered breathing or a $PETco_2$ 45 mm Hg or greater or if the polysomnogram is being used to titrate nocturnal positive-pressure ventilation (NPPV). Some authors have suggested that an unattended sleep study in the home [30] or overnight oximetry and $PETco_2$ monitoring [22] may substitute for overnight laboratory polysomnography. The sensitivity and specificity of these portable tests are undetermined in this patient population.

Respiratory support interventions

Ventilatory support

Noninvasive ventilation

The use of noninvasive ventilation (ventilation without tracheostomy) has expanded dramatically since the 1970s because of technologic advances in the area of small, portable ventilators and inexpensive patient-ventilator interfaces (masks and mouthpieces). This expansion has been spurred by the rapid development of treatment devices for sleep apnea in the general population. Noninvasive support is now available for nocturnal and daytime use.

Hypoventilation occurs initially at night, and almost all individuals with DMD begin using noninvasive ventilation while sleeping. This ventilatory support consists in almost all cases of positive-pressure ventilation applied with a nasal or oronasal mask and a pressure support or a volume cycled ventilator. Table 1 lists most interfaces currently available in the United States along with manufacturers and contact information. The pressure support–type machines all should be equipped with backup rate capability. That is, if the patient does not initiate a breath, the machine automatically delivers a breath. Individuals with DMD often have significant central sleep apnea in which no breaths are initiated. In the authors' experience, most patients with DMD require NPPV with a backup rate.

Table 1
Interfaces for noninvasive ventilation

Nasal masks		
ComfortGel	Respironics, Inc	www.respironics.com/ products_library
ComfortClassic		
ComfortSelect		
ComfortLite (nasal shell)		
Contour		
Profile Lite		
Simplicity		
Mirage	ResMed Corp	www.resmed.com
Mirage Vista		
Ultra Mirage		
Mirage Activa		
SoftFit Ultra	Puritan-Bennett, Inc	www.puritanbennett.com/prod/ product
Breeze DreamSeal		
Phantom Nasal Mask	SleepNet Corp	www.sleep-net.com
IQ Nasal Mask		
Mini Me		
FlexiFit 405	Fisher & Paykel Healthcare	www.fphcare.com/osa/interfaces
FlexiFit 407		
Alizes	Hans Rudolph, Inc	www.rudolphkc.com
Twilight	Invacare Corp	www.invacare.com
FlexAire	DeVilbiss, Sunrise Medical	www.sunrisemedical.com.au/products
Serenity		
Advantage	Tiara Medical Systems, Inc	www.tiaramed.com_shop
SOMNOmask	Weinmann	www.weinmann.de/framesets
SOMNOplus		
Comfo-seal	VacuMed	www.vacumed.com/zoom/product
Facemasks		
ComfortFull	Respironics, Inc	www.respironics.com/product_library
Total Face Mask		
Mirage Series II	ResMed Corp	www.resmed.com
Ultra Mirage Series III		
7500 VIP Series	Hans Rudolph, Inc	www.rudolphkc.com
7600 Series V Mask		
FlexiFit 431	Fisher & Paykel Healthcare	www.fphcare.com/osa/interfaces
Fleximask	B&D Medical	www.bdemed.fsnet.co.uk/mask
Full Face Mask	VacuMed	vacumed.com/zcom/product
Nasal pillows		
ADAM circuit	Purritan Bennett	www.puritanbennett.com/prod/ Product
Breeze		
Aura	AEIOmedical	www.aeiomed.com
ComfortLite	Respironics Corp	www.respironics.com/product_library

(continued on next page)

Table 1 (*continued*)

Infinity 481	Fisher & Paykel Healthcare	www.fphcare.com/osa/interfaces
Lyra Spiritus	VIASYS Healthcare	www.viasyhc.com/prod_serv/prod
Mirage Swift	ResMed Corp	www.resmed.com
Nasal-Aire II	InnoMed Technologies, Inc	www.innomedinc.com/content
Nasal –PAP Freestyle		
SNAPP	Tiara Medical Systems, Inc	www.tiaramed.com_shop
Oral interface		
Oracle 452	Fisher & Paykel Healthcare	www.fphcare.com/osa/interfaces

Negative-pressure ventilation, such as that provided by an iron lung, cuirass, or "poncho"-style ventilator, is not employed often because the devices are more cumbersome, and their use has been associated with worsening of obstructive sleep apnea [16,31]. Some authors have reported the use of an oral interface that can be held between the teeth in concert with a nose clip [32,33]. In addition to the pressure support type of ventilators, NPPV also can be delivered with a volume-cycled ventilator. Bach [34,35] suggested that volume-cycled, rather than pressure-cycled ventilation may be more effective for nocturnal ventilation for individuals with DMD because it allows delivery of a greater volume (and pressure) breath to the patient with better maintenance of ventilation. NPPV is titrated to an effective level by careful follow-up assessment of symptoms of sleep-disordered breathing and either home oximetry and PETco_2 monitoring or titration in the sleep laboratory. Because breathing muscle weakness is progressive, ventilator settings often need to be adjusted to increase the effective inflation pressure over time. Symptom assessment, oximetry, measurement of PETco_2, and polysomnography are tools to assess adequate home ventilation.

Daytime support with noninvasive ventilation can be accomplished with mask ventilation; however, patients may find the mask interferes with communication and is uncomfortable to wear. A method of mouthpiece or "sip" ventilation has been available for decades [36] and has shown a resurgence in use [33,37,38]. With this technique, a bent mouthpiece attached to a ventilator circuit and volume-cycled ventilator can be accessed by the patient on a demand basis (Fig. 2). When the patient takes a "sip" from the mouthpiece, a full tidal breath is delivered by the machine. The patient may take as few or as many breaths per minute as desired. There is no tracheostomy, so the risks of tracheostomy potentially are avoided. One significant advantage of the mouthpiece NPPV is that the patient may take more than one breath ("breath stacking"), which allows the stored elastic energy in the lung and chest to assist the patient in coughing [19,39]. Table 2 lists all volume-cycled ventilators that can support mouthpiece ventilation currently available in the United States. Reported disadvantages of the mouthpiece style of ventilation include a "less secure" method of ventilation and no direct access to the airway for suctioning [22]. One of the major limitations to

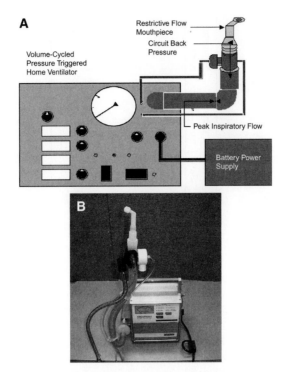

Fig. 2. (*A*) Diagram of setup for mouthpiece ventilation showing ventilator, connecting tubing, and mouthpiece. (*B*) HT-50 volume cycled ventilator with mouthpiece attachment for mouthpiece ventilation.

the application of mouthpiece NPPV may be a lack of centers with the expertise to provide this treatment modality. In the most recent survey available of Muscular Dystrophy Association clinics, only 20% of clinics were offering daytime ventilation with a mouthpiece device, although 88% offered NPPV via mask [40].

Another form of noninvasive ventilatory support that can be used is the pneumobelt [41–44]. The pneumobelt is a rubber bladder enclosed in a canvas belt worn around the waist that can be inflated repeatedly with a positive-pressure generator. The inflation of the belt results in inward movement of the abdomen and the exhalation of air. When the bladder deflates, gravity acts to drop the abdominal contents, and the lungs inflate passively. This device is used less frequently now.

Glossopharyngeal breathing is a method whereby an individual with reduced respiratory muscle strength can ventilate by using the muscles of the oropharynx to "gulp" boluses of air into the lungs [45,46]. It can be used as an adjunct in concert with other methods of NPPV to allow the individual time off mechanical support.

Table 2
Volume-cycled ventilators available in the United States that support mouthpiece ventilation

Ventilator brand and model	Ventilator weight (lb)	Ventilator dimensions (inches)	A/C mode apnea duration (s)	Peak inspiratory flow control	Minimum pressure alarm (cwp)	Minimum breaths/min
Respironics						
PLV100	28.2	9 H × 12.25 W × 12.25 D	15	Flow	2	4
Respironic						
PLV Continuum	22.2	7.25 H ×	15	Flow	3	4
Mallinckrodt						
Achieva	32	10.75 H × 13.3 W × 15.6 D	10	1 time	3	6
Pulmonetics						
LTV800	14.2	12 H × 10 W × 3 D	60 (adjustable)	1 time	0 (adjustable)	1
Newport HT50	15	10.2 H × 10.6 W × 7.9 D	30	1 time	2	3
Uni-vent Eagle 754	13	11.5 H × 8.87 W × 4.5 D	15	1 time	0 (adjustable)	4

Invasive (tracheostomy) ventilation

Some individuals with DMD use tracheostomy with full-time ventilator support. Placement of the tracheostomy involves a surgical procedure and a period of hospitalization. Risks of tracheostomy include infection, bleeding, and impaired speech and swallowing and tracheostomy tube occlusion with mucus [47–51]. The ATS Consensus Statement recommends that tracheostomy be offered to individuals when expertise in mouthpiece ventilation is unavailable; when contraindications to NPPV exist, such as severe bulbar muscle weakness and inability to control secretions; or when the patient prefers tracheostomy.

Cough support

A crucial and often overlooked aspect of respiratory support in DMD is cough support and secretion management. Effective airway clearance is crucial to prevention of pneumonia, which can lead to respiratory failure and death. Early intervention seems to reduce the incidence of pneumonia and hospitalization [18]. As noted earlier, cough flow correlates well with the ability to clear secretions [52]. Many techniques are available to increase cough flow rates in individuals who have impaired cough function, including manual and mechanically assisted techniques. Manual techniques involve increasing the breath volume by having the patient use glossopharyngeal breathing or a self-inflating resuscitator bag (Fig. 3) to take in one or more breaths that are larger than they would be able to take in spontaneously maximal insufflation capacity (MIC). This breath stacking or MIC maneuver increases the inspiratory capacity, the volume of the chest, and the elastic recoil pressure of the chest wall and lung, which allows a more forceful cough to be performed [53–56]. This maneuver can be combined

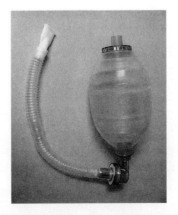

Fig. 3. Resuscitator bag with mouthpiece attached used to augment maximum insufflation capacity and peak cough flow rates.

with abdominal thrusts or lateral rib cage compression ("quad cough") to increase PCF further.

Mechanical assistance for cough is available with mechanic insufflation-exsufflation, a technique developed in the 1950s for polio patients. The Cough Assist (Emerson, Cambridge, Massachusetts) is a commercially available device that is widely used (Fig. 4). It mimics cough function by providing positive pressure through a mask or mouthpiece to inflate the respiratory system followed by a rapid switch to a negative pressure that clears the airway of secretions. Repeated applications are often needed to clear the airway adequately. Research has looked at the ability of the various techniques to augment PCF, and breath stacking, manual cough assistance, and the Cough Assist all seem to be effective in increasing the PCF levels to produce effective secretion removal [56]. The ATS Consensus Panel Statement recommends implementation of cough assistance when the PCF decreases to less than 270 L/min or the maximum expiratory pressure is less than 60 cm H_2O.

Numerous devices that oscillate the lung and chest wall and are designed to loosen respiratory secretion from the airways are available. Essentially no data looking at the use of these devices in DMD are available, so a recommendation as to their use cannot be made [22]. The major issue with individuals with DMD is generating adequate cough flow, however, a problem that these devices do not address.

Data concerning ventilatory support and Duchenne muscular dystrophy

Respiratory insufficiency and pneumonia is the most frequent cause of death in individuals with DMD [1,2,4,5]. Numerous studies of NPPV using volume ventilators have shown that daytime $Paco_2$ can be improved and symptoms of fatigue, daytime hypersomnolence, and morning headaches can be reduced significantly by nocturnal ventilation in patients with

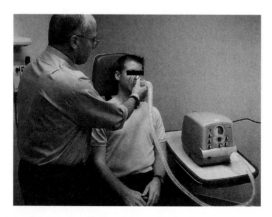

Fig. 4. Mechanic insufflation-exsufflation delivered by assistance with Cough Assist device.

neuromuscular restrictive thoracic disorders, including many patients with DMD [57–65]. Application of nocturnal ventilation when appropriate also improves survival. No randomized controlled trials have been performed because many investigators believe that it is ethically unacceptable to randomize a patient to no therapy [66]. Many studies, such as that of Vianello et al [67], in which five patients with DMD who accepted NPPV were alive after 2 years compared with none of five similar patients who declined therapy, strongly suggest improved survival with NPPV. A British study reported survival rates of 85% at 1 year and 73% at 5 years with treatment with NPPV [68]. Studies reporting brief withdrawal of NPPV in patients who had been successfully treated for nocturnal hypoventilation showed a return of symptoms of sleep-disordered breathing and desaturation and hypercapnia during sleep [69,70].

Many clinics seem to be offering their patients nocturnal ventilation. In a survey published in 2000, 80% of Muscular Dystrophy Association clinics were offering nocturnal support to individuals with DMD [40]. There seem to be consensus, both published (ATS and Chest Consensus) and in practice, regarding this aspect of ventilatory support. This is not the case, however, when ventilatory failure progresses to the point of requiring daytime ventilatory support. Bach [18,33,71–74] has vigorously argued that noninvasive ventilatory support during the day (predominantly mouthpiece ventilation) coupled with nocturnal support with nasal, oronasal, or mouthpiece volume ventilation is the most effective method to prolong survival and maintain quality of life. Other authors have suggested, however, that when reliance on noninvasive ventilation meets or exceeds 16 hours per day this may indicate a need to consider tracheostomy ventilation [66,75]. In many countries, including the United States, full-time ventilation with either mouthpiece or tracheostomy is not offered to individuals with DMD on a routine basis [40,68,76]. The reasons are unclear, although this practice may be partly due to the health care provider's perception of the ventilator user's quality of life [76]. One important point that is raised in the ATS Consensus Panel Statement is that all individuals with DMD should be informed of the potential treatments for nocturnal and diurnal respiratory failure, and that the risks and benefits of these should be discussed with the individual and his or her family in advance of an emergency situation [22].

Support of ventilation alone is inadequate to maintain respiratory health in individuals with DMD. Cough support likely plays an equal role in health maintenance in individuals with DMD. No prospective controlled clinical trials have been performed looking at the independent effect of cough support on survival, hospitalizations, or quality of life; however, physiologic data [19,52,56] and numerous cohort studies [18,77,78] strongly support the use of cough assistance with mechanic inexsufflation, breath-stacking maneuvers, or manually assisted cough in patients with neuromuscular disease, some of whom had DMD. The ATS Consensus Panel Statement correctly underscores the necessity of assessing cough function frequently and implementing cough augmentation therapy when the value for PCF decreases to less than 270 L/min or maximum expiratory pressure is less than 60 cm H_2O.

Summary

Excellent respiratory assessment and support are necessary to maintain quality of life, extend duration of survival, and avoid emergency situations for individuals with DMD. A program of assessment and intervention at appropriate points during the progression of the disease has been outlined and should help standardize respiratory management across centers. More work needs to be done to ensure that all individuals with DMD have access to proper ongoing assessment and the full range of respiratory support methods.

References

[1] Vignos PJ Jr. Respiratory function and pulmonary infection in Duchenne muscular dystrophy. Isr J Med Sci 1977;13:207–14.

[2] Rideau Y, Gatin G, Bach J, Gines G. Prolongation of life in Duchenne's muscular dystrophy. Acta Neurol (Napoli) 1983;5:118–24.

[3] Mukoyama M, Kondo K, Hizawa K, Nishitani H. Life spans of Duchenne muscular dystrophy patients in the hospital care program in Japan. J Neurol Sci 1987;81:155–8.

[4] Inkley SR, Oldenburg FC, Vignos PJ Jr. Pulmonary function in Duchenne muscular dystrophy related to stage of disease. Am J Med 1974;56:297–306.

[5] Brooke MH, Fenichel GM, Griggs RC, et al. Duchenne muscular dystrophy: patterns of clinical progression and effects of supportive therapy. Neurology 1989;39:475–81.

[6] McDonald CM, Abresch RT, Carter GT, et al. Profiles of neuromuscular diseases: Duchenne muscular dystrophy. Am J Phys Med Rehabil 1995;74(Suppl):S70–92.

[7] Jenkins JG, Bohn D, Edmonds JF, Levison H, Barker GA. Evaluation of pulmonary function in muscular dystrophy patients requiring spinal surgery. Crit Care Med 1982;10:645–9.

[8] Phillips MF, Quinlivan RC, Edwards RH, Calverley PM. Changes in spirometry over time as a prognostic marker in patients with Duchenne muscular dystrophy. Am J Respir Crit Care Med 2001;164:2191–4.

[9] Baydur A, Gilgoff I, Prentice W, Carlson M, Fischer DA. Decline in respiratory function and experience with long-term assisted ventilation in advanced Duchenne's muscular dystrophy. Chest 1990;97:884–9.

[10] Kurz LT, Mubarak SJ, Schultz P, Park SM, Leach J. Correlation of scoliosis and pulmonary function in Duchenne muscular dystrophy. J Pediatr Orthop 1983;3:347–53.

[11] Estenne M, Heilporn A, Delhez L, Yernault JC, De Troyer A. Chest wall stiffness in patients with chronic respiratory muscle weakness. Am Rev Respir Dis 1983;128:1002–7.

[12] Gibson GJ, Pride NB, Davis JN, Loh LC. Pulmonary mechanics in patients with respiratory muscle weakness. Am Rev Respir Dis 1977;115:389–95.

[13] Phillips MF, Smith PE, Carroll N, Edwards RH, Calverley PM. Nocturnal oxygenation and prognosis in Duchenne muscular dystrophy. Am J Respir Crit Care Med 1999;160:198–202.

[14] Smith PE, Calverley PM, Edwards RH. Hypoxemia during sleep in Duchenne muscular dystrophy. Am Rev Respir Dis 1988;137:884–8.

[15] Smith PE, Edwards RH, Calverley PM. Ventilation and breathing pattern during sleep in Duchenne muscular dystrophy. Chest 1989;96:1346–51.

[16] Goldstein RS, Molotiu N, Skrastins R, et al. Reversal of sleep-induced hypoventilation and chronic respiratory failure by nocturnal negative pressure ventilation in patients with restrictive ventilatory impairment. Am Rev Respir Dis 1987;135:1049–55.

[17] Gozal D. Pulmonary manifestations of neuromuscular disease with special reference to Duchenne muscular dystrophy and spinal muscular atrophy. Pediatr Pulmonol 2000;29:141–50.

[18] Bach JR, Ishikawa Y, Kim H. Prevention of pulmonary morbidity for patients with Duchenne muscular dystrophy. Chest 1997;112:1024–8.

[19] Bach JR. Mechanical insufflation-exsufflation: comparison of peak expiratory flows with manually assisted and unassisted coughing techniques. Chest 1993;104:1553–62.

[20] Bach JR, Smith WH, Michaels J, et al. Airway secretion clearance by mechanical exsufflation for post-poliomyelitis ventilator-assisted individuals. Arch Phys Med Rehabil 1993;74:170–7.

[21] Szeinberg A, Tabachnik E, Rashed N, et al. Cough capacity in patients with muscular dystrophy. Chest 1988;94:1232–5.

[22] Finder JD, Birnkrant D, Carl J, et al. Respiratory care of the patient with Duchenne muscular dystrophy: ATS consensus statement. Am J Respir Crit Care Med 2004;170:456–65.

[23] Leith DE, Butler JP, Sneddon SL, Brain JD. Cough. In: Handbook of physiology: the respiratory system, vol. III. Bethesda (MD): American Physiologic Society; 1990. p. 315–36.

[24] Bach JR, Saporito LR. Criteria for extubation and tracheostomy tube removal for patients with ventilatory failure: a different approach to weaning. Chest 1996;110:1566–71.

[25] Lindahl SG, Yates AP, Hatch DJ. Relationship between invasive and noninvasive measurements of gas exchange in anesthetized infants and children. Anesthesiology 1987;66:168–75.

[26] Janssens JP, Laszlo A, Uldry C, Titelion V, Picaud C, Michel JP. Non-invasive (transcutaneous) monitoring of PCO2 (TcPCO2) in older adults. Gerontology 2005;51:174–8.

[27] McBride ME, Berkenbosch JW, Tobias JD. Transcutaneous carbon dioxide monitoring during diabetic ketoacidosis in children and adolescents. Paediatr Anaesth 2004;14:167–71.

[28] Garcia E, Abramo TJ, Okada P, Guzman DD, Reisch JS, Wiebe RA. Capnometry for noninvasive continuous monitoring of metabolic status in pediatric diabetic ketoacidosis. Crit Care Med 2003;31:2539–43.

[29] Hukins CA, Hillman DR. Daytime predictors of sleep hypoventilation in Duchenne muscular dystrophy. Am J Respir Crit Care Med 2000;161:166–70.

[30] Kirk VG, Flemons WW, Adams C, Rimmer KP, Montgomery MD. Sleep-disordered breathing in Duchenne muscular dystrophy: a preliminary study of the role of portable monitoring. Pediatr Pulmonol 2000;29:135–40.

[31] Bach JR, Penek J. Obstructive sleep apnea complicating negative-pressure ventilatory support in patients with chronic paralytic/restrictive ventilatory dysfunction. Chest 1991;99:1386–93.

[32] Bach JR, Alba AS. Sleep and nocturnal mouthpiece IPPV efficiency in postpoliomyelitis ventilator users. Chest 1994;106:1705–10.

[33] Bach JR, Alba AS, Saporito LR. Intermittent positive pressure ventilation via the mouth as an alternative to tracheostomy for 257 ventilator users. Chest 1993;103:174–82.

[34] Bach JR. Mechanical exsufflation, noninvasive ventilation, and new strategies for pulmonary rehabilitation and sleep disordered breathing. Bull N Y Acad Med 1992;68:321–40.

[35] Bach JR. Ventilatory support alternatives to tracheostomy and intubation: current status of the application of this technology. Conn Med 1991;55:323–9.

[36] Round Table Conference on Poliomyelitis Equipment. New York City, May 28–29, 1953. White Plains (NY): National Foundation for Infantile Paralysis, March of Dimes; 1953.

[37] Bach JR, Alba AS, Bohatiuk G, Saporito L, Lee M. Mouth intermittent positive pressure ventilation in the management of postpolio respiratory insufficiency. Chest 1987;91:859–64.

[38] Bach JR, Alba AS. Noninvasive options for ventilatory support of the traumatic high level quadriplegic patient. Chest 1990;98:613–9.

[39] Bach JR. Mechanical insufflation/exsufflation: has it come of age? A commentary. Eur Respir J 2003;21:385–6.

[40] Bach JR, Chaudhry SS. Standards of care in MDA clinics. Muscular Dystrophy Association. Am J Phys Med Rehabil 2000;79:193–6.

[41] Dettenmeier PA, Jackson NC. Chronic hypoventilation syndrome: treatment with non-invasive mechanical ventilation. AACN Clin Issues Crit Care Nurs 1991;2:415–31.

[42] Hill NS. Clinical applications of body ventilators. Chest 1986;90:897–905.

[43] Miller HJ, Thomas E, Wilmot CB. Pneumobelt use among high quadriplegic population. Arch Phys Med Rehabil 1988;69:369–72.

[44] Yang GF, Alba A, Lee M, Khan A. Pneumobelt for sleep in the ventilator user: clinical experience. Arch Phys Med Rehabil 1989;70:707–11.

[45] Bach JR, Alba AS, Bodofsky E, et al. Glossopharyngeal breathing and non-invasive aids in the management of post-polio respiratory insufficiency. Birth Defects 1987;23:99–113.

[46] Baydur A, Layne E, Aral H, et al. Long term non-invasive ventilation in the community for patients with musculoskeletal disorders: 46 year experience and review. Thorax 2000;55: 4–11.

[47] Sue RD, Susanto I. Long-term complications of artificial airways. Clin Chest Med 2003;24: 457–71.

[48] Durbin CG Jr. Early complications of tracheostomy. Respir Care 2005;50:511–5.

[49] Epstein SK. Late complications of tracheostomy. Respir Care 2005;50:542–9.

[50] Baydur A, Kanel G. Tracheobronchomalacia and tracheal hemorrhage in patients with Duchenne muscular dystrophy receiving long-term ventilation with uncuffed tracheostomies. Chest 2003;123:1307–11.

[51] Sanada Y, Kojima Y, Fonkalsrud EW. Injury of cilia induced by tracheal tube cuffs. Surg Gynecol Obstet 1982;154:648–52.

[52] King M, Brock G, Lundell C. Clearance of mucus by simulated cough. J Appl Physiol 1985; 58:1776–82.

[53] Hardy KA, Anderson BD. Noninvasive clearance of airway secretions. Respir Care Clin N Am 1996;2:323–45.

[54] Niranjan V, Bach JR. Noninvasive management of pediatric neuromuscular ventilatory failure. Crit Care Med 1998;26:2061–5.

[55] Gomez-Merino E, Sancho J, Marin J, et al. Mechanical insufflation-exsufflation: pressure, volume, and flow relationships and the adequacy of the manufacturer's guidelines. Am J Phys Med Rehabil 2002;81:579–83.

[56] Kang SW, Bach JR. Maximum insufflation capacity: vital capacity and cough flows in neuromuscular disease. Am J Phys Med Rehabil 2000;79:222–7.

[57] Bach JR, Alba AS. Management of chronic alveolar hypoventilation by nasal ventilation. Chest 1990;97:52–7.

[58] Bach JR, Alba A, Mosher R, Delaubier A. Intermittent positive pressure ventilation via nasal access in the management of respiratory insufficiency. Chest 1987;92:168–70.

[59] Carroll N, Branthwaite MA. Intermittent positive pressure ventilation by nasal mask: technique and applications. Intensive Care Med 1988;14:115–7.

[60] Goldstein RS, De-Rosie JA, Avendano MA, Dolmage TE. Influence of noninvasive positive pressure ventilation on inspiratory muscles. Chest 1991;99:408–15.

[61] Gay PC, Patel AM, Viggiano RW, Hubmayr RD. Nocturnal nasal ventilation for treatment of patients with hypercapnic respiratory failure. Mayo Clin Proc 1991;66:695–703.

[62] Heckmatt JZ, Loh L, Dubowitz V. Night-time nasal ventilation in neuromuscular disease. Lancet 1990;335:579–82.

[63] Leger P, Jennequin J, Gerard M, Lassonnery S, Robert D. Home positive pressure ventilation via nasal mask for patients with neuromusculoskeletal disorders. Eur Respir J Suppl 1989;7:640s–4s.

[64] Kerby GR, Mayer LS, Pingleton SK. Nocturnal positive pressure ventilation via nasal mask. Am Rev Respir Dis 1987;135:738–40.

[65] Ellis ER, Bye PT, Bruderer JW, Sullivan CE. Treatment of respiratory failure during sleep in patients with neuromuscular disease: positive-pressure ventilation through a nose mask. Am Rev Respir Dis 1987;135:148–52.

[66] Mehta S, Hill NS. Noninvasive ventilation. Am J Respir Crit Care Med 2001;163:540–77.

[67] Vianello A, Bevilacqua M, Salvador V, Cardaioli C, Vincenti E. Long-term nasal intermittent positive pressure ventilation in advanced Duchenne's muscular dystrophy. Chest 1994; 105:445–8.

[68] Simonds AK, Muntoni F, Heather S, Fielding S. Impact of nasal ventilation on survival in hypercapnic Duchenne muscular dystrophy. Thorax 1998;53:949–52.

[69] Hill NS, Eveloff SE, Carlisle CC, Goff SG. Efficacy of nocturnal nasal ventilation in patients with restrictive thoracic disease. Am Rev Respir Dis 1992;145(2 Pt 1):365–71.

[70] Jimenez JFM, de Cos Equin JS, Vicente CD, Valle MH, Otero FF. Nasal intermittent positive pressure: analysis of its withdrawal. Chest 1995;107:382–8.

[71] Bach JR, Campagnolo DI, Hoeman S. Life satisfaction of individuals with Duchenne muscular dystrophy using long-term mechanical ventilatory support. Am J Phys Med Rehabil 1991;70:129–35.

[72] Bach JR. Noninvasive ventilation is more than mask ventilation. Chest 2003;123:2156–7.

[73] Bach JR. Why be limited to nocturnal noninvasive IPPV? Chest 1997;111:1471–2.

[74] Bach JR. You need more than nocturnal NIPPV to manage Duchenne's muscular dystrophy. Chest 1995;107:592.

[75] Branthwaite MA. Noninvasive and domiciliary ventilation: positive pressure techniques. Thorax 1991;46:208–12.

[76] Gibson B. Long-term ventilation for patients with Duchenne muscular dystrophy: physicians' beliefs and practices. Chest 2001;119:940–6.

[77] Bach JR, Rajaraman R, Ballanger F, et al. Neuromuscular ventilatory insufficiency: effect of home mechanical ventilator use v oxygen therapy on pneumonia and hospitalization rates. Am J Phys Med Rehabil 1998;77:8–19.

[78] Tzeng AC, Bach JR. Prevention of pulmonary morbidity for patients with neuromuscular disease. Chest 2000;118:1390–6.

ELSEVIER
SAUNDERS

Phys Med Rehabil Clin N Am
16 (2005) 1141–1169

PHYSICAL MEDICINE
AND REHABILITATION
CLINICS OF
NORTH AMERICA

Cumulative Index 2005

Note: Page numbers of article titles are in **boldface** type.

A

Abdominal muscles, development of, in runners, 671–674

Acetaminophen, for pain, in disabled adults, 70

Achilles tendonitis, in runners, 794–796

Acupuncture, for pain, in disabled adults, 75–76

Acute disseminated encephalomyelopathy, diagnosis of, 371

Adaptive devices, for chronic pain, in Duchenne muscular dystrophy, 1119

Adaptive reasoning, multiple sclerosis and, 421

Air displacement plethysmography, of obesity, in neuromuscular diseases, 1054–1055

Alcohol abuse, in multiple sclerosis, 566–567

Alzheimer's disease, with traumatic brain injury, 170–171

Amantadine
  for cognitive impairment, in multiple sclerosis, 423
  for fatigue, in multiple sclerosis, 493
  for post-polio syndrome, 210

Amenorrhea, in female runners, 701–703
  and stress fractures, 759–760

Aminopyridines, for fatigue, in multiple sclerosis, 496

Amputation, aging with, **179–195**
  and physical activity, 47–48
  diagnostic tests before, 184
  energy expenditure in, 181–182
  epidemiology of, 179–180
  future research on, 190
  heel ulcers and, 188
  impact of, 188–189
  level of function before, 182

pain management in, 58, 63, 80
pre- and postoperative care for, 181–184
predicting further limb loss in, 187–188
prevention of, 188
prosthetic phase in, 184–187
  complications of, 186–187
  K-modifiers scale in, 186
  predicting outcome of, 186
  socket designs in, 185
rehabilitation for, 277
risk factors for, 184
versus revascularization and limb salvage, 181

Amyotrophic lateral sclerosis
  fatigue in, 1064, 1074–1075, 1107
  management of, 1085, 1095
  microgenomics of, **909–924**
    blood-brain barrier in, 919–920
    difficulties in, 917–918
    investigational difficulties in, 912–914
    laser-based tissue microdissection in, 914
    literature review on, 920–921
    microarray analysis in, 916–917
    molecular Trojan horses in, 919–920
    motor neuron degeneration and apoptosis in, 911
    RNA amplification in, 914–916
    RNA interference in, 918–919
    RNA quality in, 912
  microglial cells in, **1081–1090**
    as mediators of neuroinflammation, 1082–1083
    superoxide dismutase, 1082, 1084, 1085
  neuropathology of, 910–911
  neurotrophic factors in, 1000, 1002–1007
  risk factors for, 1092
  single muscle fiber physiology in, 959–960
  skeletal muscle in, **1091–1097**

Amyotrophic (*continued*)
    therapeutic implications of,
      1094–1096
    transgenic models of, 1092–1094
      SOD1, 1092–1094

Anesthetics, local, for pain, in disabled
    adults, 73

Angiotensin II, in skeletal muscle size,
    931–932

Ankle injuries, in runners, 787–797
    anatomy in, 787–788
    anterior ankle pain, 793–794
    biomechanics of, 787–788
    epidemiology of, 787
    lateral ankle pain, 789–793
      ligamentous sprains and,
        789–792
      osteochondral talus injuries and,
        793
      peroneal tendinopathy and,
        792–793
      sinus tarsi syndrome or subtalar
        ligament sprain and, 793
      soft tissue impingement and, 792
    medial ankle pain, 794
    posterior ankle pain, 794–797
      Achilles tendonitis and, 794–796

Ankle joint, and running gait, 604–605

Ankles
    flexibility of, and overuse injuries, in
      runners, 659
    open kinetic chain assessment of, in
      runners, 725–726

Anorexia nervosa, in female runners
    and stress fractures, 758–759
    signs and symptoms of, 697

Anterior cruciate ligament injuries, in
    female runners, 695

Anterior drawer test, for ankle sprains, in
    runners, 790

Anterior horn cell disorders, single muscle
    fiber physiology in, 959–960

Anthracycline analogs, for multiple
    sclerosis, 229

Anthropometric variables, in overuse
    injuries, in runners, 658–659

Antibiotics, tetracycline, for amyotrophic
    lateral sclerosis, 1085

Anticonvulsants, for spinal cord injury, 81

Antidepressants
    for cognitive impairment, in multiple
      sclerosis, 423–425

for fatigue, in multiple sclerosis,
    495–496
for pain, in disabled adults, 72

Antiepileptics, for pain, in disabled adults,
    72

Antioxidant activity, age-related changes in,
    20

Antioxidant defenses, in endurance exercise,
    866

Aquatic exercise, for post-polio syndrome,
    212–213

Aricept, for cognitive impairment, in
    multiple sclerosis, 423

Arrhythmias, cardiac, and collapse, in
    runners, 837–838

Arthritis, cerebral palsy and, 238

Articular cartilage, age-related changes in,
    27–29

Articular cartilage procedures, for
    patellofemoral pain syndrome, in
    runners, 769

Artificial nutrition and hydration, for
    end-stage cancer, 296–297

Ashworth Scale, to assess mobility, in
    multiple sclerosis, 534

Assistive devices, for chronic pain, in
    Duchenne muscular dystrophy, 1119

Asthenia, and rehabilitation and palliative
    care, for end-stage cancer,
    287–288

Atherosclerosis, and amputation. *See*
    Amputation.

Atrogin/MAFbx, in skeletal muscle
    dysfunction, 930–931

Attentional tasks, multiple sclerosis and,
    418–419

Avonex, for multiple sclerosis, 229, 355,
    455–456

Azathioprine, for multiple sclerosis, 229

B

Baclofen
    for pain, in disabled adults, 73
    for spasticity
      in multiple sclerosis, 474,
        476–477, 535
      in neuromuscular diseases,
        1106–1107

Balance, development of, in runners, 684, 686–687

Balance tests, in injured runners, 630–632

B cells, in multiple sclerosis, 353

Behavioral activation approaches, for depression, in multiple sclerosis, 444

Behavioral dyscontrol, with traumatic brain injury, 171–172

Betaferon, for multiple sclerosis, 454–455

Betaseron, for multiple sclerosis, 229, 355, 454–455

Biomechanical variables, in overuse injuries, in runners, 659–660

Biopsy, muscle, in muscular dystrophy, needle electromyography in, 985–986

Bisphosphonates, for osteoporosis, in female runners, 706

Bladder complications
    of cerebral palsy, 241
    of multiple sclerosis, 225–226

Body mass index, in neuromuscular diseases, 1054

Bone marrow-derived cells, in skeletal muscle repair, 895–897

Bone mineral density, and stress fractures, in runners, 756

Bones, age-related changes in. See Musculoskeletal system.

Bosu Balance Trainer, in core strengthening program, in runners, 687

Botulinum toxin
    for pain, in disabled adults, 78
    for spasticity, in multiple sclerosis, 473

Bowel complications, of multiple sclerosis, 226

Braces
    for patellofemoral pain syndrome, in runners, 768
    pneumatic, for stress fractures, in runners, 764

Brain-derived neurotrophic factor, in neuromuscular diseases, 1003–1004

Brain lesions, in multiple sclerosis
    magnetic resonance imaging of, 388–389
    neuropsychological evaluation of, 416–417

Breast-feeding, in runners, 693

Brief Fatigue Inventory, to measure fatigue, in elderly, 97–98

Bulimia nervosa, in female runners, signs and symptoms of, 698

C

Cachexia
    and rehabilitation and palliative care, for end-stage cancer, 297
    reactive oxygen species in, 926–931

Caffeine with histamine, for fatigue, in multiple sclerosis, 496

Calcaneal stress fractures, in runners, 783

Calcium intake, and stress fractures, in runners, 758

Calf pain, in Duchenne muscular dystrophy, 1116–1117

Cannabinoids, for chronic pain, in neuromuscular diseases, 1106

Capacitance coupling, for stress fractures, in runners, 764

Capsaicin, for pain, in disabled adults, 73

Capsular hip dysfunction, in runners, management of, 730

Carbon dioxide levels, in Duchenne muscular dystrophy, 1127–1128

Cardiac disease
    and collapse, in runners. See Downed runners.
    multiple sclerosis and, 228

Cardiac dysfunction, oxidative stress in, 935–936

Cardiac muscle function, magnetic resonance imaging of, 1045–1046

Cardiomyopathy, hypertrophic, and collapse, in runners, 837

Cardiopulmonary disease, **251–264**
    and collapse, in runners, 837
    epidemiology of, 252
    pathophysiology of, 251–252
    rehabilitation for
        exercise in, 258
        exercise training studies in, 259
        future research in, 261–262
        patient factors in, 259–260
        pulmonary function in, 260–261
        risk stratification in, 257
    risk factors for, 253–258
        diabetes mellitus, 255
        hypertension, 253–254

Cardiopulmonary (*continued*)
    lipids, 254–255
    metabolic syndrome, 256, 258
    psychologic factors, 256
    smoking, 255–256

Cardiopulmonary resuscitation, for
    end-stage cancer, 296

Cardiorespiratory endurance, in elderly, 101

Cardiovascular complications
    of cerebral palsy, 240
    of spinal cord injury, 139–141

Cardiovascular disease, osteoporosis and, in
    female runners, 706–707

Cardiovascular stress test, in rehabilitation,
    for multiple sclerosis, 538

Cartilage, articular, age-related changes in,
    27–29

Catheterization, for genitourinary
    complications
    of multiple sclerosis, 226
    of spinal cord injury, 145

Celecoxib, for amyotrophic lateral sclerosis,
    1085

Cell therapy, in skeletal muscle repair. *See*
    Skeletal muscle repair.

Central nervous system factors, and fatigue,
    in multiple sclerosis, 485–486

Cerebellar complications, of multiple
    sclerosis, 225

Cerebral autosomal dominant arteriopathy,
    with subcortical infarcts and
    leukoencephalopathy, versus multiple
    sclerosis, 376–377

Cerebral palsy, aging with, **235–249**
    cardiovascular changes in, 240
    dental disease in, 242–243
    epidemiology of, 235–236
    fatigue in, 239
    fractures in, 238–239
    future research on, 246
    gastrointestinal changes in, 240–241
    genitourinary changes in, 241
    hearing and vision impairment in, 243
    life expectancy in, 245–246
    loss of function in, 239
    management of
        adaptive equipment in, 245
        exercise in, 243–244
    musculoskeletal changes in, 237–238,
        241
    nerve entrapment and overuse
        syndromes in, 238

    neurologic changes in, 241–242
    nutrition in, 243
    pain management in, 81, 236–237
    reproductive changes in, 242
    resources for, 246–247
    respiratory changes in, 240
    social issues in, 244–245
    speech and swallowing difficulty in,
        243

Cerebrospinal fluid abnormalities, in
    multiple sclerosis, 365

Charcot-Marie-Tooth disease
    chronic pain in, 1100, 1103–1104
    electrodiagnostic studies of, **967–979,**
        983–984
        PMP-22 in, 968–969, 973
        trembler and *trembler-j* mouse
            models in, 969–970,
            973–974
        nerve conduction studies in,
            970–971
        stimulated single fiber
            electromyography in,
            971–972, 975
    neurotrophic factors in, 1002

Chicago Multiscale Depression Inventory,
    in multiple sclerosis, 441

Chondrocytes, age-related changes in, 29

Chronic intermittent hypoxia, oxidative
    stress in, 935–936

Chronic pain. *See also* Pain management.
    in multiple sclerosis, **503–512**
        and depression, 506
        and fatigue, 487
        biopsychosocial factors in,
            507–508
        demographics of, 507–508
        etiology of, 503–504
        impact of, 506–507
        management of, 508–509
            cognitive behavioral
                therapy in, 509
        nature and scope of, 504–506
    in neuromuscular diseases, **1099–1112**
        Charcot-Marie-Tooth disease,
            1100, 1103–1104
        Duchenne muscular dystrophy,
            1113–1124
            assessment of, 1115–1116
            calf pain, 1116–1117
            contractures and, 1117
            fractures and, 1117–1118
            gastrointestinal, 1118
            growing pains, 1118
            management of,
                1118–1120

fascioscapulohumeral muscular
dystrophy, 1100
Guillain-Barré syndrome,
1099–1100
management of, 1105–1109
flexibility and range of
motion in, 1108
nutrition and weight control
in, 1108–1109
pharmacologic, 1105–1107
rehabilitation in, 1107–1108
muscle weakness with, 1105
myotonic dystrophy type 2,
1100–1101

Ciliary neurotrophic factor, in
neuromuscular diseases, 1004

Closed kinetic chain exercises
for overuse injuries, in runners,
726–734
for patellofemoral pain syndrome, in
runners, 767

Cognitive behavioral therapy
for chronic pain
in disabled adults, 73
in Duchenne muscular
dystrophy, 1120
in multiple sclerosis, 509
for depression, in multiple sclerosis,
442–443

Cognitive dysfunction
and physical activity, with aging, 47
evaluation of. See Neuropsychological
evaluation.
in multiple sclerosis, 224
rehabilitation for, 537, 542–543

Cold therapy, for pain, in disabled adults, 74

Colorectal cancer, spinal cord injury and,
148

Communication tasks, multiple sclerosis
and, 419–420

Computed tomography, of stress fractures,
in runners, 763

Concentration tasks, multiple sclerosis and,
418–419

Constipation
multiple sclerosis and, 226, 565–566
spinal cord injury and, 146–148

Contraceptives, oral, and stress fractures, in
female runners, 758

Contractures
and chronic pain
in Duchenne muscular
dystrophy, 1117

in neuromuscular diseases, 1108
and physical activity, with aging,
45–46
spinal cord injury and, 137

Cooling programs, in multiple sclerosis
and exercise tolerance, 525–527
for fatigue, 492

Copaxone, for multiple sclerosis, 229, 355,
357, 458–459

Core mobility tests, in runners, 717–720

Core musculature, in runners, **669–689**
eccentric-concentric control of,
720–721
imbalances in, 675–679
postural versus phasic muscles in,
676, 678–679
role of, 670–675
development of abdominal
muscles, 671–674
strengthening program for, 679–681
balance and motor control in,
684, 686–687
functional movement training in,
687–688
lumbo-pelvic stability in, 681–684
stretching exercises in, 680
warm-up in, 681
tight and inhibited muscles in, 670

Core stability assessment, in injured
runners, 631–632, 640–641

Coronary artery disease. See
Cardiopulmonary disease.

Coronary heart disease. See
Cardiopulmonary disease.

Cough Assist device, for Duchenne
muscular dystrophy, 1133

Cough support, in Duchenne muscular
dystrophy, 1133–1136

COX-2 inhibitors, for pain, in disabled
adults, 70

Cyclophosphamide, for multiple sclerosis,
229

Cytokines
and fatigue, in elderly, 96
in multiple sclerosis, 352–353
in skeletal muscle dysfunction,
927–929

D

Dantrolene, for spasticity, in multiple
sclerosis, 475

Dehydroepiandrosterone, for age-related musculoskeletal problems, 25

Delirium, and rehabilitation and palliative care, for end-stage cancer, 290–292

Dementia, and falls, in elderly, 113

Dental complications, of cerebral palsy, 242–243

Depression
  in disabled adults, 13–14
  in multiple sclerosis, 223–224, **437–448**
    and fatigue, 487
    chronic pain and, 506
    definitions in, 437–439
    diagnosis of, 440–441
      Chicago Multiscale Depression Inventory in, 441
      Patient Health Questionnaire in, 440
    impact of, 439–440
    management of, 441–444
      cognitive behavioral therapy in, 442
      exercise in, 443–444
      future directions in, 444
      interpersonal therapy in, 444
      selective serotonin reuptake inhibitors in, 442
      sertraline in, 442
    prevalence of, 439
  spinal cord injury and, 149
  with fatigue, in neuromuscular diseases, 1069

Dermatomyositis, single muscle fiber physiology in, 961–962

Devic's syndrome, versus multiple sclerosis, 377

Diabetes mellitus
  and cardiopulmonary disease, 255
  metabolic syndrome and, 1058

Diabetic neuropathies, neurotrophic factors in, 1000–1002

Diazepam, for spasticity, in multiple sclerosis, 475–476

Dietary programs
  for fatigue, 492
  for multiple sclerosis, 565–566

Diffuse axonal injury, and traumatic brain injury, 166

Disability, aging with, **1–18**
  and physical activity, **41–56**
    asymmetrical weakness in, 45

barriers to, 53
cognitive dysfunction in, 47
contractures in, 45–46
disability exacerbation in, 46
endurance training in, 50–51
fatigue and chronic pain in, 47
impact on health and function, 42–44
instruments for measuring, 51, 53
limb loss in, 47–48
muscle function in, 46
National Center on Physical Activity and Disability in, 53–54
need for future research in, 48–53
overuse injuries in, 51
progressive disability, 45
public health recommendation in, 49
record-keeping in, 46–47
reduced joint flexibility in, 45–46
resistance training in, 52
responders versus non-responders in, 49
sensory nerve damage in, 46
spasticity in, 45
  co-morbidities and, 2–3, 8–9
  coping with, 11–12
  elder law issues in, **305–313**
    defenses to liability claims, 312–313
    guardianship, 309–310
    health care proxies, 305–308
    lack of family, 310
    liability for accidental versus intentional actions, 310–311
    living will, 306
    nursing home liability and *respondeat superior*, 311–312
    power of attorney, 308–309
  functional issues in, 10–12
  life expectancy and, 2
  loss of capacity and, model for, 5–7
  pain management in. *See* Pain management.
  physical changes and, 7–10
  psychosocial issues in, 12–15
    depression, 13–14, 149, 223–224
    long-term care, 14–15
    quality of life, 12–14
  rehabilitation for, **265–282**
    Acute Care for the Elderly Program in, 268
    acute inpatient systems for, 269
    acute medical/surgical hospital units in, 267–268
    Adult Day Health Care in, 272–273

amputation, 277
case management in, 279
financial issues in, 277–278
formal home care in, 274–275
future research on, 279
Geriatric Assessment units in,
270
Geriatric Day Hospital in, 273
Geriatric Evaluation and
Management units in,
269–270
home-based primary care in, 274
hospice care in, 272
informal home care in, 274
inpatient systems for, 267
long-term care residential
programs in, 273–274
multiple sclerosis, 277
outcomes of, 279
outpatient programs in, 273
post-polio syndrome, 277
preventive, 278
Program for All Inclusive Care of
the Elderly in, 272
respite care in, 271
skilled nursing facilities in,
270–271
spinal cord injury, 276
subacute care facilities in, 271
tele-home health care in, 275–276
telemedicine in, 275
theoretically achievable goal in,
266–267
traumatic brain injury, 276
reserve capacity and, 4
versus non-disabled people, 7–9

Dithiothreitol, in skeletal muscle
dysfunction, 937

Dizziness, and falls, in elderly, 113

Donepezil hydrochloride, for multiple
sclerosis, 423

Downed runners, **831–849**
cardiac causes of, 836–838
arrhythmias, 837–838
coronary artery disease, 837
hypertrophic cardiomyopathy,
837
exercise-associated, 838–839
heat generation and, 839–841
hyperthermia and heat stroke,
839–841
hypothermia and, 841
medical support for, 832–836
differential diagnosis in,
833–836
organization of medical tent,
832–833

Drug abuse, in multiple sclerosis, 566–567

Dual energy absorptiometry scans
of obesity, in neuromuscular diseases,
1054
of osteoporosis, in female runners, 705

Duchenne muscular dystrophy
chronic pain in. See Chronic pain.
clinical features of, 1114–1115
gene therapy for, 880–882
muscle regeneration in, cell therapy in,
889–890
respiratory complications of,
1125–1126
respiratory muscle function in,
1126–1128
carbon dioxide levels, 1127–1128
peak cough flow rate, 1127
respiratory support in, **1125–1139**
cough support, 1133–1136
invasive (tracheostomy)
ventilation, 1133
noninvasive ventilation, 1128,
1130–1131, 1133, 1135
sleep assessment in, 1128

Dyna Disk, in core strengthening program,
in runners, 687

Dynamic electromyography, of running
gait, 618

Dysphagia
in multiple sclerosis, 544
in post-polio syndrome, 209

Dyspnea, and rehabilitation and palliative
care, for end-stage cancer, 289–290

E

Eating disorders, in female runners. See
Female runners.

Electrical stimulation
for age-related musculoskeletal
problems, 24
for pain, in disabled adults, 74

Electrodiagnostic automation, **1015–1032**
data analysis in, 1018–1019
data collection in, 1018
data reporting in, 1019
future directions in, 1027–1029
historical aspects of, 1016–1018
limitations of, 1023–1026
children, 1025
elderly patients, 1024
misdirected or incomplete
technology, 1023–1024
physician and technician
challenges, 1024–1025

Electrodiagnostic (*continued*)
    predesigned electrode
      configuration, 1025
    reporting and decision support,
      1023
    NC-stat in, 1019–1023
      components of, 1020
      motor responses in, 1020–1021
      onCall report in, 1022–1023
      supramaximal stimulus intensity
        in, 1020
      waveform analysis in, 1021–1022
    validation of, statistical issues in,
      1026–1027

Electrodiagnostic studies
    of Charcot-Marie-Tooth disease. *See*
      Charcot-Marie-Tooth disease.
    of muscle function, versus magnetic
      resonance imaging, 1037–1043
    of muscular dystrophy. *See* Muscular
      dystrophy.
    of post-polio syndrome, 199–200
    of primary muscle disease, 1047

Embryonic stem cells, in skeletal muscle
    repair, 892–893

Encephalomyelopathy, acute disseminated,
    diagnosis of, 371

End-stage cancer, rehabilitation and
    palliative care for, **283–303**
    artificial nutrition and hydration in,
      296–297
    asthenia and, 287–289
    cachexia syndrome and, 297
    cardiopulmonary resuscitation in, 296
    case study of, 298–300
    delirium and, 290–292
    dyspnea and, 289–290
    ethical dilemmas in, 293
    Functional Independence Measure in,
      288
    future challenges in, 300
    goal-setting in, 294
    historical aspects of, 285–287
    informed consent and
      decision-making capacity in,
      294–296
    pain management in, 289
    similarities between, 283–284

Endocrine complications, of spinal cord
    injury, 139–141

Endocrine factors, and fatigue, in multiple
    sclerosis, 486

Endothelial growth factor, for amyotrophic
    lateral sclerosis, 1095

Endurance exercise. *See* Exercise training.

Endurance training
    in disabled adults, 50–51
    versus endurance exercise, 866

Energetic measurements, of running gait,
    618–619

Energy conservation, for fatigue, in multiple
    sclerosis, 492, 539–540

Entrapment neuropathy, post-polio
    syndrome and, 213

Epidural steroid injections, for pain, in
    disabled adults, 78–79

Epley maneuver, to prevent falls, in elderly,
    116–117

Erectile dysfunction, spinal cord injury and,
    144

Essential fatty acids, in multiple sclerosis,
    565

Estrogen replacement therapy, for age-
    related musculoskeletal problems, 25

Excursion tests, in injured runners, 630

Executive tasks, multiple sclerosis and, 421

Exercise
    and collapse, in runners, 838–839
    closed kinetic chain, for overuse
      injuries, in runners, 726–734
    for chronic pain, in Duchenne
      muscular dystrophy, 1119–1120
    for disabled adults
      in pain management, 74–75
      to prevent falls, 116
      with cardiopulmonary disease,
        258–259
      with cerebral palsy, 243–244
      with fatigue, 100–103
      with musculoskeletal problems,
        23–24
      with post-polio syndrome,
        212–213
      with spinal cord injury, 135,
        140–141
    in multiple sclerosis, 427, 559–560. *See*
      also Rehabilitation.
      for depression, 443–444
      for fatigue, 491–492
      for spasticity, 471–472

Exercise training, skeletal muscle
    adaptation in, **859–873**
    endurance exercise, 864–866
      aerobic ATP generation in,
        864–866
      antioxidant defenses in, 866
      FOXO1 in, 865
      MTI-III proteins in, 866

PDK4 in, 864–865
PGC1α in, 864
PPARδ in, 865
signals and pathways in, 869
upregulated genes in, 868
versus endurance exercise, 866
genomics in, 863
microarray analysis in, 863
protein adaptations in, 861
resistance exercise, 867–869
signals and pathways in, 869
SREBP-2 in, 867–869
upregulated genes in, 868
transcriptional level in, 862–863

F
_____

Facilitation therapy, for multiple sclerosis,
532–533

Falls
in elderly, **109–128**
and hip fractures, 110
caretaker advice on, 120–121
case study of, 119–120
clinical pearls on, 123
community-dwelling versus
institutionalized, 111
diagnosis of, 114–115
dizziness and, 113
environmental hazards and, 114
epidemiology of, 110
management of, 115–119
environmental
modifications in, 117
exercise in, 116
hip protectors in, 117
medication management in,
118
monitoring devices in,
118–119
physical restraints in, 118
vestibular therapy in,
116–117
resources on, 122
risk factors for, 111–113
syncope and, 113
transfers and, 113–114
vision impairment and, 112, 114
wheelchair-related, 113–114
multiple sclerosis and, 227–228

Family Medical Leave Act, and
employment issues, in multiple
sclerosis, 576

Fascioscapulohumeral muscular dystrophy
aging with, pain management in, 59
chronic pain in, 1100
single muscle fiber physiology in, 961

Fast-twitch muscles, versus slow-twitch,
age-related changes in, 19–20, 22

Fat pad contusions, in runners, 783

Fatigue
in cancer, 1064
in elderly, **91–108**
definition of, 92
diagnosis of, 99
differential diagnosis of, 99
epidemiology of, 92–93
management of, 99–103
exercise in, 100–103
measurement of, 96–99
Brief Fatigue Inventory in,
97–98
Fatigue Assessment
Instrument in, 98–99
Fatigue Questionnaire in,
98
Fatigue Severity Scale in, 97
Fatigue Symptom
Inventory in, 98
Multidimensional Fatigue
Inventory in, 98
Piper Fatigue Scale in, 98
pathophysiology of, 93–96
central versus peripheral,
95–96
in all age groups, 94
in specific disorders, 94
with cerebral palsy, 239
with multiple sclerosis, 223
with post-polio syndrome, 202
in multiple sclerosis, **483–502,** 1065
central nervous system factors in,
485–486
clinical features of, 484
definition of, 483–484
depression and, 487
employment issues in, 574
endocrine factors in, 486
immune dysregulation and,
484–485
management of, 491–496,
521–523, 530
amantadine in, 493
aminopyridines in, 496
antidepressants in,
495–496
cooling programs in, 492
diet in, 492
energy conservation in, 492,
539–540
exercise in, 491–492
modafinil in, 493, 495
pemoline in, 495
Prokarin in, 496
measurement of, 487–490, 522

Fatigue (*continued*)
    Fatigue Assessment
      Inventory in, 490
    Fatigue Descriptive Scale
      in, 490
    Fatigue Impact Scale in, 490
    Fatigue Severity Scale in,
      490, 522
    visual analog scale in, 488,
      490
  medications and, 487
  neurotransmitter dysregulation
    and, 486
  pain and, 487
  physical deconditioning and, 486
  sleep dysfunction and, 486–487
in neuromuscular diseases, **1063–1079**
  amyotrophic lateral sclerosis,
    1064, 1074–1075, 1107
  depression with, 1069
  measurement of, 1066–1069
    Fatigue Severity Scale in,
      1067
    in laboratory, 1069–1071
    McGill Quality of Life
      questionnaire in, 1074
    motor evoked potentials in,
      1072–1073
    Multidimensional Fatigue
      Inventory in,
      1067–1068
    Piper Fatigue Scale in, 1067,
      1068, 1076
    transcranial magnetic
      stimulation in,
      1071–1074
    twitch interpolation in,
      1071–1075
    Visual Analogue Scale of
      Fatigue in, 1067–1069
  Parkinson's disease, 1065
  post-polio syndrome, 1076
  pulmonary dysfunction with,
    1069
  sleep disorders with, 1069

Fatigue Assessment Instrument, to measure
  fatigue, in elderly, 98–99

Fatigue Questionnaire, to measure fatigue,
  in elderly, 98

Fatigue Severity Scale
  to measure fatigue
    in elderly, 97
    in neuromuscular diseases, 1067

Fatigue Symptom Inventory, to measure
  fatigue, in elderly, 98

Feet, open kinetic chain assessment of, in
  runners, 725–726

Feldenkreis technique, for multiple
  sclerosis, 533

Female athlete triad, and stress fractures, in
  runners, 759–760

Female runners, **691–709**
  adolescent, 692
  aging, 694–695
    stress fractures in, 694–695
    stress urinary incontinence in,
      694
  anterior cruciate ligament injuries in,
    695
  breast-feeding, 693
  eating disorders in, 696–701
    and stress fractures, 758–759
    anorexia nervosa, signs and
      symptoms of, 697
    bulimia nervosa, signs and
      symptoms of, 698
    definition of, 696–697
    iron deficiency anemia with, 701
    management of, 700–701
    medical complications of, 699
    psychologic issues in, 698
    red flags for, 699–700
  groin pain in, 695
  low back pain in, 695
  menstrual dysfunction in, 701–704
    amenorrhea, 701–703
      management of, 703
    and stress fractures, 757,
      759–760
  osteoporosis in, 704–707
    and cardiovascular disease,
      706–707
    bisphosphonates for, 706
    dual-energy absorptiometry
      scans of, 705
    hormone replacement therapy
      for, 706
    menstrual dysfunction with, 705
    nutritional status and, 704–705
    parathyroid hormone for, 706
    weight-bearing activity for, 704
  patellofemoral pain and dysfunction
    in, 695
  pregnant, 692–693
  stress fractures in
    eating disorders and, 758–759
    menstrual dysfunction and, 757,
      759–760
    screening for, 760–761
  upper extremity injuries in, 695–696
  versus male runners, anatomic and
    biomechanical differences in,
    691–692

Fibroblast growth factor-I, in
  neuromuscular diseases, 1008

Fibroblasts, in skeletal muscle repair, 897

Flexibility, in elderly, 103

Flexibility tests, in footwear evaluation, in runners, 821

Foot care, in prevention, of amputation, 188

Foot deformities, cerebral palsy and, 237

Foot injuries, in runners, 779–787
anatomy in, 780–781
biomechanics of, 780–781
epidemiology of, 779–780
forefoot pain, 785–787
extensor and flexor tendonitis and, 786
first metatarsophalangeal disorders and, 786–787
interdigital neuromas and, 787
metatarsal stress fractures and, 785–786
metatarsalgia and, 786
midfoot pain, 784
anterior tarsal tunnel syndrome and, 784
navicular stress fractures and, 784
peroneal tendinopathy and, 784
posterior tibial tendinopathy and, 784
rearfoot pain, 781–783
calcaneal and talar stress fractures and, 783
fat pad contusions and, 783
plantar fasciitis and, 781–783
tarsal tunnel syndrome and, 783

Footwear, for runners. See Runners, footwear and orthoses for.

Force plate analysis, of running gait, 617–618

Forefoot pain, in runners. See Foot injuries.

FOXO1, in endurance exercise, 865

Fractures
and chronic pain, in Duchenne muscular dystrophy, 1117–1118
cerebral palsy and, 238
falls and, 110
post-polio syndrome and, 208–209
spinal cord injury and, 137–138
stress. See Stress fractures.

Functional Independence Measure, and rehabilitation and palliative care, for end-stage cancer, 288

Functional magnetic resonance imaging of multiple sclerosis, 393–394, 403

of muscle function, 1043–1045

Functional reach test, in neuromuscular assessment, of elderly, 115

G

Gabapentin, for spasticity, in multiple sclerosis, 476

Gait analysis
for footwear, in runners, 814–815
in injured runners, 645, 648

Gait cycle, in running. See Running gait.

Gallstones, spinal cord injury and, 148

Gastrointestinal complications
of cerebral palsy, 240–241
of spinal cord injury. See Spinal cord injury.

Gastrointestinal complications, of Duchenne muscular dystrophy, 1118

GDF-8, in gene transfer, for skeletal muscle enhancement, 883–884

Gene therapy
for age-related musculoskeletal problems, 24
for amyotrophic lateral sclerosis, 1095–1096

Gene transfer, in skeletal muscle enhancement. See Skeletal muscle enhancement.

Genitourinary complications
of cerebral palsy, 241
of spinal cord injury. See Spinal cord injury.

Get up and go test, in neuromuscular assessment, of elderly, 115

Glasgow Outcome Scale, of function, after traumatic brain injury, 168–169

Glatiramer acetate, for multiple sclerosis, 229, 355, 357, 458–459

Glial cell line-derived neurotrophic factor, in neuromuscular diseases, 1004–1005

Gray matter, in multiple sclerosis, magnetic resonance imaging of, 391–392

Groin pain, in female runners, 695

Ground reaction forces, and overuse injuries, in runners, 653–655

Growing pains, in Duchenne muscular dystrophy, 1118

Growth factors
    for amyotrophic lateral sclerosis,
      1095
    in skeletal muscle repair, 894

Growth hormone, for age-related
    musculoskeletal problems, 25–26

Guardianship, for disabled adults,
    309–310

Guillain-Barré syndrome
    aging with, pain management in, 59
    chronic pain in, 1099–1100

H

Hallus dorsiflexion, in footwear evaluation,
    in runners, 817–818

Hamstring injuries, in runners, management
    of, 731–732

Health care proxies, for disabled adults,
    305–308

Hearing impairment, cerebral palsy and,
    243

Heart disease, post-polio syndrome and,
    213

Heart failure, oxidative stress in, 936–937

Heat intolerance, multiple sclerosis and, 227

Heat stroke, and collapse, in runners,
    839–841

Heat therapy, for pain, in disabled adults,
    74

Heel ulcers, and amputation, 188

Hematomas, subdural, and traumatic brain
    injury, 165–166

Hemorrhoids, spinal cord injury and, 148

Hip dislocation, cerebral palsy and, 237

Hip fractures, in elderly, falls and, 110

Hip protectors, to prevent hip fractures, in
    elderly, 117

Hip-scapula reaction, in runners, 721–723

Hips
    examination of, in injured runners,
      639–640
    overuse injuries of, in runners. *See*
      Overuse injuries.

Histamine with caffeine, for fatigue, in
    multiple sclerosis, 496

H_2O_2, in skeletal muscle dysfunction,
    936–937

Hormonal factors, and stress fractures, in
    runners, 757–758

Hormone replacement therapy
    and stress fractures, in female runners,
      761
    for age-related musculoskeletal
      problems, 25
    for menstrual dysfunction, in female
      runners, 703
    for osteoporosis, in female runners,
      706

Hyaluronic acid, for pain, in disabled
    adults, 77

Hypertension, and cardiopulmonary
    disease, 253–254

Hyperthermia, and collapse, in runners,
    839–841

Hypertrophic cardiomyopathy, and
    collapse, in runners, 837

Hypothermia, and collapse, in runners, 841

Hypovitaminosis D, and falls, in elderly,
    111–112

Hypoxia, chronic intermittent, oxidative
    stress in, 935–936

I

Iliotibial band friction syndrome, in
    runners. *See* Knee injuries.

Immune dysregulation, and fatigue, in
    multiple sclerosis, 484–485

Immune response, in skeletal muscle repair.
    See Skeletal muscle repair.

Immune tolerance, in skeletal muscle repair,
    892

Immunomodulatory agents, for multiple
    sclerosis, 355, **449–466**
    and cognition, 423, 459
    central nervous system myelin disease
      and, 451
    clinical trials of, 398–401
    diagnostic criteria and, 451–452
    efficacy of, 459–460
    future directions in, 461
    glatiramer acetate, 355, 357, 458–459
    interferons, 355, 356, 454–458
    long-term effects of, 458–459
    mechanisms of action of, 453–454
    neutralizing antibodies, 355–357,
      456–457
    rationale for, 452–453
    relapsing remitting disease course and,
      450

suboptimal response to, 460
T-cell mediated inflammation and, 451

Immunosuppressants
for multiple sclerosis, 229, 354–355
to suppress host immune reaction, in skeletal muscle repair, 891–892

Impact force, and overuse injuries, in runners, 661

Inclusion body myositis, single muscle fiber physiology in, 961–962

Infections, urinary tract, spinal cord injury and, 144–145

Information processing speed, multiple sclerosis and, 419

Injections
for pain, in disabled adults, 76–79
of donor cells, in skeletal muscle repair, 898–899

Injured runners, functional evaluation of, **623–649**
footwear assessment in, 643–645
gait analysis in, 645, 648. *See also* Running gait.
patient history in, 623–626
physical examination in, 626
prone examination in, 642–643
subtalar neutral tests in, 643
screening gait evaluation in, 626–629
gait exaggeration in, 627–628
seated examination in, 634–639
inspection and palpation in, 634–635
knee examination in, 638–639
passive range of motion of foot and ankle in, 635–638
side-lying examination in, 641–642
standing examination in, 629–634
core stability assessment in, 631–632
excursion tests in, 630
palliative tests in, 632, 634
provocation tests in, 632
single leg balance reach tests in, 631
single-legged squat in, 630
supine examination in, 639–641
core stability assessment in, 640–641
hip examination in, 639–640
inspection and palpation in, 639
knee examination in, 640
training errors in, 625–626

Innominate dysfunction, in runners, management of, 730

Insulin-like growth factor
for amyotrophic lateral sclerosis, 1095
in neuromuscular diseases, 1005–1007

Insulin-like growth factor, for post-polio syndrome, 210

Integumentary complications, of spinal cord injury, 142

Interdigital neuromas, in runners, 787

Interferons, for multiple sclerosis, 229, 355, 356, 454–458

Interferons, in skeletal muscle dysfunction, 929

Interleukins, in skeletal muscle dysfunction, 929

Interpersonal therapy, for depression, in multiple sclerosis, 444

Intracranial pressure, increased, traumatic brain injury and, 166

Intrathecal drugs, for spasticity, in multiple sclerosis, 476–477, 535

Intrathecal opioids, for pain, in disabled adults, 78–79

Inversion test, for ankle sprains, in runners, 790

Iron deficiency anemia, in female runners, eating disorders and, 701

Isometric contractile measurements, in neuromuscular diseases, 954–955

Isotonic contractile measurements, in neuromuscular diseases, 955–957

J

Joint flexibility, and physical activity, in disabled adults, 45–46

Joints, age-related changes in, 26–27, 30–32

K

Kinetic variables, in overuse injuries, in runners, 660–661, 714

K-modifiers scale, in amputation, 186

Knee deformities, cerebral palsy and, 237

Knee injuries, in runners, 764–771
iliotibial band friction syndrome, 769–771
clinical features of, 770
management of, 770–771
injections in, 771

Knee injuries (*continued*)
    rehabilitation in, 770–771
    surgical, 771
  physical examination for, 770
  patellofemoral pain syndrome, 695, 764–769
    clinical features of, 766
    diagnosis of, 766
    factors predisposing to, 765–766
    generators of, 765
    management of, 766–769
      closed kinetic chain exercises in, 767
      surgical, 769
      taping, braces, and orthoses in, 768–769
      vastus medialis oblique strengthening in, 767–768

Knees, examination of, in injured runners, 638–639, 640

Kurtzke Expanded Disability Status Scale, in multiple sclerosis, 222, 513–515

L

Language tasks, multiple sclerosis and, 419–420, 543–535

Lateral retinacular release, for patellofemoral pain syndrome, in runners, 769

Lee Silverman Voice Therapy, in multiple sclerosis, 544

Leg length discrepancy, and stress fractures, in runners, 757

Lentiviral vectors, in gene transfer, for skeletal muscle enhancement, 876–877

Liability issues, for disabled adults, 310–313

Lidocaine, for pain, in disabled adults, 73

Ligaments
  and running gait, 608
  overuse injuries of, in runners, 713
  sprains of, in runners, 789–792

Lipids, and cardiopulmonary disease, 254–255

Living wills, for disabled adults, 306

Local anesthetics, for pain, in disabled adults, 73

Low back pain, in female runners, 695

Lower extremities, and running gait, 604

Lower extremity balance and reach, in runners, 723–725

Lower extremity static alignment, in runners, 715

Lumbo-pelvic stability, in core strengthening program, in runners, 681–684

M

Macro electromyography, of muscular dystrophy, 993

Macrophages, in multiple sclerosis, 353–354

Magnetic resonance imaging
  of ankle sprains, in runners, 790
  of multiple sclerosis, 221–222, 360–362, 364–365, 366, **383–410**
    blood-brain barrier in, 384–385
    brain atrophy in, 389
    brain lesions in, 388–389
    chronic T1-hyperintense lesions in, 387–388
    clinical significance of, 396–397
    criteria for, 397–398
    disease course in, 394–396
    enhancing lesions in, 384–385
    for treatment response, 459–460
    functional imaging in, 393–394, 403
    gray matter in, 391–392
    in clinical trials, 398–401
      of immunomodulatory agents, 398–401
    magnetic resonance spectroscopy in, 391, 402–403
    magnetization transfer imaging in, 401
    neuronal tract degeneration in, 392–393
    normal-aapearing white matter in, 390–391
    primary progressive multiple sclerosis, 395–396
    spinal cord lesions in, 389–390
    T2-hyperintense lesions in, 385–387
    water diffusion-based measures in, 401
  of muscle function, **1033–1051**
    cardiac muscle, 1045–1046
    fast spin-echo proton density sequences in, 1035
    functional imaging in, 1043–1045
      after intense exercise, 1045
      automated texture analysis versus visual analysis in, 1045

in older subjects, 1044
of mass specific blood flow, 1044
image analysis in, 1036–1037
physiology of, 1034–1036
primary muscle disease, 1046–1047
short-time inversion recovery pulse sequences in, 1035–1036, 1038–1043
spin-echo pulse sequences in, 1035
T1-weighted, 1034–1043
T2-weighted, 1034–1041
techniques for, 1034
versus electrodiagnostic studies, 1037–1043
motor unit action potentials in, 1041
with magnetic resonance spectroscopy, 1047–1048
of stress fractures, in runners, 763
with electrodiagnostic studies, of muscular dystrophy, 993

Magnetic resonance spectroscopy
of multiple sclerosis, 391, 402–403
with magnetic resonance imaging, of muscle function, 1047–1048

Magnetization transfer imaging, in magnetic resonance imaging, of multiple sclerosis, 401

Major depressive disorder, in multiple sclerosis. See Depression.

Major depressive episode, in multiple sclerosis. See Depression.

Massage, for pain, in disabled adults, 76

McDonald criteria, in diagnosis, of multiple sclerosis, 360–365, 452
definitions in, 363–365

McGill Quality of Life questionnaire, in neuromuscular diseases, 1074

Mean arterial pressure, increased, traumatic brain injury and, 166

Mechanical exsufflation, for Duchenne muscular dystrophy, 1133

Mechanical ventilation
for Duchenne muscular dystrophy. See Duchenne muscular dystrophy.
for post-polio syndrome, 205–207

Medial tibial stress syndrome, versus stress fractures, in runners, 762–763

Medio-lateral forces, and overuse injuries, in runners, 655

Memory tasks, multiple sclerosis and, 419

Menstrual dysfunction, in female runners. See Female runners.

Mesenchymal stem cells, in skeletal muscle repair, 897

Metabolic syndrome
and cardiopulmonary disease, 256, 258
and neuromuscular diseases. See Neuromuscular diseases, obesity in.

Metatarsal stress fractures, in runners, 785–786

Metatarsalgia, in runners, 786

Metatarsophalangeal disorders, in runners, 786–787

Metatarsophalangeal joints, and running gait, 607

Methylphenidate, for cognitive impairment, in multiple sclerosis, 423

Microglial cells, in amyotrophic lateral sclerosis. See Amyotrophic lateral sclerosis.

Midfoot pain, in runners. See Foot injuries.

mIgf-I, in gene transfer, for skeletal muscle enhancement, 882–883

Minimal Assessment of Cognitive Function in MS, for multiple sclerosis, 426

Mini-Mental State Examination, for multiple sclerosis, 425

Minocycline, for amyotrophic lateral sclerosis, 1085

Mitogen-activated protein kinases, in skeletal muscle dysfunction, 929, 931

Mitoxantrone, for multiple sclerosis, 229, 354–355
for suboptimal treatment response, 460

Modafinil
for fatigue
in amyotrophic lateral sclerosis, 1075, 1107
in multiple sclerosis, 493, 495

Modified Ashworth Scale, to assess spasticity, in multiple sclerosis, 469, 534–535

Motion analysis, of running gait, 617

Motor control, development of, in runners, 684, 686–687

Motor evoked potentials, to measure
    fatigue, in neuromuscular diseases,
    1072–1073

Motor neuron injury
    in multiple sclerosis, 225
    in post-polio syndrome, 199

Motor neurons, age-related changes in, 20

Motor-speech impairment, multiple
    sclerosis and, 419–420

Motor unit action potentials
    in electrodiagnostic studies, of muscle
        function, 1041
    in needle electromyography, of
        muscular dystrophy, 984–986,
        991

Motor unit degeneration, in post-polio
    syndrome, 200–201

Movement training, in core strengthening
    program, in runners, 687–688

MS Functional Composite, in multiple
    sclerosis, 514

MTI-III proteins, in endurance exercise,
    866

Multidimensional Fatigue Inventory
    to measure fatigue
        in elderly, 98
        in neuromuscular diseases,
            1067–1068

Multiple sclerosis
    aging with, **219–234**
        and driving, 230–231
        and vaccinations, 228
        bladder changes in, 225–226
        bowel changes in, 226
        cardiac disease in, 228
        cerebellar changes in, 225
        classification of, 220–221
        cognitive dysfunction in, 224
        depression in, 223–224
        diagnosis of, 221–222
        epidemiology of, 220
        falls in, 227–228
        family dynamics in, 231
        fatigue in, 94, 223
        functional assessment in, 222
        heat intolerance in, 227
        management of, 228–230
            assistive devices in,
                229–230
            pharmacologic, 228–229
        motor loss and spasticity in, 225
        ophthalmologic changes in,
            224–225
        osteoporosis in, 228

    rehabilitation for, 277
    resources for, 232
    sensory disturbance and pain in,
        222–223
    sexual changes in, 227
    swallowing difficulty in, 227
    vocational issues in, 230
and life participation, **583–594**
    benefits of, 587–588
    definition of, 585
    factors influencing, 585–586
    measurement of, 586
    physician's role in, 588
    strategies for health care
        communication, 590–592
        avoid decision making in
            periods of crisis, 592
        costs/benefits of activities,
            591–592
        individualized information,
            591
        listen to person living with
            disease, 590–591
    trajectory and changes over time,
        589–590
chronic pain in. *See* Chronic pain.
depression in. *See* Depression.
diagnosis of, **359–381**
    cerebrospinal fluid abnormalities
        in, 365
    historical aspects of, 359–360
    magnetic resonance imaging in.
        See Magnetic resonance
        imaging.
    McDonald criteria for, 360–365,
        452
        definitions in, 363–365
    pitfalls in, 367–378
        errors in addressing other
            explanations, 372–373,
            375–377
        errors in definition of
            attacks, 367–368
        errors in diagnosing
            primary progressive
            multiple sclerosis,
            377–378
        errors in dissemination in
            space, 372
        errors in dissemination of
            time, 370–372
        errors in requiring objective
            findings, 370
        errors in symptom
            identification,
            368–370
    Poser criteria for, 360
    primary progressive multiple
        sclerosis, 365–367

versus cerebral autosomal
    dominant arteriopathy,
    376–377
versus neuromyelitis optica, 377
versus stroke, 375–376
employment issues in, **571–582**
    accommodations for
        employment, 573–575
        for cognitive changes, 574
        for fatigue, 574
        for heat sensitivity, 575
        for mobility restrictions,
            575
        for vision changes, 575
        requests for, 575
    decision making in, 580–581
    disability benefits, 576–577
        Family Medical Leave Act,
            576
        receiving subsidy and
            working, 577
        short- and long-term
            disability insurance,
            576
    resources for, 577–580
        Internet, 579–580
        Projects with Industry
            program, 579
        state vocational
            rehabilitation services,
            577–578
        Ticket to Work program,
            578–579
        WorkSource program, 579
epidemiology and etiology of,
    327–349
    definitions in, 327
    geographic distribution in,
        329–347
        Asia and Africa, 331–332
        epidemics in, 338–339,
            341–342, 345, 347
        Europe, 331, 336
        Faroe Islands, 339,
            341–342, 345, 347
        Iceland, 339
        Latin America, 332, 334
        migration in, 334–336, 338
        Scandinavia, 330–331
        Shetland and Orkney
            Islands, 339
        South Africa, 336
    historical aspects of, 328–329
fatigue in. See Fatigue.
health promotion in, **557–570**
    processes of, 557–558
    targets of, 558–567
        alcohol or drug abuse,
            566–567

compliance with therapies,
    564
diet and nutrition, 565–566
exercise, 559–560
social support and coping
    skills, 562–564
stress management, 561–562
immunology of, **351–358**
immunopathology of, 351–354
    B cells in, 353
    cytokines in, 352–353
    macrophages in, 353–354
    T cells in, 352
immunotherapy for, 354–357
    immunomodulatory agents in.
        See Immunomodulatory
        agents.
    immunosuppressive agents in,
        354–355
    neutralizing antibodies in,
        355–357, 456–457
management of
    amantadine in, 423, 493
    antidepressants in, 423–425
    donepezil hydrochloride in, 423
    immunomodulatory agents in.
        See Immunomodulatory
        agents.
    methylphenidate in, 423
    occupational therapy in, 427,
        539–540
    psychotherapy in, 427
    rehabilitation in. See
        Rehabilitation.
    vocational rehabilitation in, 428,
        545
neuropsychological evaluation in.
    See Neuropsychological
    evaluation.
primary progressive. See Primary
    progressive multiple sclerosis.
spasticity in. See Spasticity.

Muscle biopsy, in muscular dystrophy,
    needle electromyography in, 985–986

Muscle function
    and physical activity, in disabled
        adults, 46
    magnetic resonance imaging of. See
        Magnetic resonance imaging.

Muscle imbalances, in runners, 675–679
    postural versus phasic muscles in,
        676,678–679

Muscle relaxants, for pain, in disabled
    adults, 73

Muscle RING Finger 1, in skeletal muscle
    dysfunction, 930

Muscle strains, in runners, management of, 730–731

Muscles
abdominal, development of, in runners, 671–674
lower leg, and running gait, 609
overuse injuries of, in runners, 713

Muscular dystrophy
aging with, pain management in, 59
Duchenne. *See* Duchenne muscular dystrophy.
electrodiagnostic studies of, **981–997**
magnetic resonance imaging with, 993
needle electromyography, 984–992
depth of anesthesia in, 990–991
motor unit action potentials in, 984–986, 991
needle electrodes in, 990
to guide muscle biopsy, 985–986
nerve conduction studies, 981–982
single fiber electromyography, 992–993
surface electromyography, 982–984

Musculoskeletal complications, of cerebral palsy, 237–238, 241

Musculoskeletal system, age-related changes in, **19–39**
antioxidant activity and, 20
articular cartilage, 27–29
chondrocytes, 29
fast-twitch versus slow-twitch muscles in, 19–20, 22
inadequate dietary protein and, 21
joints, 31
management of, 23–26, 32
dehydroepiandrosterone in, 25
electrical stimulation in, 24
estrogen therapy in, 25
gene therapy in, 24
growth hormone in, 25–26
physical activity and exercise in, 23–24
testosterone in, 25
motor neuron loss, 20
muscles and soft tissues, 30–31
oxidative capacity and, 21
satellite cells and, 20
subchondral bone and synovial membrane, 30
synovial joint, 26–27
testosterone decrease and, 21–22

tumor necrosis factor and, 21
with post-polio syndrome, 208–209

Myoblast transplantation. *See* Skeletal muscle repair.

Myofibrillar calcium sensitivity, in skeletal muscle dysfunction, 937

Myopathic disorders, single muscle fiber physiology in, 960–962

Myosin heavy chain composition, in neuromuscular diseases, 957

Myostatin, in gene transfer, for skeletal muscle enhancement, 883–884

Myotonic dystrophy type 1, single muscle fiber physiology in, 960–961

Myotonic dystrophy type 2, chronic pain in, 1100–1101

N

Natalizumab, for multiple sclerosis, 461

Navicular stress fractures, in runners, 784

Needle electromyography, of muscular dystrophy. *See* Muscular dystrophy.

Nerve conduction studies
automated. *See* Electrodiagnostic automation.
of Charcot-Marie-Tooth disease, 970–971
of muscular dystrophy, 981–982

Nerve entrapment, cerebral palsy and, 238

Nerve growth factor, in neuromuscular diseases, 1000–1001

Neural stem cells, in neuromuscular diseases, 1008–1009

Neurologic complications, of cerebral palsy, 241–242

Neuromas, interdigital, in runners, 787

Neuromuscular blocks, for spasticity, in multiple sclerosis, 472–473

Neuromuscular complications, of spinal cord injury. *See* Spinal cord injury.

Neuromuscular diseases. *See also* specific diseases.
chronic pain in. *See* Chronic pain.
fatigue in. *See* Fatigue.
neurotrophic factors in, **999–1014**
brain-derived, 1003–1004
ciliary, 1004

future directions in, 1007–1009
fibroblast growth factor-I,
1008
neural stem cells, 1008–1009
pigment epithelium-derived
factor, 1008
glial cell line–derived, 1004–1005
insulin-like growth factor,
1005–1007
nerve growth factor, 1000–1001
neurotrophin-3, 1001–1002
vascular endothelial–derived
growth factor, 1007
obesity in, **1053–1062**
air displacement
plethysmography of,
1054–1055
and chronic pain, 1109
body mass index in, 1054
dual energy absorptiometry scans
of, 1054
metabolic syndrome, 1056–1058
and type 2 diabetes mellitus,
1058
definitions of, 1057
dietary modifications for,
1060
food choices and, 1059
lack of preventive care and,
1059
physical activity and,
1058–1059
prevalence of, 1057–1058
weight reduction for, 1060
nutritional aspects of, 1056
physical activity and energy
expenditure and,
1055–1056
single muscle fiber physiology in,
951–965
anterior horn cell disorders,
959–960
future directions in, 963
myopathic disorders, 960–962
skinned methodology in, 953–957
isometric contractile
measurements,
954–955
isotonic contractile
measurements,
955–957
myosin heavy chain
composition, 957

Neuromyelitis optica, versus multiple
sclerosis, 377

Neuronal tract degeneration, in multiple
sclerosis, magnetic resonance imaging
of, 392–393

Neuropathy
and falls, in elderly, 111
post-polio syndrome and, 213

Neuropsychological evaluation, in multiple
sclerosis, **411–436**, 542–543
case reports of, 428–433
early relapsing remitting multiple
sclerosis, 428–429
later relapsing remitting multiple
sclerosis, 429–430
primary progressive multiple
sclerosis, 430–432
secondary progressive multiple
sclerosis, 432–433
components of, 412–413
definition of, 412
for adaptive reasoning, 421
for attention and concentration,
418–419
for communication and language,
419–420
for complex problem solving, 421
for degree of impairment, 421–422
for executive functions, 421
for impact on brain, 416–418
for impairment patterns, 421
for information processing speed, 419
for medication effects, 423–425
with amantadine, 423
with antidepressants, 423–425
with donepezil hydrochloride,
423
with immunomodulatory agents,
423
with methylphenidate, 423
for memory function, 419
for visuoperceptual processing,
420–421
importance of, 414–416
occupational therapy with, 427
physical therapy with, 427
psychotherapy with, 427
test batteries in, 425–427
Mini-Mental State Examination,
425
Minimal Assessment of
Cognitive Function in MS,
426
vocational rehabilitation with, 428

Neurosurgery, for spasticity, in multiple
sclerosis, 478

Neurotransmitter dysregulation, and
fatigue, in multiple sclerosis, 486

Neurotrophin-3, in neuromuscular diseases,
1001–1002

Neutralizing antibodies, for multiple
sclerosis, 355–357, 456–457

Nonsteroidal anti-inflammatory drugs
     for chronic pain
          in disabled adults, 67, 69–70
          in Duchenne muscular
               dystrophy, 1119

Nonviral vectors, in gene transfer, for
     skeletal muscle enhancement, 876

Novantrone, for multiple sclerosis, 354–355
     for suboptimal treatment response,
          460

Nuclear factor-kB, in skeletal muscle
     dysfunction, 929, 930

Nursing home liability, for disabled adults,
     311–312

Nutritional complications
     of cerebral palsy, 243
     of spinal cord injury, 141–142

Nutritional factors
     and osteoporosis, in female runners,
          704–705
     and stress fractures, in runners,
          758–759

O

Obesity, in neuromuscular diseases. See
     Neuromuscular diseases.

Obstructive sleep apnea, oxidative stress in,
     934–935

Occupational therapy, for multiple sclerosis,
     427, 539–540

Omega-6 supplements, in multiple sclerosis,
     565

Ophthalmologic complications, of multiple
     sclerosis, 224–225

Opiates, for chronic pain, in Duchenne
     muscular dystrophy, 1119

Opioids, for pain, in disabled adults, 70–71,
     78–79, 81

Oral contraceptives, and stress fractures, in
     female runners, 758

Orthopedic surgery, for spasticity, in
     multiple sclerosis, 477–478

Orthoses
     for pain, in disabled adults, 75
     for post-polio syndrome, 211
     for runners. See Runners, footwear
          and orthoses for.
     to prevent hip fractures, in elderly, 117

Osteoarthritis, cerebral palsy and, 238

Osteochondral talus injuries, in runners, 793

Osteoporosis
     cerebral palsy and, 241
     in female runners. See Female runners.
     multiple sclerosis and, 228, 566
     post-polio syndrome and, 213
     spinal cord injury and, 137–139

Ottawa Ankle Rules, for imaging, of ankle
     sprains, in runners, 790

Overuse injuries
     cerebral palsy and, 238
     in disabled adults, 51
     in runners, **651–667**
          definition of, 651–652
          early management of, 661–663
               education in, 663
               footwear selection in,
                    662–663
               screening tests in, 662
          etiology of, 655–661
               anatomy, 658
               ankle flexibility, 659
               anthropometric variables,
                    658–659
               biomechanical variables,
                    659–660
               impact force, 661
               kinetic variables, 660–661,
                    714
               stretching exercises, 657
               surface and footwear, 657
               training errors, 656–657
          ground reaction forces and,
               653–655
     hip and pelvic injuries,
          711–747
          anatomy and biomechanics
               in, 712–714
          capsular and joint
               dysfunction, 730
          differential diagnosis of,
               726, 727
          functional evaluation of,
               714–715
          functional examination of,
               715–728
               core mobility tests,
                    717–720
               eccentric-concentric
                    control of core,
                    720–721
               hip-scapula reaction,
                    721–723
               lower extremity
                    balance and
                    reach, 723–725
               open kinetic chain
                    assessment of

foot and ankle, 725–726
running, 715–716
static alignment of lower extremity, 715
unilateral squat, 716–717
hamstring injuries, 731–732
kinetic variables in, 714
management of, 726–734
muscle strains and tendonitis, 730–731
muscles in, 713
orthopedic examination for, 715
performance enhancement and injury prevention in, 735–746
return to running after, 733–734
sacroiliac and innominate dysfunction, 730
sacroiliac joints in, 713
soft tissue overload, 730–733
internal forces and, 653–654
medio-lateral forces and, 655
stress-frequency curve in, 652–653

Oxidative capacity, age-related changes in, 21

Oxybutynin, for genitourinary complications, of spinal cord injury, 145

P

Pain, chronic. *See* Chronic pain.

Pain management. *See also* Chronic pain.
in disabled adults, **57–90**
acetaminophen in, 70
acupuncture in, 75–76
adverse effects of, 66–67
aging process and, 59–60
antiepileptics in, 72
botulinum toxin injections in, 78
capsaicin in, 73
cognitive behavioral modification in, 73
cold therapy in, 74
COX-2 inhibitors in, 70
drug-drug interactions in, 68–69
efficacy of, 79–81
in amputation, 80
in cerebral palsy, 81
in end-stage cancer, 289
in Parkinson's disease, 80
in post-polio syndrome, 81
in spinal cord injury, 81
in stroke, 80–81
in traumatic brain injury, 80
epidural steroid injections in, 78–79
exercise in, 74–75
heat therapy in, 74
intra-articular injections in, 76–78
local anesthetics in, 73
massage in, 76
nonsteroidal anti-inflammatory drugs in, 67, 69–70
opioids in, 70–71, 78–79, 81
orthoses in, 75
pain assessment in, 60–64
barriers to, 60
diagnostic tests in, 63–64
history in, 61
pain characteristics in, 61–62
physical examination in, 63
previous diagnostic tests in, 62
previous treatments in, 62
social history in, 63
pain epidemiology and, 57–59
amputation, 58, 63
cerebral palsy, 236–237
fascioscapulohumeral muscular dystrophy, 59
Guillain-Barré syndrome, 59
multiple sclerosis, 222–223
Parkinson's disease, 58
spinal cord injury, 134–135, 136–137
stroke, 58–59
traumatic brain injury, 58
physical therapy in, 73–74
skeletal muscle relaxants in, 73
tramadol in, 71–72
trazodone in, 72
tricyclic antidepressants in, 72

Palliative tests, in injured runners, 632, 634

Parathyroid hormone, for osteoporosis, in female runners, 706

Parkinson's disease, aging with, pain management in, 58, 80

Parkinson's disease, fatigue in, 1065

Patellofemoral pain syndrome, in runners. *See* Knee injuries.

Patient Health Questionnaire, to assess depression, in multiple sclerosis, 440

PDK4, in endurance exercise, 864–865

Peak cough flow rate, in Duchenne muscular dystrophy, 1127

Pelvis, overuse injuries of, in runners. *See* Overuse injuries.

Pemoline, for fatigue, in multiple sclerosis, 495

Peripheral neuropathies
  and falls, in elderly, 111
  neurotrophic factors in, 1000–1001

Peripheral vascular disease, and amputation. *See* Amputation.

Peroneal tendinopathy, in runners, 784, 792–793

PGC1α, in endurance exercise, 864

Phasic muscles, versus postural muscles, in runners, 676, 678–679

Phosphocreatine recovery, after exercise, magnetic resonance imaging of, 1047–1048

Physical deconditioning, and fatigue, in multiple sclerosis, 486

Physical therapy
  for multiple sclerosis. *See* Exercise; Rehabilitation.
  for pain, in disabled adults, 73–74

Pigment epithelium-derived factor, in neuromuscular diseases, 1008

Piper Fatigue Scale
  to measure fatigue
    in elderly, 98
    in neuromuscular diseases, 1067–1068, 1076

Plain films
  of patellofemoral pain syndrome, in runners, 766
  of stress fractures, in runners, 763

Plantar fascia, and running gait, 608

Plantar fasciitis, in runners, 781–783

Plethysmography, air displacement, of obesity, in neuromuscular diseases, 1054–1055

PMP-22, in Charcot-Marie-Tooth disease, 968–969, 973

Pneumatic braces, for stress fractures, in runners, 764

Pneumobelt, in ventilation, for Duchenne muscular dystrophy, 1131

Pneumococcal vaccination, in spinal cord–injured patients, 143

Polio
  aging with. *See* Post-polio syndrome.
  prior, single muscle fiber physiology in, 959

Polypharmacy, and falls, in elderly, 112

Polysomnography, in Duchenne muscular dystrophy, 1128

Poser criteria, in diagnosis, of multiple sclerosis, 360

Post-polio syndrome, aging with, **197–218**
  and dysphagia, 209
  and entrapment neuropathy, 213
  and heart disease, 213
  and musculoskeletal changes, 208–209
  and osteoporosis, 213
  and respiratory changes, 204–207
  diagnosis of, 202–204
    history in, 203
    laboratory tests in, 204
    physical examination in, 203–204
  epidemiology of, 198
  management of, 210–213
    energy conservation in, 211–212
    exercise in, 212–213
    pharmacologic, 210–211
  pain management in, 81
  pathophysiology of, 198–202
    central versus peripheral electrophysiologic, 199–200
    fatigue, 202
    historical aspects of, 198–199
    motor neuron injury, 199
    motor unit degeneration, 200–201
    persistent poliovirus, 201
  psychologic issues in, 207–208
  rehabilitation for, 277

Post-polio syndrome, fatigue in, 1076

Postnatal tissue cells, in skeletal muscle repair, 893–898

Postural changes
  and falls, in elderly, 113
  spinal cord injury and, 133

Postural muscles, versus phasic muscles, in runners, 676, 678–679

Power of attorney, for disabled adults, 308–309

PPARδ, in endurance exercise, 865

Prednisone, for post-polio syndrome, 210

Pregnancy, in runners, 692–693

Pressure ulcers, spinal cord injury and, 142

Primary progressive multiple sclerosis, diagnosis of, 365–367
  magnetic resonance imaging in, 395–396
  pitfalls in, 377–378

Problem solving tasks, multiple sclerosis and, 421

Progressive resistive exercises, for multiple sclerosis, 528–529, 533–534

Projects with Industry program, and employment issues, in multiple sclerosis, 579

Prokarin, for fatigue, in multiple sclerosis, 496

Prone examination, of injured runners, 642–643

Proprioceptive training, for ankle sprains, in runners, 791–792

Prosthetics, for amputees. See Amputation.

Protein, inadequate intake of, musculoskeletal complications of, 21

Protein adaptations, in exercise training, 861

Provocation tests, in injured runners, 632

Proximal myotonic myopathy, chronic pain in, 1100–1101

Psychotherapy, for multiple sclerosis, 427

Pulmonary dysfunction, with fatigue, in neuromuscular diseases, 1069

Pulmonary rehabilitation, for cardiopulmonary disease, 260–261

Pyridostigmine, for post-polio syndrome, 210

Q

Quality-of-life issues, in aging with disability, 12–14

R

Range of motion exercises, for spasticity, in multiple sclerosis, 471–472, 535–536

Range of motion tests, in injured runners, 630, 635–638

Real-time magnetic resonance imaging, of muscle function, 1045–1046

Rearfoot pain, in runners. See Foot injuries.

Rebif, for multiple sclerosis, 229, 355, 456

Recombinant adeno-associated viral vectors, in gene transfer, for skeletal muscle enhancement, 877–880

Recombinant viral vectors, in gene transfer, for skeletal muscle enhancement, 876

Redox mechanisms, of skeletal muscle dysfunction. See Skeletal muscle dysfunction.

Reflexology, for multiple sclerosis, 545–546

Rehabilitation
  for chronic pain, in neuromuscular diseases, 1107–1108
  in multiple sclerosis, 427, **513–555**. See also Exercise.
    assistive devices in, 540
    cardiovascular stress test in, 538
    caveats in, 537–539
    cooling programs in, 525–527
    energy conservation in, 492, 539–540
    for cognitive impairment, 537, 542–543
    for dysphagia, 544
    for fatigue, 491–492, 521–523
    inpatient, 516–521
      cost/benefit analysis of, 519
      multidisciplinary, 519
      patient expectations in, 520
      spa programs in, 519–520
    Kurtzke Expanded Disability Scale in, 513–515
    Lee Silverman Voice Therapy in, 544
    MS Functional Composite in, 514
    nursing in, 540–542
    occupational therapy in, 427, 539–540
    outpatient, 527–536
      Ashworth Scale in, 534
      baclofen in, 535
      facilitation therapy in, 532–533
      Feldenkreis technique in, 533
      for balance, 532
      for falls, 531
      for fatigue, 530
      for mobility, 531–532
      for progressive disease, 529–530
      for range of motion, 535–536
      for spasticity, 534–535
      maintenance programs in, 529

Rehabilitation (*continued*)
  modified Ashworth scale in,
    534–535
  progressive resistive
    exercises in, 528–529,
    533–534
  task-oriented therapy in,
    532–533
    versus home-based, 532
  prescription for, 536–537
  quality of life in, 514–515,
    518–519
  reflexology in, 545–546
  relapses in, 514–515
  safety of, 523–525
  speech and swallowing therapy
    in, 543–545
  spinal cord stimulation in, 545
  Unthoff phenomenon in, 523
  usage patterns in, 516
  vocational, 545

Reproductive complications, of cerebral
  palsy, 242

Resistance exercise. *See* Exercise training.

Resistance training
  for cardiopulmonary disease, 259
  in disabled adults, 52

Respiratory complications
  of cerebral palsy, 240
  of post-polio syndrome, 204–207
  of spinal cord injury, 142–143

Respiratory support, in Duchenne muscular
  dystrophy. *See* Duchenne muscular
  dystrophy.

Respondeat superior, and disabled adults,
  311–312

Retinacular release, for patellofemoral pain
  syndrome, in runners, 769

Ritalin, for cognitive impairment, in
  multiple sclerosis, 423

Rivermead Mobility Index, in multiple
  sclerosis, 531–533

Royal London Hospital Test, for Achilles
  tendonitis, in runners, 795

Runners. *See also* Running gait.
  ankle injuries in. *See* Ankle injuries.
  core musculature in. *See* Core
    musculature.
  downed. *See* Downed runners.
  female. *See* Female runners.
  foot injuries in. *See* Foot injuries.
  footwear and orthoses for, **801–829**
    and stress fractures, 753–754

decision making in, 822
  for excessive pronators, 822–824,
    826–827
  for injured runners, 643–645
    with overuse injuries, 657,
      662–663
  for neutral runners, 825
  for patellofemoral pain
    syndrome, 768–769
  for plantar fasciitis, 782
  for supinators, 824–825, 827
  normal pronation and, 803–804
  normal supination and, 804
  objective evaluation for, 814–822
    flexibility tests in, 821
    gait evaluation in, 814–815
    nonweight-bearing
      observation in,
      821–822
    standing examination in,
      816–818
    strength tests in, 819–820
    weight-bearing tests in,
      815–816
  orthosis anatomy in, 810–812
  orthosis casting technique in,
    812–813
  orthosis types in, 812
  shoe anatomy in, 805
  shoe types in, 806–810
    cushion shoes, 806–807
    motion control shoes, 808,
      810
    stability shoes, 807–808
  subjective evaluation for, 814
  subtalar/midtarsal joint
    relationship and, 801–803
  versus walking, 804–805
  injured. *See* Injured runners.
  knee injuries in. *See* Knee injuries.
  overuse injuries in. *See* Overuse
    injuries.
  stress fractures in. *See* Stress fractures.

Running gait. *See also* Runners.
  analysis of, 615–619
    dynamic electromyography in,
      618
    force plate, 617–618
    motion, 617
    observational, 616–617
    stride, 619
  anatomy and, 604–609
    ankle joint, 604–605
    ligaments, 608
    lower extremity, 604
    metatarsophalangeal joints, 607
    muscle fiber orientation, 609
    muscles, 609
    plantar fascia, 608

subtalar joint, 606–607
talocrural joint, 604
tarsometatarsal joint, 607
biomechanics of, **603–621**
energetic measurements of, 618–619
gait cycle in, 612–615
foot flat to heel-off, 613
heel-off to toe-off, 614
initial contact to foot flat,
612–613
initial swing, 614–615
terminal swing, 615
running economy in, 611
versus walking, 609–611
with increased velocity, 610–611

S

Sacroiliac joint dysfunction, in runners,
management of, 730

Sacroiliac joints, overuse injuries of, in
runners, 713

Satellite cells
age-related changes in, 20
in skeletal muscle repair, 893–895

Scoliosis, cerebral palsy and, 237, 241

Seated examination, of injured runners. *See*
Injured runners.

Seizures, cerebral palsy and, 241–242

Selective serotonin reuptake inhibitors
for cognitive impairment, in multiple
sclerosis, 424
for depression, in multiple sclerosis,
442

Semont maneuver, to prevent falls, in
elderly, 117

Sensory nerves, and physical activity, in
disabled adults, 46

Sertraline, for depression, in multiple
sclerosis, 442–443

Sexual complications, of multiple sclerosis,
227

Shin splints, versus stress fractures, in
runners, 762–763

Shock wave therapy, for plantar fasciitis, in
runners, 782–783

Shoes, for runners. *See* Runners, footwear
and orthoses for.

Shoulders, painful, management of, 77–78

Side-lying examination, of injured runners,
641–642

Side population cells, in skeletal muscle
repair, 896

Single fiber electromyography, of muscular
dystrophy, 992–993

Single leg balance reach tests, in evaluation,
of injured runners, 631

Single leg squat, in evaluation, of injured
runners, 630

Single muscle fibers, in neuromuscular
diseases. *See* Neuromuscular diseases.

Sinus tarsi syndrome, in runners, 793

Skeletal muscle, in amyotrophic lateral
sclerosis. *See* Amyotrophic lateral
sclerosis.

Skeletal muscle adaptation, in exercise
training. *See* Exercise training.

Skeletal muscle dysfunction, redox
mechanisms of, **925–949**
atrogin1/MAFbx, 930–931
cytokines, 927–929, 933
in cardiac dysfunction, 935–936
in chronic intermittent hypoxia,
934–935
in heart failure, 936–937
in myofibrillar calcium sensitivity, 937
in obstructive sleep apnea, 931–935
in sleep-disordered breathing,
934–936
interferons, 929
interleukins, 929
mitogen-activated protein kinases,
929, 931
Muscle RING Finger 1, 930
nuclear factor-kB, 929, 930
oxidative stress, 925
reactive oxygen species biology,
925–926
reactive oxygen species effects on
striated muscle, 931–934
reactive oxygen species in cachexia,
926–931
response to mechanical strain, 933–934
tumor necrosis factor-α, 928–929, 930,
931, 933
ubiquitin/proteasome pathway, 928

Skeletal muscle enhancement, gene transfer
in, **875–887**
combination therapy in, 882–884
for Duchenne muscular dystrophy,
880–882
lentiviral vectors in, 876–877
mIgf-I in, 882–883
myostatin in, 883–884
nonviral vectors in, 876

Skeletal muscle (*continued*)
    rational expression cassette and
        transgene design in, 880–882
    recombinant adeno-associated viral
        vectors in, 877–880
    recombinant viral vectors in, 876

Skeletal muscle relaxants, for pain, in
    disabled adults, 73

Skeletal muscle repair, cell therapy in,
    889–907
    cell survival in, 892–898
        bone marrow-derived cells,
            895–897
        cells from postnatal tissue,
            893–898
        embryonic stem cells, 892–893
        fibroblasts, 897
        mesenchymal stem cells, 897
        satellite cells, 893–895
        side population cells, 896
        vascular endothelial cells,
            897–898
    for Duchenne muscular dystrophy,
        889–890
    future directions in, 900–901
    immune response in, 890–892
        early, 891
        later, 891
        suppression of, 891–892
    immune tolerance in, 892
    limited dissemination in, 898–900
        cell delivery in, 898
        intramuscular migration of
            donor cells in, 899
        local injection in, 898–899
        local regeneration in, 899
        systemic delivery in,
            899–900
    microenvironment in, 900

Skilled rehabilitation, for spasticity, in
    multiple sclerosis, 471–472

Sleep apnea syndrome, spinal cord injury
    and, 142–143

Sleep assessment, in Duchenne muscular
    dystrophy, 1128

Sleep-disordered breathing, oxidative
    stress in, 934–936

Sleep disorders
    and falls, in elderly, 112
    and fatigue, in multiple sclerosis,
        486–487
    and fatigue, in neuromuscular
        diseases, 1069

Slow-twitch muscles, versus fast-twitch,
    age-related changes in, 19–20, 22

Smoking, and cardiopulmonary disease,
    255–256

SOD1, in amyotrophic lateral sclerosis,
    1092–1094

Sodium-23 magnetic resonance imaging, of
    muscle function, 1048

Soft tissue impingement, and ankle pain, in
    runners, 792

Soft tissue overload, in runners,
    management of, 730–733

Spasm Frequency Scale, in multiple
    sclerosis, 469

Spasticity
    and falls, in elderly, 112
    and physical activity, in disabled
        adults, 45
    in multiple sclerosis, 225, **467–481,**
        534–535
        evaluation of, 469–470,
            534–535
            Ashworth Scale in, 534
            Modified Ashworth Scale
                in, 469, 534–535
            Spasm Frequency Scale in,
                469
        management of, 470–478, 535
            baclofen in, 474, 476–477,
                535
            dantrolene in, 475
            diazepam in, 475–476
            gabapentin in, 476
            neuromuscular blocks in,
                472–473
            range of motion exercises
                in, 471–472, 535–536
            skilled rehabilitation in,
                471–472
            stretching in, 471–472, 535
            surgical, 477–478
            tizanidine in, 474–475
        pathophysiology of, 468–469
    in neuromuscular diseases,
        management of, 1106–1107

Speech difficulty, cerebral palsy and, 243

Speech therapy, in multiple sclerosis,
    543–545

Spinal cord injury, aging with, **129–161**
    cardiovascular and endocrine changes
        in, 139–141
        management of, 140–141
    gastrointestinal changes in, 146–148
        colorectal cancer, 148
        constipation, 146
        gallstones, 148

hemorrhoids, 148
  management of, 147–148
genitourinary changes in, 143–146
  erectile dysfunction, 144
  urinary tract infections,
    144–145
  in women, 150–151
integumentary changes in, 142
mortality and life expectancy in, 130
neuromusculoskeletal changes in,
    132–134
  and fractures, 137–138
  contractures, 137
  equipment needs in, 135–136
  lower extremity, 136–139
  management of, 134–136, 139
  osteoporosis, 137–139
  pain management in, 134–135,
    136–137
  postural changes, 133
  upper extremity, 132–134
nutrition in, 141–142
pain management in, 81
premature aging, 130–132
psychosocial issues in, 149–150
  depression, 149
  quality of life, 149–150
rehabilitation for, 276
respiratory changes in, 142–143
  management of, 143

Spinal cord lesions, in multiple sclerosis,
    magnetic resonance imaging of,
    389–390

Spinal cord stimulation
  for multiple sclerosis, 545
  for pain, in disabled adults, 79

Spinal deformities, and chronic pain, in
    neuromuscular diseases, 1108

Splints, for plantar fasciitis, in runners,
    782

SREBP-2, in resistance exercise, 867–869

Stem cells
  embryonic, in skeletal muscle repair,
    892–893
  mesenchymal, in skeletal muscle
    repair, 897

Steroids
  epidural injections of, for pain, 78–79
  for Achilles tendonitis, in runners, 796
  for multiple sclerosis, 355
  for plantar fasciitis, in runners, 783
  for post-polio syndrome, 210

Stimulated single fiber electromyography, of
    Charcot-Marie-Tooth disease,
    971–972, 975

Strength tests
  in footwear evaluation, in runners,
    819–820
  in injured runners, 630–632

Strength training, in elderly, 102–103

Stress fractures, in runners, 749–764
  aging female runners, 694–695
  basic bone science in, 749–751
    cancellous bone, 750
    lamellar bone, 750
    osteoblasts, 750
    osteoclasts, 751
    osteocytes, 751
    woven bone, 750
  bone remodeling and, 751–752
  calcaneal, 783
  conservative management of, 763–764
  diagnosis of, 761–763
    computed tomography in, 763
    magnetic resonance imaging in,
      763
    plain films in, 763
  etiology of, 752–759
    anatomy, 756–757
    biomechanical factors, 756
    demographic factors, 755–756
      activity level, 756
      age, 755
      gender, 755
      race, 755–756
    footwear, 753–754
    hormonal factors, 757–758
    leg length discrepancy, 757
    menstrual dysfunction, 757
    nutritional factors, 758–759
    oral contraceptives, 758
    training regimen, 753
    training surface, 754–755
    type of sport, 755
  female athlete triad and, 759–760
  metatarsal, 785–786
  navicular, 784
  prevention of, 760–761
  screening for, 760–761
  talar, 783
  tibial, versus shin splints, 762–763

Stress management, in multiple sclerosis,
    561–562

Stretching exercises
  and overuse injuries, in runners, 657
  for spasticity, in multiple sclerosis,
    471–472, 535
  in core strengthening program, in
    runners, 680

Striated muscle, growth and repair of,
    reactive oxygen species in, 931–934

Stride analysis, of running gait, 619

Stroke
    aging with, pain management in,
        58–59, 80–81
    versus multiple sclerosis, 375–376

Subchondral bone, age-related changes
    in, 30

Subdural hematomas, and traumatic brain
    injury, 165–166

Subtalar joint pronation, in runners,
    716–717

Subtalar joints, and running gait, 606–607

Subtalar ligament sprains, in runners, 793

Subtalar neutral tests, in injured runners, 643

Superoxide dismutase, in amyotrophic
    lateral sclerosis, 1082, 1084, 1085

Supine examination, of injured runners. See
    Injured runners.

Surface electromyography, of muscular
    dystrophy, 982–984

Swallowing difficulty
    cerebral palsy and, 243
    multiple sclerosis and, 227

Swallowing therapy, in multiple sclerosis,
    543–545

Symmetrel, for cognitive impairment, in
    multiple sclerosis, 423

Synchromed pump, for intrathecal drugs, in
    multiple sclerosis, 476–477

Syncope, and falls, in elderly, 113

Synovial joints, age-related changes in,
    26–27

Synovial membrane, age-related changes in,
    30

T

Tai Chi Chuan, to prevent falls, in elderly,
    116

Talar stress fractures, in runners, 783

Talar tilt test, for ankle sprains, in runners,
    790

Talocrural joint, and running gait, 604

Tarsal tunnel syndrome, in runners, 783,
    784

Tarsometatarsal joints, and running gait,
    607

Task-oriented therapy, for multiple
    sclerosis, 532–533

T cells, in multiple sclerosis, 352

Tendinopathy
    of ankle, in runners, 792–793
    of midfoot, in runners, 784

Tendonitis, in runners
    Achilles, 794–796
    forefoot, 786
    management of, 730–731

Testosterone levels, age-related changes in,
    21–22

Testosterone replacement therapy, for age-
    related musculoskeletal problems, 25

Tetracycline antibiotics, for amyotrophic
    lateral sclerosis, 1085

Thompson test, for Achilles tendonitis, in
    runners, 795

Tibial stress fractures, in runners, 762–763

Tibial tendinopathy, in runners, 784

Ticket to Work program, and employment
    issues, in multiple sclerosis, 578

Tizanidine
    for spasticity
        in multiple sclerosis, 474–475
        in neuromuscular diseases,
            1106–1107

Tracheostomy, in ventilation, for Duchenne
    muscular dystrophy, 1133

Tramadol, for pain, in disabled adults,
    71–72

Transcranial magnetic stimulation, to
    measure fatigue, in neuromuscular
    diseases, 1071–1074

Transcutaneous electrical stimulation, for
    pain, in disabled adults, 74

Traumatic brain injury, aging with, **163–177**
    Alzheimer's disease and, 170–171
    behavioral dyscontrol with, 171–172
    epidemiology of, 164–165
    fatigue in, 94
    outcomes of, 166–167
        mortality, 167–168
        short-term, 168–170
    pain management in, 58, 80
    pathophysiology of, 165–166
    psychiatric co-morbidities with, 171,
        173
    rehabilitation for, 172–173, 276

Trazodone, for pain, in disabled adults, 72

Treadmill, in analysis, of running gait, 616

Tricyclic antidepressants, for pain, in disabled adults, 72

Tumor necrosis factor-α, in skeletal muscle dysfunction, 928–929, 930, 931, 933

Twitch interpolation, to measure fatigue, in neuromuscular diseases, 1071–1075

Tysabri, for multiple sclerosis, 461

U

Ubiquitin/proteasome pathway, in skeletal muscle dysfunction, 928

Ulcers
heel, and amputation, 188
pressure, spinal cord injury and, 142

Ultrasonography, of Achilles tendonitis, in runners, 794–795

Unilateral squat, in functional examination, of runners, 716–717

Upper extremity injuries, in female runners, 695

Upregulated genes
in endurance exercise, 868
in resistance exercise, 868

Urinary stress incontinence, in aging female runners, 694

Urinary tract infections, spinal cord injury and, 144–145

V

Vascular endothelial cells, in skeletal muscle repair, 897–898

Vascular endothelial-derived growth factor, in neuromuscular diseases, 1007

Vastus medialis oblique strengthening, for patellofemoral pain syndrome, in runners, 767–768

VEGF-A, in gene transfer, for skeletal muscle enhancement, 879–880

Ventilation
mechanical
for Duchenne muscular dystrophy. *See* Duchenne muscular dystrophy.

for post-polio syndrome, 205–207

Vestibular therapy, to prevent falls, in elderly, 116–117

Vision impairment
and falls, in elderly, 112, 114
cerebral palsy and, 243

Visual Analogue Scale of Fatigue, to measure fatigue, in neuromuscular diseases, 1067–1069

Visuoperceptual processing, multiple sclerosis and, 420–421

Vitamin B_{12} deficiency, and falls, in elderly, 112

Vitamin D deficiency, and stress fractures, in runners, 758

Vocational rehabilitation, for multiple sclerosis, 428, 545

W

Walking gait, versus running gait, 609–611
and footwear evaluation, 804–805

Water diffusion-based measures, in magnetic resonance imaging, of multiple sclerosis, 401

Weight-bearing activity, for osteoporosis, in female runners, 704

Weight-bearing tests, in footwear evaluation, in runners, 815–816

Weight control, for chronic pain, in neuromuscular diseases, 1108–1109

Weight gain, in multiple sclerosis, 566

Wheelchair use
and falls, in elderly, 113–114
and overuse injuries, 63

White matter, in multiple sclerosis, magnetic resonance imaging of, 390–391

WorkSource program, and employment issues, in multiple sclerosis, 579

Z

Zoloft, for depression, in multiple sclerosis, 442–443